WITHDRAWN

THE NEUROSES
AND THEIR TREATMENT

THE NEUROSES
AND THEIR TREATMENT

Edited by

EDWARD PODOLSKY, M.D., F.A.P.A., F.A.P.M.

*Department of Psychiatry, Kings County Hospital,
Brooklyn, New York*

Psychiatrist, Boro Medical Center, Brooklyn, New York

PHILOSOPHICAL LIBRARY

New York

© Copyright by Philosophical Library, Inc.
15 East 40th Street, New York

PRINTED IN THE UNITED STATES OF AMERICA

FOREWORD

What is a neurosis? There are almost as many definitions as there are psychiatrists. According to L. J. Meduna: "A neurosis is a stereotyped, specific response to unspecific stimuli and is caused by connotations of the stimuli not inherent in them." Franz Alexander states: "A neurosis is an inadequate, unsuccessful attempt to restore the emotional equilibrium disturbed by the presence of unsatisfied or poorly satisfied subjective urges." Paul Schilder defined a neurosis as "a wrong attitude resulting from the interruption of the process of testing and probing." Freud was sure that a neurosis is the result of a conflict between the ego and its id. L. G. Moench declared that "A neurosis represents an inability to make a satisfactory response to certain stressful situations, either within the person or between the person and the outside world."

An individual may carry on against the burdens of his inner difficulties with only a slight impairment of his drives and energy, and yet be able to function normally and without too great difficulty. When, however, these difficulties become great and overwhelming so as to interfere with his everyday life or for a long period of time, it is at this point that a neurosis becomes manifested.

Neuroses are essentially conditioned anxiety reactions. Their emergence is automatic once they have been conditioned. They persist until the conditioning has been overcome by relevant emotional retraining processes.

In a neurosis, there is usually a diminution of energy. There is a disappearance of values and meanings, changed affects, displacement of certainty and the emergence of doubt, obsessive questioning, and unreality.

FOREWORD

The neuroses form a major portion of the emotional ills of modern life. Their diagnosis, management and treatment are of the utmost importance to every physician in active practice. It is for this reason that the present volume has come into existence. It is a collection of papers by eminent authorities in the field on all phases of the neurosis.

In a work of this sort, written by many hands and gathered from various sources, it is impossible to maintain the uniformity obtainable in a book that is the work of a single author. Since each paper is reproduced as nearly as possible in its original form, stylistic discrepancies are inevitable. Some overlapping of content is likewise unavoidable, along with a greater emphasis on some phases of the subject than on others.

The editor will welcome from serious readers any suggestions which might improve future editions of the work.

THE EDITOR

ACKNOWLEDGEMENT

The editor is grateful to the editors of the following periodicals for generous permission to reprint papers originally published in their journals:

A.M.A. Archives of Neurology and Psychiatry, for "Chronic Anxiety Symptomatology, Experimental Stress, and HCl Secretion," by George F. Mahl, Ph.D., and Eugene B. Brody, M.D.; and "An Outline of the Process of Recovery from Severe Trauma," by Harley C. Shands, M.D.

American Journal of Orthopsychiatry, for "Psychiatric Therapy in Infancy," by René A. Spitz, M.D.; and "Anxiety in Children Convalescing from Rheumatic Fever," by Irene M. Josselyn, M.D., Albert J. Simon, M.D., and Eleanor Eells.

American Journal of Psychiatry, for "Treatment of Hyperkinetic Emotionally Disturbed Children with Prolonged Administration of Chlorpromazine," by Herbert Freed, M.D., and Charles A. Peifer, B.S.; "Experimental Studies on Anxiety Reactions," by Thomas H. Holmes, M.D., and Herbert S. Ripley, M.D.; "Compulsion Neurosis with Cachexia (Anorexia Nervosa)," by Franklin S. DuBois, M.D.; "Diagnosis and Treatment of the Phobic Reaction," by Walter I. Tucker, M.D.; "The Place of Sedatives in the Treatment of Psychoneurotics," by Robert Arnot, M.D.; and "Physiological Background of the Carbon Dioxide Treatment of the Neuroses," by L. J. Meduna, M.D.

American Journal of Psychotherapy, for "A Rationale for Psychotherapy in Anxiety, Obsession and Depression," by George Winokur, M.D.

Diseases of the Nervous System, for "Occupation Neuroses: A Study in Dependency Reaction," by John W. Bick, Jr., M.D.;

"The Meaning of Anxiety," by Edward Podolsky, M.D.; "A Type of Post Partum Anxiety Reaction," by Murray DeArmond, M.D.; and "The Grantham Lobotomy for the Relief of Neurotic Suffering," by Frank J. Ayd, Jr., M.D.

Geriatrics, for "The Addition of Chlorpromazine to the Treatment Program for Emotional and Behavior Disorders in the Aging," by Benjamin Pollack, M.D.

International Journal of Psycho-Analysis, for "Anxiety in Infancy: A Study of Its Manifestations in the First Year of Life," by René A. Spitz, M.D.; "Impairment of the Sense of Reality as Manifested in Psychoneurosis and Everyday Life," by George Frumkes, M.D.; and "Trauma and Symptom Formation," by Max M. Stern, M.D.

International Record of Medicine and General Practice Clinics, for "Treatment of Anxiety States with Meprobamate (Miltown)," by Walter A. Osinski, M.D.

Journal of Clinical and Experimental Psychopathology and Quarterly Review of Psychiatry and Neurology, for "The Carbon Dioxide Treatment," by L. J. Meduna, M.D.

Journal of Nervous and Mental Diseases, for "Allergy and Psychoneuroses," by Frank C. Metzger, M.D.; "The States of Being and Awareness in Neurosis and Their Redirection in Therapy," by Bernard Zuger, M.D.; and "The Mode of Action of Carbon Dioxide Treatment in Human Neuroses," by L. J. Meduna, M.D.

Medical Annals of the District of Columbia, for "Reassurance," by Paul Chodoff, M.D.

The Nervous Child, for "Clinical Features of Hysteria in Children," by Eli Robins and Patricia O'Neal; "Cases of Hysteria in Childhood," by Marynia F. Farnham; and "The Psychoanalysis of a Case of 'Grand Hysteria of Charcot' in a Girl of Fifteen," by Lydia G. Dawes.

Northwest Medicine, for "Some Symptoms and Signs of Anxiety States," by Ovid O. Meyer, M.D.

Psychiatric Quarterly, for "The Neuroses of Everyday Living," by David C. Wilson, M.D.; "Instinct of Self-Preservation and Neurosis," by Siegfried Fischer, M.D.; "Factors Involved in the Genesis and Resolution of Neurotic Detachment," by Montague Ullman, M.D.; and "Emotional Problems of the Middle-Aged Man," by Otto Billig, M.D., and Robert Adams, M.D.

Psychosomatic Medicine, for "Coexisting Organ Neuroses," by Peter L. Giovacchini, M.D.; "Separation Reaction in Psychosomatic Disease and Neurosis," by Henry H. Brewster, M.D.; and "Evaluation of Psychotherapy, with a Follow-up Study of 62 Cases of Anxiety Neurosis," by Henry H. W. Miles, M.D., Edna L. Barrabee, M.S., and Jacob E. Finesinger, M.D.

CONTENTS

Foreword v

Acknowledgment vii

Anxiety in Infancy: A Study of Its Manifestations in the First Year of Life 3
RENÉ A. SPITZ, M.D.

Psychiatric Therapy in Infancy 15
RENÉ A. SPITZ, M.D.

Clinical Features of Hysteria in Children, with a Note on Prognosis. A Two to Seventeen Year Follow-up Study of 41 Patients 30
ELI ROBINS AND PATRICIA O'NEAL

Cases of Hysteria in Childhood 66
MARYNIA F. FARNHAM

The Psychoanalysis of a Case of "Grand Hysteria of Charcot" in a Girl of Fifteen 74
LYDIA G. DAWES

Anxiety in Children Convalescing from Rheumatic Fever 126
IRENE J. JOSSELYN, M.D., ALBERT J. SIMON, M.D., AND ELEANOR EELLS

Treatment of Hyperkinetic Emotionally Disturbed Children with Prolonged Administration of Chlorpromazine 141
HERBERT FREED, M.D., AND CHARLES A. PEIFER, B.S.

On Treatment by Hydroxyzine of Nervous Conditions During Childhood 152
J. BAYART, M.D.

CONTENTS

Impairment of the Sense of Reality as Manifested in Psychoneurosis and Everyday Life — 158
GEORGE FRUMKES, M.D.

The Neuroses of Everyday Living — 178
DAVID C. WILSON, M.D.

Occupational Neuroses: A Study in Dependency Reaction — 192
JOHN W. BICK, JR., M.D.

Instinct of Self-Preservation and Neurosis — 200
SIEGFRIED FISCHER, M.D.

Factors Involved in the Genesis and Resolution of Neurotic Detachment — 213
MONTAGUE ULLMAN, M.D.

The Meaning of Anxiety — 226
EDWARD PODOLSKY, M.D.

Chronic Anxiety Symptomatology, Experimental Stress, and HCl Secretion — 229
GEORGE F. MAHL, PH.D., AND EUGENE B. BRODY, M.D.

Allergy and Psychoneuroses — 247
FRANK C. METZGER, M.D.

Trauma and Symptom Formation — 255
MAX M. STERN, M.D.

Coexisting Organ Neuroses: A Clinical Study — 289
PETER L. GIOVACCHINI, M.D.

Some Symptoms and Signs of Anxiety States — 299
OVID O. MEYER, M.D.

Experimental Studies on Anxiety Reactions — 307
THOMAS H. HOLMES, M.D., AND HERBERT S. RIPLEY, M.D.

Compulsion Neurosis with Cachexia (Anorexia Nervosa) — 324
FRANKLIN S. DU BOIS, M.D.

CONTENTS

Diagnosis and Treatment of the Phobic Reaction — 341
WALTER I. TUCKER, M.D.

Separation Reaction in Psychosomatic Disease and Neurosis — 353
HENRY H. BREWSTER, M.D.

Emotional Problems of the Middle-Aged Man — 366
OTTO BILLIG, M.D., AND ROBERT ADAMS, M.D.

A Type of Post Partum Anxiety Reaction — 378
MURRAY DE ARMOND

The Addition of Chlorpromazine to the Treatment Program for Emotional and Behavior Disorders in the Aging — 386
BENJAMIN POLLACK, M.D.

An Outline of the Process of Recovery from Severe Trauma — 397
HARLEY C. SHANDS, M.D.

Reassurance — 411
PAUL CHODOFF, M.D.

A Rationale for Psychotherapy in Anxiety, Obsession and Depression — 420
GEORGE WINOKUR, M.D.

The States of Being and Awareness in Neurosis and Their Redirection in Therapy — 426
BERNARD ZUGER, M.D.

The Place of Sedatives in the Treatment of Psychoneurotics — 441
ROBERT ARNOT, M.D.

Evaluation of Psychotherapy, with a Follow-up Study of 62 Cases of Anxiety Neurosis — 453
HENRY H. W. MILES, M.D., EDNA L. BARRABEE, M.S., AND JACOB E. FINESINGER, M.D.

The Carbon Dioxide Treatment: A Review 502
L. J. MEDUNA, M.D.

The Mode of Action of Carbon Dioxide Treatment in Human Neuroses 525
L. J. MEDUNA, M.D.

The Grantham Lobotomy for the Relief of Neurotic Suffering 529
FRANK J. AYD, JR., M.D.

Treatment of Anxiety States with Meprobamate (Miltown) 539
WALTER A. OSINSKI, M.D.

Abreaction—Catharsis: A Critical Reappraisal 549
HAROLD PALMER, M.D.

THE NEUROSES
AND THEIR TREATMENT

ANXIETY IN INFANCY: A STUDY OF ITS MANIFESTATIONS IN THE FIRST YEAR OF LIFE

René A. Spitz, M.D.

Limitations of space force me to omit references to authors who have investigated anxiety in infancy, such as S. Freud, Anna Freud, Greenacre, Melanie Klein, Odier, and many others. I must also omit definitions and quotations as well as the larger part of the theoretical conclusions arising from my findings. I will present mainly, in telegraphic style, the behaviouristic description of these empirical findings. They are gathered from observational material on 239 babies observed from the age of ten days to the age of one year; and on forty-five babies delivered without anaesthetic and observed from delivery to the tenth day.

At and immediately after delivery discharge phenomena can be observed in the newborn. They are in the nature of unpleasure, but strikingly brief and mild.

Immediately after birth the neonate's reaction to various stimuli is inconsistent, diffuse and unspecific. Even the famous Watson experiment of dropping the infant mostly does not elicit anything that could be qualified as anxiety. As for the provocation of rage (Watson) by restricting the infant's movements, that is a statement which belongs to the realm of fable and is based on improper observational technique.

I believe therefore that if we are to describe the psychological correlate of what we can observe in the way of emotions at birth and in the first weeks, we shall have to limit ourselves to the categories of unpleasure and quiescence only. At that early stage anxiety cannot be observed in the behaviour of the infant, and neither can pleasure. The system is regulated by the Nirvana-principle which aims at the reduction of tension. To make the experience of pleasure possible, at least some rudimentary form of Ego must be present.

At this stage at which the Ego is still nonexistent, its defence functions are partly replaced by an exceedingly high perceptive threshold which acts as a biological stimulus barrier. This makes it difficult, if not impossible, to get any but the most diffuse response to stimulations which, to be effective at all, have to be violent. Hartmann has suggested in his recent papers that this stimulus barrier will serve later as a model for certain Ego functions in the nature of defence, more specifically those on the lines of repression. But before that can come to pass the threshold must be progressively reduced and finally disappear, to be replaced by Ego functions. This process takes several months.

The rest of the Ego's functions of defence as well as the Ego's functions of adaptation and mastery are safeguarded by a quasi-biological unity of mother and child, called by us the mother-child binomial, an expression borrowed from the Spanish pediatrician Morchio. It is this unity of mother and child which ensures survival.

In the following weeks, reliably stimulus-specific reactions are set up according to the pattern of the conditioned reflex. One of the first of these, in response to an equilibrium stimulus, is the child's turning towards the breast when put into the feeding position.

In the course of the second and third months, the first responses in the nature of pleasure can be distinguished. They are connected with innumerable expectancies (Gesell) implanted by the only actual person existing in the infant's life, its mother. It is as a consequence of these expectancies that the infant develops in the third month the social smile (Ch.

Bühler) in response to the face of the adult seen straight on (Kaila, Spitz).

During the same period the unpleasure responses became more specific. The stimuli which provoke them are not connected any longer nearly exclusively to inner sensations. Neither are these unpleasure responses any more the fleeting and short-lasting discharge phenomena of the first days. Memory traces have been laid down. They are evident in the social response of recognition manifested in the smile; their effectiveness is equally evident in the longer duration of unpleasure responses to perceptions of a psychological nature.

Therefore, in the third month, the infant is not only able to manifest pleasure when beholding its human partner, but also to produce long-lasting unpleasure reactions when deprived of him. These two responses are the greatest advance in discriminatory development at this age. No such discrimination can be demonstrated in respect to toys or even to food at the same period. This is a finding which certainly will not come as a surprise to psychoanalysts.

There are, however, exceptions. We find children in the first five months who react to the adult's face by crying. We have invariably found in our material that in these cases a particularly painful mother-child relationship existed. The expectancies created in these children by the human partner, by the mother, were those of unpleasure, and every human being, therefore, provokes the same unpleasure reaction. This atypical response is the sign of a psychopathological process.

In these cases we have the impression that the unpleasure is much more specific than what we have discussed up to now. The physiognomical expression of these infants is really one which might be qualified as anxiety. For the first time in the infant's development we can see here reactions in the nature of flight in response to psychological stimulations, for up to this point flight reactions occurred only in response to physical stimuli.

It is at the next stage that we are inclined to recognize anxiety proper. After the sixth month, in an age range varying from the seventh to the tenth month, the normal child shows a fundamentally changed attitude towards the human partner. Whereas between the third and the sixth month it would smile at *any* human being approaching it in the appropriate manner (that is frontally), in this new stage of emotional development it will show definite signs of anxiety, with drastic flight reactions, when approached by a stranger. This behaviour has many individual variations. Accordingly it has been described in various ways by psychologists. The child may simply "act coy," turning its head away; it may hide its head in its mother's clothes. It may hide its face in the blankets, it may begin to weep. It may scream. We have called this anxiety of the child the "eight-months' anxiety" after the period at which it is most frequently manifested.

The phenomenon has another rather strange corollary. It is very easy to overcome, though few people are familiar with the device we have introduced for this purpose. This device consists in turning one's back on the child, remaining motionless in close proximity to it. Within a very brief time, usually a few seconds, the tears will cease and the child will reach out to take hold of the stranger's hands or clothes.

From here on the pattern of anxiety branches out. It becomes difficult to say what is normal and what is not. We know that the eight-months' anxiety subsides in the first quarter of the second year, only to reappear, generally much stronger, towards the end of the second year and in the subsequent two or three years.

On the other hand, the second half of the first year is the time at which we have been able to distinguish certain psychopathological syndromes. It is also the period at which varied objects may unexpectedly and unaccountably elicit anxiety reactions in children.

One of these psychopathological syndromes we have found is marasmus in children who, about the third month, were separated from their mother without the provision of a substitute, and remained separated. At the stages of this condition where anxiety was still present, it was manifested as a response to every stimulus and impresses the observer as a defence of the organism serving to husband the ever-vanishing energies.

In this function it seems to be a regression to the state of the neonate who reacts with unpleasure to any stimulus perceived. Perhaps the apathy which develops later in these children represents a further regression to the neonate's high threshold against stimuli which act as stimulus barrier.

In children who were separated from their mother in the *second* half of the first year and who remained separated from her for a period not exceeding three to, at most, five months, a behaviour develops which resembles depression in grown-ups; as described elsewhere, the condition is fundamentally different from the adult psychiatric condition of depression, and was therefore called by us "anaclitic depression." During the first two months of separation anxiety at the approach of a stranger shows an increasingly violent pattern. The uninitiated might confound this anxiety with the eight-months' anxiety. The difference is a quantitative one. While eight-months' anxiety can be overcome by adequate behaviour, as mentioned above, such is not the case in the anxiety of depression. No approach succeeds in calming the child. In extreme cases the desperate screaming will go on for hours; we ourselves have witnessed cases going on for two to three hours without pause.

These attacks of anxiety in anaclitic depression are accompanied by conspicuous autonomous manifestations. Tears are common in the anaclitically depressed child. In the anxiety attack heavy salivation, profuse perspiration, uncontrolled trembling, dilation of pupils and other signs of panic are often present.

Another syndrome which we have seen and in which anxiety plays a prominent rôle is coprophagia in the first year of life. As we have demonstrated elsewhere ("Autoerotism") this condition is manifested in children whose mothers show long-range mood swings.

Distressing as the picture of the anaclitically depressed child is, that of coprophagic anxiety is worse. In this condition the children appear to be sitting in a daze. They cannot be interested in anything but in their coprophagic activity. They show a suspicious behaviour, an expression which one is accustomed to see in the disturbed ward of psychiatric hospitals amongst severe paranoiacs.

This concludes the description of the phenomena of anxiety in the first year as we have been able to observe them. We will add a few theoretical considerations.

Theoretical Considerations

Why do the first unmistakable manifestations of *anxiety proper* take place in the third quarter and not earlier? We believe the reasons are structural on one hand, libido-theoretical on the other.

1. *The Structural Reason*

Freud states: "Anxiety is an affective state which can of course be experienced only by the Ego." ". . . the Ego is the real seat of anxiety." I wish to add from my observations that anxiety proper cannot be produced before the Ego is differentiated from the Id.

No Ego is present at birth; its first outline is laid down and progressively organized in the course of the second and third quarter.

At birth and in the weeks that follow *physiological* states of tension correspond to what later, when the Ego comes into existence, will be experienced *psychologically* as anxiety. Lacking an Ego, the immature personality of the infant cannot deal with these tension states. They are dealt with by diffuse, neuro-muscular discharge characterized by the phenomenon of overflow; the overflow in itself demonstrates that the coordinating function of the Ego is lacking.

Before the formation of the Ego psychological tension-states can arise only: from conflict between the drives themselves or between their component parts; from conflict between the whole system and environmental demands or environmental frustration.

After the formation of the Ego a new source of conflict becomes possible, the conflict between the Ego and the Id. This is the stage at which anxiety proper is manifested.

2. *The libido-theoretical Reason*

Psychoanalytical theory claims that the first part of infancy is characterized by the narcissistic stage. Phenomenological and experimental observations confirm and limit this statement to the first three months. During this period environmental perception takes place only in function of the presence of a need-configuration directed towards this perception. The object, which at this period is to be considered a part object, is perceived only in function of the internal need. Therefore this period has to be considered objectless.

The second quarter is a transitional period in which a slow emergence takes place from a narcissistic to a pre-objectal stage. The part objects are organized into pre-objects in the shape of the human partner's face. The laying down of memory traces, the formation of the Preconscious, the first differentiation of the Ego are concomitant, inter-related and simultaneous processes. Once they have taken place object-libidinal cathexes can be directed towards memory traces.

Prior to this the pre-objects are interchangeable, for they are lacking in object attributes. Their characteristics are not objective. They are characterized by the capacity to fulfill the exact requisites of a given need-configuration. The objects at this period do not have a face, they have a function.

It is in the third quarter that true objects appear for the first time. They now have a face, but they still retain their function of a constituent part of the child's recently established Ego. The loss of the object is therefore a diminution of the Ego at this age and is as severe a narcissistic trauma as a loss of a large part of the body. The reaction to it is just as severe. Anxiety is the affect evoked by the threatening imminence of such a loss. This affect is produced in a constant flux during the daily contacts of the mother with the child. The child is assuaged when the mother is near it, when it sees her or hears her, it becomes anxious when she leaves it. The repeated anxiety attacks are short-lived; perhaps hallucinations replace the mother during her absence.

Whether hallucination has this rôle or not, the approaching stranger will be confronted with the memory traces of the mother's face. For the face which was the first visual sign by which the child recognized a partner as such remains also the leading perception in the further establishment of the libidinal object. This remains true even for the grown-up.

The approach of a face evokes the child's hope that "mother is returning"; the stranger's unfamiliar face and gesture destroy this hope by confirming "this is not mother, mother is gone." The anxiety which the stranger's approach thus evokes might therefore be a reactivation of the anxiety experienced by the child when mother left it. This conclusion is in close agreement with Freud's assumption that the stranger-phobia of early childhood is a reaction to the danger of object-loss.

This does not explain the question why this anxiety can be so easily overcome by turning one's back on the child. That, however, is now no longer difficult to explain. Reactivation of anxiety because of being left by the mother is in itself not a very serious emotion. To keep it up it has to be nourished by the manifest contrast between the stranger's features and those of the mother; when the stranger does not present his face actively to the child the memory of this contrast will fade, the reactivated affect of anxiety will spend itself.

When therefore the approaching stranger has provoked anxiety in the child by his approaching face, but withdraws the distinctive signal of the face for an appreciable time, the child will be confronted with something which is no longer either its object, the mother, or the proof of the mother's absence, the stranger's face. It is confronted with "something which moves" and excites its curiosity. It reaches out and pulls at it to see what it is; it sees a hand and grabs it. When now the stranger cautiously returns his face the child's libidinal cathexis is already engaged and drained in the new activity of which the stranger has become a part. Anxiety, if developed at all, will be fleeting and insignificant.

It is from these modest beginnings that anxiety will rapidly develop, by becoming a signal for the approach of danger situations; situations, that is, in which a break-through from the inside or outside threatens the integrity of the Ego. The anxiety signal for the threatening break-through of the stimulus barrier, that is of the Ego, becomes the most powerful motivating force in human life, the power which organizes the character, the defences, the neuroses.

It is not accidental that at the anxiety signal's first inception we find the threat of a breakdown to the Ego through the loss of its constituent part, the mother. It is not accidental that it is at the same period that we find the first traces of clinically distinguishable psychiatric diseases, each of them motivated by special configurations of the object relations, of that object which is already libidinal object on one hand, but still a constituent part of the Ego on the other. It is at this turning-point of the development that the basic security and the basic insecurity of the child and later on of the adult is laid down. Here is the beginning of so many severe neurotic and psychotic conditions, and it is therefore here that we have to take our stand: *principiis obsta*.

Appendix

The foregoing paper suffers from the condensation imposed by the time limit usual at congresses. It was felt therefore that some of the more important arguments for classifying as "anxiety proper" the phenomena of unpleasure at the approach of strangers in the third quarter of the first year of life should be elaborated in greater detail.

Three stages were distinguished in the course of the development in the first year. They are:

(1) Physiological tension leading to diffuse discharge phenomena;
(2) unpleasure responses in the nature of fear to both physical and psychological stimulation, resulting in flight;
(3) unpleasure responses in the nature of anxiety proper.

Our task is to distinguish clearly state No. 2 from state No. 3. For this purpose we propose to discuss in somewhat greater detail our usage of terms, though it conforms essentially with that of Freud.

We call fear the emotion of unpleasure which we experience when we are confronted with a perceived physical or with a perceived psychological *threat*. A prerequisite of this reaction is that the threat be "recognized" as such. The term "recognized" implies that the threatening perception has been experienced previously and has led to painful consequences.

In stage No. 2 the physical or, as the case may be, the psychological stimuli which provoke the unpleasure response of flight during the first six months of life are in the nature of a previously experienced, remembered and "recognized" threat. This involves a certain elementary function of the ego as described by Freud most recently in his article, 'A Disturbance of Memory on the Acropolis' (*Int. J. Psycho-Anal.*, 22, 1941, and *Collected Papers*, Vol. 5) as follows: ". . . what may be termed the normal method of warding off what is painful or unbearable, by means of recognizing it, considering it, making a judgment upon it and taking appropriate action about it . . ." Such known and recognized physical experiences are the painful or even simply annoying stimulations to which an avoidance response will be produced. In the psychological field they consist mainly in the infant being left or disappointed by its partner; in other terms in the loss of the love object. In both cases an actual threat, an actual danger is involved. In both cases, physical and psychological, a repetitive experience of this actual danger has conveyed to the infant the "learning" necessary for the *recognition* of this danger. It is a form of learning which takes place *in analogy* to learning according to the formula of the conditioned reflex.

We may incidentally conclude that one of the very earliest ego-organizations to appear in the course of development is the capacity of learning in analogy to the mechanism of the conditioned reflex. Learning through conditioning is a process which appears already well before any traces of conscious ego functioning can be demonstrated, that is on an essentially physiological level, without involving conscious memory. But around the third month, in the process of establishing the ego (which involves conscious memory) the mechanism of the conditioned reflex is taken over and used in a similar manner, but applied to conscious memory traces. In parallel with this, as I have demonstrated elsewhere, a new method of learning which I called "learning according to the human pattern" is introduced. It could also be called learning through insight; it takes place through the process of thinking as described by Freud, that is a trial-action with the help of minimal quantities of energy displaced from memory trace to memory trace (Freud, *The Unconscious*, 1915). This then would be another of the earliest ego-organizations to come into being. It represents the prerequisite of the phenomena described in stage No. 3.

Anxiety on the other hand is a danger signal which is produced in certain specific circumstances. The circumstances in question are the threat of a breakthrough of the protective barrier against stimuli.

The two situations which characterize fear and anxiety show certain similarities; but while in the case of fear the threat is referred to a conscious memory, in the case of anxiety the danger refers to the unconscious prototype of the experience of birth, in which the whole personality was swamped by stimuli with which it could not deal.

If this concept is applied to the eighth month anxiety we find that the appearance of a stranger could never have been experienced actually as a danger by the child, for the overwhelming majority of our subjects certainly never had any bad experiences with strangers. But just as certainly they did have a number of unpleasant experiences with their own mothers, as every child must inevitably have them in the course of growing up. Nevertheless the mother's approach was reassuring, but the stranger's approach anxiety provoking for all these infants. It follows that their emotion of unpleasure cannot have been conditioned by their previous experience, by their memories.

We have attempted to explain this unpleasure response to the stranger's approach in stage No. 3 by assuming that the child confronts the stranger's face with the memory trace of the libidinal object. On finding that the stranger is not the object, the child concludes: "This is not mother, she does not return, I have lost mother!" The stranger's face thus becomes the cue for the apperception of a rising tension between id-demands and inadequate ego-strength.

The id-demands consist in object-libidinal strivings towards the mother, who has achieved the full status of a libidinal object by this age. These libidinal strivings are reinforced by powerful narcissistic needs. For at this age the mother has still a two-fold function: although she has already become an actual libidinal object, she is still a complementary part of the infant's immature ego. Her loss thus involves the participation of a much larger part of the infant's drives *and* of its still immature personality than would be the case at a later age. The loss not only frustrates its libidinal needs, but also threatens its total system of security. It actually is a vital threat and experienced as such.

This is an internal perception; the threat is to the ego. It is the internal threat that the ego will be swamped by uncontrollable stimuli with which it cannot deal; it is the threat of a breakthrough of the protective shield against stimuli, in analogy to its prototype in the trauma of birth. It is this aspect of the fear of strangers in the third quarter of the first year of life which made me feel justified in qualifying the phenomenon as anxiety proper, as a danger signal.

PSYCHIATRIC THERAPY IN INFANCY

René A. Spitz, M.D.

Psychiatrists rarely think of applying their science to the first year of life. The reason for this is that our present dynamic approach in psychiatry is based on the verbal behavior of our patients, even though nonverbal behavior is not only taken into consideration, but forms an important part of the clinical picture and even of the methods of approach to psychiatric disease.

Nevertheless, a moment's reflection will show that the verbal behavior of the patient—the patient's verbal interpretations of his conditions, emotions, sensations, experiences, wishes, urges, etc.—is the principal source on which we draw in our understanding as much as in our description and in our treatment of psychiatric conditions in adults.

In the infant this source fails us completely. It fails us so completely that we hardly even have a way of knowing when the infant is suffering. It is certainly one of the great handicaps of pediatrics that the manifestations of displeasure observed in the infant may or may not be in a one-to-one correlation with any detectable cause of these manifestations. Accordingly, we have a wealth of such statements as: "The infant screams because it has gas pains," leading to a quasi-religious ritual of "bubbling" indulged in in the British Isles; "Screaming is a necessary exercise for the infant," frequently leading to a shocking disregard of the infant's needs; "Baby is wet," and so on. All these statements may be quite correct at times; but mostly they betray simply our ignorance of what goes on in the infant.

From the psychiatric point of view this situation puts the

infant on the level at which we think about animals. Psychiatric disturbance is not considered a possibility; if it is considered at all, it is considered in terms of congenital or inherited somatic malformation or deficiency of the central nervous system. The era of organicism in psychiatry is still very close to us and it seems to us that the preverbal stage of infancy is the last stronghold of this school.

Of course, logically, there is no reason for assuming that psychiatric disturbance is only possible when language has been acquired. There is no jump between the preverbal stage and the later phases. The development of the psyche is a smooth, uninterrupted process in which each step is predicated on the preceding one. This is a fact which was most self-evident to academic psychologists who followed up development genetically. Theoretically at least, psychoanalytic thinking based itself on this proposition. In psychoanalytic writing, this resulted mostly in applying findings made on older children, adolescents and adults to the more elementary general phenomena of infant life.

Our approach to the problem was a different one. We reasoned that, as the psychoanalytic technique of verbal exploration is not feasible with infants, we would have to use the approach of experimental psychology. The problems to be investigated and the principles according to which experimental psychological methods could be applied were based on the propositions furnished by psychoanalytic theory.

It was in an endeavor to elaborate this idea that our research was started fifteen years ago. In its course, with the help of methods described elsewhere, we have established certain norms of development which can be correlated to extensive experimental psychological research done by others as well as by us. Our own material on the subject covers long-term observations of 366 infants. In the course of these observations we have not only been able to establish a first approach to the criteria of normal psychological development at different age levels of infancy, but we have also been able to distinguish certain nosological entities which we are inclined to classify as "psychiatric disturbances of infancy." Of these we will speak later. We will first have to discuss the fundamental differences which we have slowly come to perceive between the human being in the preverbal stage and the human being after the acquisition of language.

These differences are both of a quantitative and a qualitative nature; they apply to the most varied sectors of personality. In our approach we have used the Hetzer-Wolf Babytests which enable us to differentiate between six sectors of the infantile personality: (1) Perceptive Mastery, (2) Body Mastery, (3) Social Relations, (4) Mastery of Memory and Imitation, (5) Manipulative Ability, and (6) Intelligence.

Brief reflection shows that in all these sectors there is an enormous gap between the capacities of the child and those of the adult. As regards the last-mentioned one, Intelligence, everybody realizes that it has to develop. But the same applies to Manipulative Ability, to Memory, to the Mastery of Social Relations, to Bodily Activities, and to Perception. All are undeveloped at birth and take a long time to reach a level where their functioning is in any way comparable to that of adults.

These are facts which can be, and have been, demonstrated by experimental psychological methods. The infant has a quantitatively and qualitatively differentiated function from that of the individual at a later stage of life; it follows that the infant's experience of his environment, perceptive and otherwise, will be profoundly different from that of the older individual.

This holds true also of that sector of the personality with which psychiatry is most intimately concerned, namely, the emotions. Emotions in the infant are not easily evaluated or classified. What we can observe is apt to be confusing; one fact stands out: at birth, like every other function of the infant, the emotions are undifferentiated and unorganized. A slow process of development in the course of the first year differentiates emotions first into two great classes, the "positive" and the "negative" emotions. From these then progressively the emotions of fear, anxiety, anger, rage, jealously, cupidity, love, affection, etc., are differentiated in the course of the first year, leading in the next few years to progressively finer subdivision.

In terms of psychoanalytic theory, we can say that the infant at birth does not possess an ego, that is, a central steering organization. Starting around the third month, a rudimentary beginning of an ego will be delimited from the rest of the personality. In the course of the first year it will develop progressively; but even at the end of the first year it will be far from completely organized. This is a task which will take many more years.

In the first year of life the different part organizations of the ego will still be largely undifferentiated. We have already referred to the ego organizations which can be observed during the first year: we described them as the six sectors of the personality. Even these six sectors, however, are still quite undifferentiated; they merge not only with each other, but also with their somatic counterparts in a much more intimate manner than in the adult. The result of this lack of differentiation is that traumata, be they psychic or somatic, will be received by an organism which can respond to them mainly in a generalized, unspecific manner. Furthermore, the consequence of the qualitative difference between the functioning of the infant and the adult is that traumata which to the adult may represent little or nothing can be extremely serious in the infant. On the other hand, the infant may not even perceive experiences which for the adult are seriously traumatic.

The traumata to which the infant is exposed in different areas of his personality are related to emergencies of survival. Such emergencies of survival refer to the infant's needs; these can be classified into somatic needs and emotional needs.

The somatic needs are easily understood. They refer to the infant's humoral balance, to his thermic balance, to his hygiene, his bodily integrity, his nutrition. There are surely others; for instance, it is our belief that a minimum of stimulation is one of the somatic needs of the infant, though it remains a moot question whether this is not equally an emotional need.

The question whether to gratify or not to gratify the emotional needs of the infant has had many, and often antithetical, answers. The most striking interference with emotional needs was the Watsonian idea of treating the infant more or less as a machine for intake and excretion, with no emotional interchange. This approach, which, we are convinced, has surely done much harm in the course of the last thirty years, is going out of fashion now. It has been recognized that the infant does have emotional needs.

It should further be stressed that the emotional needs of the infant are much greater than those of the adult; they vary according to the age level which is under consideration. The survival value of their gratification is in direct proportion with the infant's biological helplessness, with his lack of specific responses and his lack of preformed behavior patterns. Accordingly, the infant's emotional needs will be greatest in the beginning and will diminish progressively in the course of the first year.

This is a statement which appears to be contradicted by everyday experience. The contradiction, however, is only apparent, for the issue is beclouded by the special conditions under which the newborn lives. At birth the infant spends close to 89 per cent of the twenty-four hours of the day in sleeping or dozing; and even at three months he spends 69 per cent of the day thus. The remaining time is to a large extent taken up by providing the infant with the food, hygiene, etc., which must be forthcoming if he is not to die in short order. During these ministrations it is almost impossible to exclude a large amount of emotional interchange between the nursing person and the infant.

Accordingly, infants in their first three months will rarely suffer from a lack of emotional interchange. This should not mislead us into the assumption that their emotional needs are small—we should recognize that nature has insured that the newborn gets the necessary minimum in this respect, just as nature has provided him with an admirable protection against the hazards of extrauterine life. This protection, which decreases slowly in the course of the first few months, is the infant's extraordinarily high threshold for environmental stimuli, on the one hand, and the long period of sleep which fills his days on the other. But after this first period wakefulness increases and perception becomes more acute. In the second, third, and fourth trimester of the first year the emotional gratification offered during the period of bodily care becomes inadequate. Thus it would seem as if the quantity of emotional gratification required by the child at this time is greater than in the beginning. Actually it is only the much longer waking periods, without an increase in obligatory handling of the child, which increase the over-all requirements.

Toward the end of the first year a further change is brought into the picture of the child's emotional needs. The first steps into the outside world are taken. The child ceases to be the passive recipient of emotional gratification that he was up to the acquisition of locomotion. He sallies forth, actively to demand assuagement of his emotional demands. This activity, this independence, has to be encouraged by a decrease of the emotional manifestations of the environment which by now would become cloying to the child.

In this process of development the six sectors of the personality, as well as the emotional sphere, are so closely interrelated as to be indistinguishable from each other. They represent the progressive coordination of one part of the child's personality into a steering organization for the whole, into the ego, as it is called by Freud. Thus is an ego structure laid down in the course of the first year.

It is here that the problem with which we are dealing is situated. For psychiatric diseases, by and large, are diseases of the ego, or of the relations of the ego to the other spheres, be they the superego, the id, or the environment. Therefore, when we speak of psychiatric disease in infancy, we are making the assumption that some disturbances have occurred in some part of the rudimentary ego or that some deficiency in the factors necessary for its development is present. In the latter sense those child analysts who think of psychiatric diseases in infancy in terms of development are correct.

Any therapeutic measures for such disturbances will have to compensate for the possible deficiencies in the very limited world of the infant. These deficiencies may be in the nature of the lack of necessary factors; they may be in the nature of too much of certain factors; and they may be, and mostly are, in the nature of an imbalance between the factors needed.

In considering such therapeutic measures, we must once again return to the picture we have drawn of the infant. The outstanding factors in this picture were a lack of differentiation, a lack of organization, a lack of discrimination. This discriminative inadequacy results in a generalization both in the afferent and in the efferent sectors of the psychic apparatus. This generalization is conclusively shown by a number of psychological experiments the description of which would lead us too far afield. It is manifested by the infant's reaction to total situations rather than to single stimuli. But the generalization is not limited to the infant's psyche; as already mentioned, experiences in the somatic sector show an overflow into the psychic sector and vice versa.

Imbalance in the psychic sector of the infant's personality will occur through the infant's perceptions, visual, auditory, tactile, etc. We believe that an important sense organ of the infant is to be found in deep sensibility, the functioning of which has as yet been insufficiently explored. These modes of perception will provide us with the approaches for the psychiatric treatment of the infant; they are, after all, also our avenue of approach in the treatment of the adult. The difference in our approach will be that we cannot use verbal methods of communication; no agreement between infant and adult on signals and cues is possible except on a very elementary level.

We possess, however, another avenue, more elementary, to the treatment of psychiatric disturbances in infancy. As already stated, psychiatric disturbances will be the consequence of deficiency in the gratification of the infant's needs, be these needs somatic or emotional. By deficiencies we do not necessarily mean the absence of gratifications; imbalance in the gratification of the need pattern, or the surfeit of one or the other need, may be just as pathogenic. With this in mind, we realize that one approach to therapy will consist in the removal of environmental obstacles which represent an impediment in the gratification of the infant's urges or drives; or the approach will consist in the proper adjustment of those environmental stimuli which are responsible for an overstimulation of one or several of these urges and drives.

Having thus defined the field in which any therapeutic measure of infant psychiatry can be undertaken, we will review the clinical pictures which we have thus far been able to isolate in our observations on psychiatric disturbances in infancy, and we will discuss specific measures of treatment.

1. *Marasmus*. This is a condition in which the infant's physical development is first arrested, and then shows a regression of a specific type, leading in a large percentage of the cases to mental impairment or death.

2. *Anaclitic depression*. The picture is that of a depression with a quite striking symptomatology including weeping, unappeasable screaming at the approach of strangers, withdrawal, eating disturbances and sleeping disturbances as well as developmental arrest.

3. *Motor restlessness*. This is the picture of children in the first year of life whose main activity consists in rocking in the knee-elbow position.

4. *Coprophagia*. We have given this name to the syndrome because of its most outstanding presenting symptom. The children subject to this condition, besides rejecting all toys, except their own feces, show a deeply disturbed expression which often goes to the point of paranoid suspiciousness.

5. *Eczema*. This condition could be considered a purely

somatic one were it not for the fact that the mental development of infants subject to eczema shows a circumscribed specific difference from the mental development of children who are not affected by this disease. The outstanding characteristics of the picture are a reflex irritability already present at birth, a conspicuous retardation in the capacity for negative responses in the field of social perceptive discrimination, and an equally conspicuous retardation in the field of imitation and learning. The whole picture is one of severe disturbance in the formation of object relations on the basis of identification.

6. *The "three months colic."* This is a condition on which we have relatively little material and information, but which is acknowledged by pediatricians as a disturbance of psychogenic origin.

On the basis of the concept of the infant's psychic structure and its peculiarities described above, a certain number of etiological factors can be isolated as underlying these conditions either singly or in various combinations. The factors we have isolated are as follows:

1. *Emotional starvation of the infant.* This condition can be subdivided into several components which will influence the resulting clinical picture. In the first place, emotional starvation can occur in degrees varying as to severity, from the emotional neglect to which children in foster homes and particularly in broken homes may be subjected, to extremes like those described by Kingsley Davis. A second component in the picture of emotional starvation is also quantitative. This is the length of time during which the infant is subjected to emotional deprivation. A third and equally important component is the developmental period of the child's life at which emotional starvation is inflicted. According to the way in which these components are varied the resulting picture will vary also. All the results, however, can be considered as emotional deficiency diseases falling within the framework of infant psychiatry.

2. *Withholding of age-adequate stimulation.* This also can be classified as a deficiency disease and is usually a concomitant

of emotional starvation. We have yet to see a case in which age adequate stimulation was withheld without concomitant emotional deprivation.

3. *Maternal hostility to the infant*. This can be classified under two aspects: overt hostility and repressed hostility. The latter may take the form of either overprotection or rejection. Both headings have to be subjected to closer terminological definition, as various forms of maternal behavior can be observed in each of them.

With these we have the prerequisites for our discussion of the possible therapeutic approaches to psychiatric conditions in infancy. We have suggested four such approaches: (1) prophylactic measures; (2) restitutive measures; (3) substitutive measures; (4) modifying measures.

1. *Prophylaxis*. It is strange that in psychiatry the concept of prevention plays such a subordinate role. The term "Preventive Psychiatry" is one which hitherto has hardly been used in our science, notwithstanding the fact that we are more and more aware of the preventive nature of many of our measures in the fields of social work, child guidance, etc. It is regrettable that the preventive measures in these fields have been concentrated until now mainly on remedying psychiatric disease which had already become manifest. The measures therefore were preventive only insofar as they prevented the solid establishment and the dangerous sequels which would develop from a process already begun.

Our concept of preventive psychiatry is different from this. We do not believe, of course, that preventive psychiatry will obviate any and all outbreaks of psychiatric conditions. We believe that certain environmental factors in infancy will lead to psychiatric disease, either immediately or by establishing a predisposition in the individual which favors its later outbreak. The prophylactic measures we have in mind can best be compared with dental prophylaxis which has the purpose of removing environmental conditions leading to dental caries. Equally, psychiatric prophylaxis will make suggestions regarding the

PSYCHIATRIC THERAPY IN INFANCY

avoidance of factors which have been shown to lead to psychiatric disease.

Our prophylactic suggestions are of the simplest and like so much of psychiatry correspond to the dictates of common sense. They are:

a) During the first year of life depriving infants of emotional interchange for prolonged periods should be strenuously avoided. Infants should under no circumstances be deprived of their love object during the second half of the first year for a period of more than three months without an adequate substitute. The practice of pediatric hospitals of forbidding parents to visit their sick infants in the hospital or, as is the case with some hospitals, of permitting parents to visit only when the infants are asleep, cannot be condemned too severely.

b) Depriving infants in their first year of life of toys, that is, of age-adequate stimuli, with the usual hygienic motivation, should be strenuously avoided. The toys provided should be age-adequate. They should not be chosen from the point of view of grownups who fancy a "cute" toy. They should be chosen as an incentive for the child to develop his activities toward the age level immediately following the one at which he is at the given moment. For example, up to six months rattles are adequate toys. After six months hollow blocks should be added. Toys fancied by adults are frequently a source of anxiety to children. We have observed, for instance, that dolls frequently provoke the most violent anxiety, even panic, on the part of certain children in the second half of the first year.

c) Providing the infant with age-adequate stimulation includes also the necessity to provide, beginning at the latest at six months, the fullest opportunity for locomotion. Both hospitals and other institutions for the housing of infants disregard this need flagrantly. It is one which is important from other aspects, too, which we will discuss under therapy.

2. *Restitution*. When infants have been deprived either of their love object or of age-adequate stimulation during the first year, and a disturbance develops, a reliable cure for this

disturbance will be achieved if the love object and the stimuli are restored within a maximum of three months.

3. *Substitution.* In a number of cases neither prophylaxis nor restitution is possible. The love object, the mother, may die, or may suffer prolonged illness and hospitalization, etc. In such cases it is imperative to attempt the substitution of another love object for the original one. In this process utmost flexibility must be observed. In the course of the substitution the infant should be encouraged as far as possible to choose his preferred love object and to manifest his likes and dislikes and should be closely observed for such manifestations. If the substitute is disliked, a replacement should be provided. It is a great advantage if at this point the infant has already achieved locomotion, whether erect or on all fours. If that is the case, locomotion should be encouraged as much as possible. This enables the infant, on the one hand, to divert a portion of his libidinal drive into the field of motor activity. On the other hand, it enables the infant to use this activity in first selecting his love object, or in manifesting his preference and then approaching his new love object whenever he feels like it.

It is gratifying to note that our findings on the emotional needs of infants during their first year have recently been confirmed for the first time by experimental psychological studies on animals. Our findings on infants have sometimes encountered opposition on the part of laymen or physicians who insist that the damage we observed in emotionally severely deprived infants must be due either to some physical impairment or to a congenital inadequacy in their inherited or inborn equipment. These persons were unable to accept the destructive nature of emotional starvation. Of course one cannot counter such objections by experiments—they are inadmissible on infants. Our results were arrived at by careful observation of infants in existing life situations or institutions and by systematic analysis of the different factors involved. It is doubly gratifying to find that in his observations on the conditioned reflex Henry Liddell has been able to demonstrate on goats during their infancy phenomena exactly similar to those we have observed in infants, In the case of animals such experiments are possible and the factors involved can be rigidly controlled.

We mention this in connection with substitutive therapy, because it is in this field that another measure, that of putting infants who have lost their love object together with other infants, is confirmed by the animal experimenter. Indeed the animal experimenter, in this case Dr. Jules H. Masserman, has quite independently introduced this measure in the treatment of experimental neurosis in cats.

In institutions and hospitals for infants, such a measure is considered "unhygienic" and is usually rejected. It is for this reason that we have regularly found the sickest children in the isolated cubicles of the most "hygienic" institutions. In contrast children on the common wards of less "hygienic" institutions were a much healthier, lustier lot.

It should be repeated here again that children deprived of their love objects must be provided with age-adequate toys. We do not mean that children deprived of their love object, or any other children for that matter, should be showered with expensive toys of the most varied kinds. Measured by adult standards, variety in itself is neither perceived nor appreciated by the child of this age, except in its grossest degrees. Nor do we wish to imply that the infant's love object can be replaced by toys. But the least we can do for a child who has been deprived of his mother is to provide for his most obvious needs as she would have done.

It should be noted that all coprophagic children and most deprived children tend to throw every object they can out of their cribs, including sheets, pillows, articles of dress and even mattresses. One toy at least should therefore be suspended above the child in such a manner that, though he can reach it, he cannot throw it out.

Within the field of therapy proper, there are a number of other measures which suggest themselves but on the effectiveness of which we have thus far relatively little information.

Such measures consist of the forcing of stimulation in the case of children who have been deprived of their love object. The first of these stimulations is the handling of the child, the offering of tactile stimulation and of stimulation of the sense of equilibrium. We have observed surprising results in deprived children whom the nurses had been instructed routinely to take in their laps and fondle for appreciable periods. This has been confirmed by personal communications from Dr. Harry Bakwin of Bellevue.

Another field of stimulation is the auditory one and experiments should be made in offering deprived children auditory perceptions. We have observed the avid eagerness with which deprived children react to the human voice even when they do not see the person. It seems, on the other hand, self-evident that if we want a child to learn to talk, then that can take place only with the help of a person who will talk with the child. A quantitative proof of this statement can be found in our publication "Hospitalism, a Follow-up Report"; children in an institution where they were not offered these auditory stimulations were almost without exception unable to talk by the age of four years. We would therefore wish to introduce into the life of deprived children periods at which routinely somebody would talk and sing to them.

Visual stimulation, by and large, is the one of which least need be said. But we cannot conclude the discussion of these stimuli without mentioning that hospitals as a matter of course offer visual stimulation at its lowest through their arid, whitewashed, colorless and "hygienic" equipment. This could easily be remedied. We want also to call the attention of all those interested in child welfare to a practice common to hospital nurses, namely, that of hanging sheets over the bedrails to get the children to sleep and to be quiet. In one such institution we found that the sheets sometimes remained there all day, limiting the child to a view of a little part of the ceiling. That we cannot speak of normal development under such circumstances need hardly be said.

4. *Modification.* We have up to this point spoken mainly of measures to be taken in the case of deficiency diseases of the infant's psyche. In the cases in which the child's love object, the mother, offers inappropriate stimulation, whether it be too much stimulation or unbalanced stimulation, an environmental manipulation will have to take place. This environmental manipulation can take two forms: (a) removing a fundamentally inappropriate mother and replacing her by a substitute; (b) modifying the personality of the mother with the help of psychotherapy.

After all we have said about the undesirability of depriving children of their love object, the suggestion that the mother should be removed may strike the reader as contradictory. However, there are a certain number of exceptions in which this is the best course. It will frequently be so when the mother is psychotic. As an example we may mention a case which has been described in one of our publications—the case of a manic-depressive mother observed by us who regularly performed cunnilingus on her child. The result was an extremely severe disturbance of the child, who obviously would have fared better even with a poor substitute.

We shall not discuss the modification of the mother's attitude through psychotherapy. Suffice it to say that the psychotherapy to be applied, which may go from counseling to long-term psychoanalysis, will be as varied as the cases in question. It is a field in which excellent results have been observed by us.

To summarize: The sum total of our findings on psychotherapy in the preverbal stage is that this has to consist in an environmental manipulation, both in regard to love objects and inanimate objects. The needs of the child are simple and an intelligent observation of the child's environment will readily disclose which of these needs is unsatisfied. For its satisfaction no elaborate measures, but only those of the simplest type, need be taken.

CLINICAL FEATURES OF HYSTERIA IN CHILDREN, WITH A NOTE ON PROGNOSIS. A TWO TO SEVENTEEN YEAR FOLLOW-UP STUDY OF 41 PATIENTS

Eli Robins and Patricia O'Neal

Grateful acknowledgment is made to Dr. Alexis Hartmann, physician-in-chief, St. Louis Children's Hospital, for his kindness in making available these records, and to Miss Shelley Ball and Mrs. Mildred Bernard for their time spent in working with the records.

Hysteria in childhood was probably first mentioned by Lepois in 1618. From the middle of the nineteenth century until 1915, the clinical description of the characteristics of childhood hysteria was the subject of numerous monographs and papers. Following 1915, interest in the clinical aspects of childhood hysteria almost disappeared. For example, Jensen & Wert report only 16 references in the Index Medicus between 1930 and 1944. A personal search of the Index Medicus for 1945 through 1950 revealed only six additional references.

In the Academic Lecture before the American Psychiatric Association in 1951, D. M. Levy ably reviewed in part the historical reasons behind this sudden cessation of interest in the clinical aspects of psychiatric diseases, including hysteria, in children. These reasons have to do with, in Levy's words, "the major influence in the United States (of) the child guidance movement." As a result of this movement, there has developed, according to Levy, "an antidiagnostic attitude, a pooh-poohing of diagnosis and history-taking. . . ." He goes on to say, "If you examine such . . . child guidance clinics in which a philosophy of treatment has departed from or is inconsistent with the discipline of classification and of diagnostic thinking, you may find a lack of interest, in fact, even a protest against follow-up studies designed to test the value and the outcome of therapeutic procedures. The result is then a checkmate on scientific values for patient and profession." This emphasis on clinical psychiatry as a fundamental necessity in the study of childhood psychiatric diseases had been voiced earlier by other experienced clinicians in the field. For example, Harms has stated (speaking particularly of childhood hysteria and schizophrenia), "There may be raised the objection that the label with which a case is tagged is only a problem of doctors' files. There is involved, however, not only a name, but with the name, a whole method and technique and cure. Thus the diagnosis of a case becomes fundamental in the task of psychiatry, the helping of the diseased individual."

The clinical method in medicine, of which child psychiatry is a part, has had a long and honorable history. The use of the clinical method is especially important in investigating the diseases in which the cause is not known. Since hysteria is one of the diseases in which the cause is not known, it would seem that a return to the investigation of this aspect of childhood hysteria is in order. The following objectives of this study are an attempt to effect this return to the clinical method in the investigation of hysteria. (1) To ascertain the approximate frequency with which the diagnosis of hysteria was given in a large children's hospital over a period of years. (2) To discover the present status of health in a number of persons diagnosed hysteria on admission to a children's hospital some years previously. (3) To discover how many of these children diagnosed hysteria turned out to have some other illness at follow-up. (4) To learn something about the course of hysteria in childhood from the cases that had hysteria at follow-up. (5) To describe the clinical picture of hysteria in children in a way that will (a) enable the clinician to diagnose hysteria using the standard techniques of diagnostic pediatrics; (b) define a homogeneous clinical group for further research in childhood hysteria.

Method of Study

Selection of Patients. The patients for this study were selected by the following procedure: (1) All diagnostic cards, including those of private and ward patients, with a final diagnosis of psychiatric disease of children admitted to a metropolitan children's hospital (age limits, birth to 14, inclusive) from January 1, 1935 to March 31, 1950 were reviewed; (2) Any child with a diagnosis of hysteria, hypochondriasis, or mixed psychoneurosis with a manifestation of pain, vomiting, paralysis, amnesia, fits, urinary retention, blindness, trances or aphonia was included. The diagnoses of hypochondriasis and mixed psychoneurosis (with the special symptoms already noted) were included in order to avoid overlooking any possible case of hysteria. It is an impression of the authors, previously stated by one of them, that what is usually called hypochondriasis is indistinguishable from hysteria as defined in that paper. The diagnosis of mixed psychoneurosis was included if any of the so-called "classical" symptoms of hysteria, according to textbooks and general clinical usage, above noted were listed as a manifestation. Forty-one patients were found who fulfilled these criteria. During the $15\frac{1}{4}$-year period covered by this study, 51,311 patients were admitted to the hospital. Of these 51,311 patients, 1,029 (2.09%) received a psychiatric diagnosis, including 597 cases of mental deficiency. The 41 cases selected here represented 0.08% of the total patients admitted. 4.0% of all patients admitted with a psychiatric diagnosis, and 8.3% of all psychiatric patients, excluding those with mental deficiency.

Locating the Patients. The patients were located by means of letters, telephone calls and visits to patients' homes or former neighborhoods. In addition, physicians, real estate companies, churches, and other hospitals were contacted. By these means 37 patients—90.2% of the total—were located (Table 1). Twenty-three patients were given a personal interview and examination. Fourteen patients or their parents were contacted by letter or telephone or both.

TABLE 1
Status of Forty-one Patients Followed After Two to Seventeen Years

	Number	Per Cent
Status of All Patients—41		
Located	37	90.2
Not Located	4	9.8
Total	41	100.0
Located Patients—37		
Examined	23	62.2
Not Examined but Contacted	14	37.8
Total	37	100.0

Characteristics of Group Selected. The group of 41 children consisted of 16 boys and 25 girls, ranging in age from three to 14 at the time of hospitalization (Table 2). The 23 patients interviewed personally consisted of 9 boys and 14 girls, ranging in age from three to 14 at the time of hospitalization. The 14 patients contacted by letter or telephone consisted of six boys and eight girls, ranging in age from seven to 15. The length of follow-up ranged from two to 17 years and averaged about nine years. The duration of the illness at the time of hospitalization ranged from one day to seven years. The duration of the illness was calculated from data in the hospital chart as the time elapsed from the onset of the earliest annoying or persistent symptom to the time of admission to the hospital.

Sources of Data About the Patients. Of the 24 patients living within 50 miles of St. Louis, 23 were personally interviewed and examined. No patient living further than 50 miles from St. Louis was seen personally. Five patients of the 23 examined had additional neurologic, otologic, orthopedic, surgical or ophthalmologic consultation. One patient received bone x-rays; another received esophageal and gastric x-rays. No other laboratory studies were done. The data on the 23 patients interviewed privately were obtained by asking first for a history of their original illness since the time of original hospitalization.

TABLE 2

Characteristics of Group Selected for Follow-up

	Total Group (41)	Patients Located (37)	Patients Examined (23)	Patients Contacted But Not Examined (14)	Patients Lost (4)
Sex					
Boys	16	15	9	6	1
Girls	25	22	14	8	3
Age at Hospitalization (Mean, years)	10.0	9.9	9.6	10.5	10.0
Age at Follow-up (Mean, years)	—	18.6	18.4	19.0	—
Length of Follow-up (Mean, years)	—	8.6	8.7	8.5	—
Length of Follow-up (Median, years)	—	9.0	10.0	8.0	—
Diagnosis at Hospitalization					
Hysteria	31	27	16	11	4
Hypochondriasis	6	6	3	3	0
Mixed Psychoneurosis	4	4	4	0	0
Diagnosis at Follow-up					
Hysteria	—	5	4	1	—
Anxiety Neurosis	—	7	5	2	—
Other Disease*	—	4	3	1	—
Other Disease* + Anxiety Neurosis	—	3	3	0	—
Well	—	6	2	4	—
Undiagnosed	—	12	6	6	—

* Other than hysteria or anxiety neurosis.

The psychiatrist then asked a standard 114-item questionnaire. This questionnaire included questions about chief complaint, symptoms, operations, hospitalizations, school history, job history, marital history, personal and social history, family history, manner and attitude during examination and specific questions concerning the course of the illness. A detailed list of some of the topics covered in this portion of the questionnaire may be found elsewhere. In addition, the patient was asked fifteen questions concerning his psychologic status, his relationships to members of his family and his psychologic reactions to various life events. The questionnaire was designed to elicit the history and symptoms, if present, of hysteria, anxiety neurosis, psychopathic personality, schizophrenia, manic-depressive psychosis, phobic neurosis and obsessive compulsive neurosis, and to learn about the presence of "maladjustment" and the possible presence of non-psychiatric diseases. The patient was interviewed in every one of these 23 cases and, in addition, in 15 of the 23 cases at least one parent was interviewed.

There were 14 patients who were located but not interviewed personally. The patients or their parents were contacted by letter or telephone or both. In four cases the patient was contacted directly; in the other cases a parent was contacted. The standard questionnaire could not be used for these telephone or mail contacts. Because these 14 patients were not seen personally, the diagnosis made at follow-up must necessarily be less definite than those made in the 23 patients examined.

Criteria for the Diagnosis made at the Time of Follow-up. Criteria were set up prior to the study for the positive diagnosis of hysteria, anxiety neurosis, psychopathic personality, schizophrenia and manic-depressive psychosis. The problem of diagnosis of schizophrenia, and manic-depressive psychosis did not arise. The criteria for the diagnosis of hysteria were based on a study of Purtell, *et al.*; those for the diagnosis of anxiety neurosis were based on a study of Wheeler *et al.* The differentiation of hysteria and anxiety neurosis is of particular interest in a follow-up study of hysteria because of the striking differences in the course of the two diseases. Patients with hysteria tend to have an excessive number of hospitalizations and an excessive number of major operations, while patients with anxiety neurosis show no differences in these respects from the normal population. There are further important differences, including amount of disability, personal and social distress, and amount and kinds of symptoms.

The criteria for the diagnosis of hysteria at the time of follow-up were the following: (1) The patient had to have a minimum of 18 of the following symptoms distributed among at least seven of these ten groups of symptoms: Group I—Headache; Group II—Blindness, diplopia, aphonia, urinary retention, paralysis, fits, trances, hallucinations (in the absence of a psychosis), amnesia; Group III—Blurring of vision, weakness, lump in throat, urinary frequency, paresthesias, faints, nervous chills, fatigue; Group IV—Breathing difficulty, palpitation, anxiety attacks, chest pain, dizziness; Group V—Anorexia, food dyscrasia, constipation, diarrhea, marked variation in weight, nausea; Group VI—Abdominal pain, vomiting; Group VII—Dysmenorrhea, menstrual irregularity, menstrual hemorrhage, menstrual lapses greater than three months; Group VIII—Sexual indifference, sexual frigidity, dyspareunia, story of attempted or successful rapes, vomiting beyond fourth month of pregnancy, story of difficult labor, impotence, premature ejaculation; Group IX—Back pain, joint pain, pain in extremities; Group X—Nervousness, cries easily, depressed feelings, unhappiness, suicidal ideas. (2) A dramatically and vaguely told medical and personal history or a history of more than one major operation or more than two hospitalizations by the age of 21. (3) No other diagnosis could be made to explain the symptoms.

The criteria for the diagnosis of anxiety neurosis at the time of follow-up were the following: (1) At least one symptom in three of the following four groups: Group I—Breathing trouble; Group II—Palpitation, chest pain; Group III—Nervousness, dizziness, faintness, anxiety attacks; Group IV—Feelings of fatigue, tiredness or limitation of activity. (2) No other disease, including hysteria, could be present to explain these symptoms.

Criteria for the diagnosis of psychopathic personality at the time of follow-up were the following: (1) The occurrence of positive findings in at least five of these seven groups: (a) arrests (b) truancy from school (c) expulsion or suspension from school (d) inability to hold a job for longer than one year (e) vagrancy and waywardness (f) excessive fighting (g) unexplained, bizarre medical symptoms. (2) No other diagnosis could be made to explain the symptoms.

Non-psychiatric diseases were diagnosed with the help of the appropriate consultants. When a patient with symptoms did not have a diagnosable psychiatric disease and the consultant could not make a diagnosis, the patient was placed in the undiagnosed category. In two cases, a psychiatric illness and a non-psychiatric disease were present together.

Method of Evaluating Health and Amount of Disability at Time of Follow-up. The patients were asked if they thought themselves well or not well and, if not well, whether they had no disability, mild disability, or moderate to severe disability from their symptoms. These four categories were defined as follows:

Well—No symptoms or at most 2 symptoms in the past two years with no complaint or disability.

Symptoms, no disability—Symptoms were present but they did not cause the patient to seek medical advice or to refrain from any pleasure or business pursuit.

Symptoms, mild disability—Symptoms were present and caused patient to seek medical advice or to limit job, social or personal life but in such fashion that there was no significant interference with schooling, work, family or social life.

Symptoms, moderate to severe disability—Symptoms were present and caused patient to seek medical advice or to limit job, social or personal life in such a way that job, social or personal life was seriously affected. He may also have sought medical advice repeatedly.

Results

The detailed presentation of results will describe the 23 patients who were interviewed and examined. These 23 patients represented 56.1% of the original sample of 41 patients and 62.2% of the 37 patients located. The 14 patients who were contacted by letter or telephone will be discussed later. This latter group of patients in general showed the same present status (Table 2) as did the patients interviewed.

The Clinical Description of the Patients. Group I. Four Patients with Hysteria (Table 3): Of the 23 patients examined, four had hysteria at the time of follow-up. All four of these

TABLE 3

Symptoms, Ages at Original Hospitalization and at Follow-up and Original Diagnosis in 23 Examined Patients Grouped According to Diagnosis at Follow-up

Pt. No.	Sex	Age at Hospitalization	Age at Follow-up	Original Diagnosis at Hospitalization	Original Symptoms Disappeared	Original Symptoms Persisted	Newly Recorded Symptoms	Disability
Group I, Hysteria (4 Patients)								
1	F	12	29	Hysteria	3,9,46,50,59	53	1,2,5,6,7,8,11,13,15,21,23,24,34,35,37,38,49,54,55,58	Severe
2	F	13	27	Hysteria	39	5,7,9,13,15,53,54	1,2,6,8,10,12,19,21,22,25,26,28,29,37,45,49,55,56	Severe
3	F	10	23	Hysteria	39,40,48	1,5,7,9,34,37,41	2,6,8,10,13,14,21,25,28,29,42,49,50,53,54,59	Mild
4	F	14	24	Hysteria	—	13,21,35,37,44,48,49,53,54	1,2,5,6,7,8,10,11,14,15,16,20,38,34,45,55	Severe
Group II, Anxiety Neurosis (5 Patients)								
5	F	12	29	Hysteria	—	11,13,16	1,5,6,7,8,10,24,28,53	Mild
6	F	4	8	Hysteria	37,41,54	—	1,8,11,44,49,53	None
7	M	11	25	Hysteria	2,4,8,51,53	1,5,7,11	6,10,14,16,45,49,55	Mild
8	M	9	13	Hysteria	35,41,51	53	1,6,8,10,44,54	Mild

TABLE 3 (Continued)

Pt. No.	Sex	Age at Hospitalization	Age at Follow-up	Original Diagnosis at Hospitalization	Original Symptoms Disappeared	Original Symptoms Persisted	Newly Recorded Symptoms	Disability
Group II, (Continued)								
9	M	10	14	Hypochondriasis	13,51	—	1,5,7,8,9,17,35, 42,44,53,55	None
Group III, Other Disease (3 Patients)								
10	F	12	22	Hysteria	—	1,3	8,44	Severe
11	F	10	18	Hysteria	15	9,50,53	1,8,16,44,54,56	Severe
12	M	11	14	Hysteria	4,41,48	1,13,15	14,46	Severe
*Group IV,** Other Disease plus Anxiety Neurosis (3 Patients)*								
13	F	8	18	Hysteria	—	39,53	1,5,38,42,44,55	Mild
14	M	2	17	Mixed Psychoneurosis	36	35,37	2,7,8,9,10,11, 34,42,53	None
15	M	12	26	Hysteria	39,40	—	1,4,5,7,8,10, 13,38,44,49	Mild
Group V, Undiagnosed (6 Patients)								
16	F	12	22	Hypochondriasis	44	1	9,14,27,37,45, 53,55	Mild
17	F	12	24	Mixed Psychoneurosis	5,38,49, 53	1	6,16,21	None
18	F	14	23	Hypochondriasis	13,14,15	1	8,22,23,53	Mild

TABLE 3 (Continued)

Pt. No.	Sex	Age at Hospitali- zation	Age at Follow-up	Original Diagnosis at Hospi- talization	Original Symptoms Disappeared	Original Symptoms Persisted	Newly Recorded Symptoms	Disability
Group V, (Continued)								
19	F	10	13	Hysteria	—	53,59	1,6,13,14,33, 44,47,54,55,56	Severe
20	F	7	10	Mixed Psychoneurosis	—	18,15	8,14,53	None
21	M	9	11	Hysteria	—	13,14,15, 37,44,48	1,36,40	Mild
Group VI, No Disease—Well (2 Patients)								
22	M	3	7	Hysteria	13	—	51,52	None
23	M	3	7	Mixed Psychoneurosis	8,9,13, 15,37,51	—	—	None

* Patients in Group III had the following diseases at the time of follow-up:
Patient 10—Macular degeneration, both eyes, cause unknown.
Patient 11—Cardiospasm.
Patient 12—Psychopathic personality.
** Patients in Group IV had the following diseases, in addition to anxiety neurosis, at the time of follow-up:
Patient 13—Idiopathic epilepsy.
Patient 14—Congenital orthopedic disease manifested by severe limitation of flexion of lumbar spine and of flexion and extension of the hips.

Patient 15—Alcoholic addiction.

In this table the patients were categorized into six groups according to the diagnosis made at the follow-up interview and examination. The amount of disability was rated as described under Methods. Symptoms that were present during the original hospitalization but that disappeared within the following year are listed in the column headed Original Symptoms Disappeared. Symptoms that were present during the original hospitalization and were still present within one year of the time of the follow-up interview are listed in the column headed Original Symptoms Persisted. Symptoms italicized in these two columns were the chief complaints at the time of original hospitalization. Symptoms that were noted for the first time at the follow-up interview are listed in the column headed Newly Recorded Symptoms. The first and second columns list all the symptoms recorded during the original hospitalization; the second and third columns list all the symptoms present at the time of the follow-up interview. The numbers in these three columns refer to the following list of symptoms:

1. Headache
2. Blurring of vision
3. Blindness
4. Diplopia
5. Dizziness
6. Lump in throat
7. Breathing difficulty
8. Palpitation
9. Chest pain
10. Anxiety attacks
11. Anorexia
12. Food dyscrasia
13. Abdominal pain
14. Nausea
15. Vomiting
16. Constipation
17. Diarrhea
18. Marked variation in weight
19. Urinary retention
20. Urinary frequency
21. Dysmenorrhea
22. Menstrual lapses greater than three months
23. Menstrual irregularity
24. Menstrual hemorrhage
25. Vomiting beyond the 4th month of pregnancy
26. Difficult labor
27. Sexual indifference
28. Sexual frigidity
29. Dyspareunia
30. Story of rape
31. Impotence
32. Premature ejaculation
33. Paralysis
34. Paresthesias
35. Back pain
36. Joint pain
37. Pain in extremities
38. Faints
39. Fits
40. Trances
41. Hallucinations or delusions
42. Nervous chills
43. Tremors
44. Fatigue
45. Insomnia
46. Difficulty in opening mouth
47. Difficulty in opening eyes
48. Difficulty in walking
49. Weakness
50. Dysphagia
51. Many episodes of fever
52. Many sore throats
53. Nervousness
54. Cries easily
55. Depressed feelings
56. Unhappiness
57. Suicidal ideas
58. Amnesia
59. Aphonia
60. Obsessions
61. Compulsions
62. Phobias

had been diagnosed hysteria originally. The ages of onset of hysteria in these four patients were five years, 13 years, nine years, and twelve years. These patients had the following chief complaints at the time of hospitalization: Patient 1—Difficulty in opening her mouth, dysphagia and aphonia; Patient 2—Fits; Patient 3—Fits and difficulty in walking; and Patient 4—Difficulty in opening her mouth. These four patients had five, 8, 10 and 9 symptoms, respectively, at the time of admission to the hospital. Three of the four patients had more symptoms than any other patient in the total series of 23 at the time of hospitalization. The fourth patient with five symptoms, ranked third in number of symptoms among the other 19 patients without hysteria at follow-up. These data indicated that apparently hysteria did not become serious enough to warrant hospitalization when only a single symptom was present.

The original symptomatic picture of hysteria in these children showed (Table 3) multiple symptoms. These included obvious nervousness, occurrence of one of the "classical" pseudoneurologic symptoms or at least of unexplained difficulty in walking without actual paralysis, and symptoms usually thought indicative of "anxiety"—headache, dizziness, fatigue, weak feelings, and paresthesias of the fingertips. The symptomatic picture in these children at the time of follow-up, after reaching adulthood, corresponds to the picture described in detail elsewhere. They gave a history of unnecessary hospitalizations and surgical operations for symptoms of hysteria. Two patients had already had two major surgical operations each for symptoms of hysteria by age 26 and another patient had had one by age 20. Two patients had each had one non-surgical hospitalization for symptoms of hysteria (other than the hospitalization in the children's hospital). Also fitting the clinical picture of hysteria in adults is the fact that three of the four patients gave their histories, medical and personal, in a highly dramatic fashion.

An analysis of the duration of the illness of these patients prior to hospitalization revealed an interesting difference between the patients who had hysteria at time of follow-up and those who did not. Every one of the patients who had hysteria at time of follow-up had already had symptoms for at least nine months before her original hospitalization. Only one-third (32%) of the other 19 patients examined had symptoms of such long standing at the time of original hospitalization. This finding might be helpful in making the differential diagnosis of hysteria in a questionable case. If a hospitalized child reports only recently acquired symptoms, one might suspect that he does not have hysteria.

At time of follow-up, all four patients diagnosed hysteria showed a clinically significant amount of disability (Table 3). Three patients suffered a severe disability, and one was mildly disabled. This suggests that hysteria beginning in childhood and continuing into adulthood with the typical clinical picture is likely to be a disabling illness.

All four of these patients with hysteria at follow-up were females; none of the males followed had hysteria. This absence of hysteria in boys at the time of follow-up cannot be explained by an excess of boys in the Undiagnosed Group (Group V). Actually, as shown in Table 3, five girls were undiagnosed and only one boy. Therefore, an excess of boys in the undiagnosed group did not explain the absence of any boy with hysteria. Of the 10 girls originally diagnosed hysteria, 40% (4 patients) had a positive diagnosis of hysteria at the time of follow-up and an additional 10% (1 undiagnosed girl) could possibly have had hysteria. Whereas of the six boys originally diagnosed hysteria, only one could not be given a positive diagnosis, and therefore not more than 17% (1 undiagnosed case) could possibly have had hysteria. This would indicate that the diagnosis of hysteria in a boy is likely to turn out to be incorrect.

Finally, it should be noted that at the time of original hospitalization the examining physicians had noted the symptom of obvious nervousness or the so-called somatic symptoms of "anxiety"—dizzy spells, difficulty in breathing, chest pains, paresthesias of the fingertips and nervous chills, among others —in each of the four patients diagnosed hysteria at the time of the follow-up. Apparently these symptoms, which hysteria patients have in common with patients with anxiety neurosis, occur early and are as characteristic of childhood hysteria as they are of adult hysteria.

Group II. Five Patients with Anxiety Neurosis: Of the five patients diagnosed anxiety neurosis at the time of follow-up, four had been diagnosed hysteria and one hypochondriasis at the time of the original hospitalization. At time of follow-up, they all had clear-cut examples of anxiety neurosis as defined under Methods and more fully described elsewhere.

An important question to ask was whether these particular cases of anxiety neurosis, who had been originally diagnosed hysteria or hypochondriasis, were so atypical or so undeveloped when first seen that the diagnosis of anxiety neurosis could not reasonably have been made. Patient 5 did not present enough symptoms of anxiety neurosis at the time of hospitalization to permit a diagnosis at that time; however, at follow-up the symptoms of anxiety neurosis caused the patient's disability. Patient 6 was ill for only one day with an acute illness which looked clinically like a drug delirium. It was noted by the doctors at the time of hospitalization that the patient seemed to cry excessively. This coupled with the sudden cessation of the symptoms and absence of any fever might have led to the diagnosis of hysteria. The patient at follow-up had none of these symptoms seen in the hospital and had only the symptoms of a very mild anxiety neurosis. Patient 7 at the time of hospitalization had chiefly symptoms of anxiety neurosis, except for his difficulty in walking and fever. It was thought possible by the authors that the latter two symptoms might be associated and that the patient had two diseases at the time of hospitalizaion: an acute disease with fever and weakness giving him trouble walking, and a chronic anxiety neurosis which persisted and was present at follow-up. Patient 8 was receiving a series of anti-rabies shots, and the differential diagnosis of an encephalitis due to rabies vaccine or hysteria was seriously considered throughout. The patient presented a picture of delirium, but once this cleared, the physicians noted the child was "nervous" and "sensitive". This latter observation was valid. At the time of follow-up the patient did have an anxiety neurosis. However, in retrospect one might have guessed that the patient had an encephalitis and a separate, and chronic, disease—anxiety neurosis. Patient 9 was diagnosed hypochondriasis, although on entry to the hospital he had a fever associated with his abdominal pain.

Of the records of these five cases who later turned out to have anxiety neurosis, only one (the record of Patient 7) presented sufficient description of the patient's "nervousness" to make a clear retrospective diagnosis of anxiety neurosis possible. Of course, at the time of the original diagnosis of hysteria or hypochondriasis in these patients, the clinical criteria used in the follow-up for diagnosing anxiety neurosis and hysteria had not been developed. But this confusion between these diagnoses at the time of the original hospitalization demonstrates how necessary such clinical criteria are for the differential diagnosis of anxiety neurosis and hysteria.

In contrast with the four patients diagnosed hysteria at follow-up (Group I), these patients with anxiety neurosis were of both sexes—two female, three male—and the amount of disability was significantly less. Two patients had no disability and three patients had only mild disability.

Group III. Three Patients with Other Disease: Three patients were diagnosed hysteria at the time of hospitalization but at time of follow-up had neither hysteria nor anxiety neurosis. Patient 10 was a girl who at time of follow-up had a macular degeneration of both eyes, cause undetermined. The ophthalmologic consultant described the macular degeneration and obtained confirmatory evidence by visual field examinations. Patient 11 was diagnosed as having cardiospasm within two months after leaving the hospital. Roentgenograms at follow-up revealed a grossly dilated esophagus. Swallowing had continued to be so difficult that the patient never had swallowed at the table, but after each meal had gone to the bathroom and spent five or more minutes forcing the food from her esophagus to her stomach. Patient 12 was diagnosed psychopathic personality at the time of follow-up examination by the criteria listed under Methods. The occurrence of medical symptoms and "neurotic" symptoms in patients with psychopathic personality has been commented on elsewhere.

Group IV. Other Disease Plus Anxiety Neurosis: Group IV consists of three patients who, at time of follow-up, had another disease in addition to their anxiety neurosis. Patient 13 had been admitted to the hospital a number of times previous to the admission during which she was diagnosed hysteria, for multiple congenital genito-urinary anomalies. She began having convulsions, and these were diagnosed as hysterical convulsions. At a later hospitalization in the same hospital the diagnosis of true idiopathic epilepsy was made. This diagnosis of epilepsy was confirmed at the time of follow-up. The presence of an anxiety neurosis was an incidental finding not related to the epilepsy and it is not known whether the anxiety symptoms were present when the diagnosis of hysteria was made. Patient 14 at the time of follow-up was diagnosed by the orthopedic consultant as having a congenital orthopedic disease manifested by severe limitation of flexion of the lumbar spine and of flexion and extension of both hips. In the opinion of the authors and the orthopedic consultant this could have accounted for the back, joint, and leg pain the patient had at the time of the original hospitalization. The presence of the anxiety neurosis was again not related to the orthopedic disease, nor were anxiety symptoms reported in the original record. Patient 15 at the time of follow-up was diagnosed as an alcohol addict. In addition, he had an anxiety neurosis. The patient was diagnosed as an addict because he was intoxicated more than once a week and he had already been court-martialed for intoxication. The present diagnoses did not help clarify the clinical picture presented when admitted to the hospital originally.

Group V. Six Patients with Symptoms but in Whom a Diagnosis Could Not be Made: Patient 16 at the time of follow-up could not be diagnosed as having specific illness. She most nearly fitted into the ill-defined group regarded as having "tension headaches". She had a family history of headache, was nervous, had headaches when nervous, and became nauseated only with her headaches. Her clinical picture at the time of original hospitalization would not be inconsistent with this. Patient 17 at the time of follow-up had no diagnosable illness and no disability but she did have headaches perhaps of the "tension" headache type. The clinical picture at the time of original hospitalization was probably most consistent with an anxiety neurosis. Patient 18 at the time of follow-up most nearly fitted into the "tension headache" group. However, this diagnosis would not help to explain the symptoms such as nausea and vomiting, present at the time of hospitalization. Patient 19 could possibly have had hysteria at the time of follow-up. She did not fit the criteria noted under Methods. On the other hand, three years after the initial hospitalization she still has aphonia. It is possible that this child may turn out to have schizophrenia. It might be pointed out here that so-called "hysterical" symptoms may occur in schizophrenia and psychopathic personality, as well as in hysteria. Patient 20 at the time of follow-up still had occasional periumbilical pain associated sometimes with nausea and vomiting. The pain had been occurring about twice a year at the time of follow-up. She described herself as nervous, but doubted that this was related to her abdominal pain. Patient 21 at the time of follow-up, only two years after hospitalization, presented a puzzling picture essentially similar to that presented at the time of hospitalization. He presented a combination of recurrent abdominal pain and vomiting associated with difficulty in walking. He did not fulfill the criteria for the diagnosis of any of the diseases here considered and the neurologic consultant could not make a neurologic diagnosis.

Group VI. Two Patients Who Were Well: Patient 22 had abdominal pain for six weeks before his entry into the hospital. About a week after leaving the hospital this pain disappeared and had not returned at the time of follow-up. A tonsillectomy one year before the follow-up interview cured his recurrent sore throats and fever. Patient 23 had an attack of illness at the time of original hospitalization lasting six months. This attack was characterized by the symptoms noted in Table 3 and a 40-pound weight loss. He became well without known reason, and at the time of follow-up was in excellent health and doing well in school.

Reasons for Diagnosing the Patients Hysteria at the Time of Original Hospitalization. The hospital charts of all 16 patients originally diagnosed hysteria (Table 3) were reviewed carefully in order to find any statements explaining why the patients were so diagnosed. There were apparently two reasons why the diagnosis was entertained in all of the 16 patients. These reasons might or might not have been stated explicitly in the chart of any individual patient. These were that the physical findings were negative or were not sufficient to "explain" the extent and severity of the symptoms, and that at least one of the symptoms the patient had was one of the "classical" neurologic symptoms of hysteria or abdominal pain or vomiting. In addition to these two reasons, the charts of all of the patients except two contained at least one reason why a diagnosis of hysteria was made or explaining the onset of the hysterical attack. A few examples of these reasons for each patient follow. Patient 1—Attack of aphonia came on when couldn't answer a question in school; she is too large and mature—already menstruating—to be in the fifth grade. Patient 2—Has reprimanding, despotic stepfather; fits are bizarre. Patient 3—She has a nervous unstable father who made a suicidal attempt; she was recently baptized and the seriousness of sinning impressed on her. Patient 4—Grandmother has pernicious anemia, has trouble walking and child imitated her; mother and father are sickly. Patient 5—Attack came on following an examination in school. Patient 6—Patient observed a cousin pass a worm per rectum; child became worse when observed. Patient 7—Having trouble in school; shy and sensitive child. Patient 8—Patient quieted down when talked with sympathetically; sensitive child. Patient 10—(No reason given.) Patient 11—Patient dislikes home town to which she recently moved; mother began to work full-time outside the home shortly before trouble started; father had gastro-intestinal complaints. Patient 12—Day before symptoms began patient was hit on head by snow ball. Patient 13—Mother thought fits were a result of nervousness; patient had no fits while happy on a ward for a few days; patient unhappy and discouraged because of anal and genitol-urinary anomalies. Patient 15—(No reason given.) Patient 19—Dreamed her hair was burned off in an apartment house fire the night before her symptoms began; after being in the hospital two days she suddenly started to talk. Patient 21—Father thinks boy is pretending and has whipped him; mother had bad ankle and foot pains and gastro-intestinal symptoms; gait disturbance is variable; smiles and sighs when sore ankles are pressed.

These were examples of the explanations listed in the hospital records of these patients. They were obviously very diverse and it was not possible to find any characteristic pattern that these reasons presented. Many of them seemed to be a short summary of some of life's less pleasant experiences common to much of, if not all of, mankind. There was no clear difference in the reasons given for the four patients who had hysteria at the time of follow-up as contrasted with the 12 patients who did not have hysteria at the time of follow-up.

Psychologic and Social Findings at the Time of Follow-up. Of the 23 patients interviewed for this study, 5 (22%) were the children of divorced parents. Of the 11 patients over 20 years of age at time of follow-up, 6 (55%) were married, and 4 (36%) had children of their own. One of these patients (9%) had been divorced and remarried. Average length of schooling of interviewed patients over 20 years of age was 9.7 years. Average monthly income of the patient or (if a married woman) her spouse was $222.00. Patients diagnosed hysteria at time of follow-up did not differ significantly from the total group of interviewed patients in their income, marital status, their parent's marital status, or their schooling. There are insufficient data to state whether these patients differed from a normal population in these respects, but a consideration of some of the personal difficulties of individual patients seems to indicate a striking amount of maladjustment, particularly among patients with hysteria.

Group I. Four Patients with Hysteria: Patient 1 reported many problems in her childhood. She had had congenital angiomata of her tongue and cheek which had to be treated with radium. Her mother was very over-solicitous and took her to a doctor with the slightest illness. The patient reported an unhappy childhood and a long history of "nervousness." She married at 20 and had had three children. During the war while her husband was gone, she tried to live alone with her children. She grew to hate the house, finally had a "nervous breakdown" and went to live with her mother. At the time of follow-up she had many problems with her husband, his family, and her family. She and her husband constantly bickered. He was unsympathetic to her nervousness. Her husband's parents and two sisters had come to live with her. This had upset the patient greatly and caused an increase in her symptoms. She argued constantly with her own mother about her husband and about her younger sisters. These arguments made her feel heartless and cruel and made her feel remorseful. She described herself now as being indecisive, as having an excessive sense of responsibility without being able to do anything about it, and as being an extremely nervous and unhappy woman. Patient 2 had had an unhappy childhood. Her parents were divorced when she was very young. Her mother remarried, and her stepfather was a cruel and tyrannical man. He and his wife made the patient's life miserable with excessive demands for work, and with unfeeling punishment if she did not perform her household tasks. At about age 10, the patient became extremely nervous, quarrelsome and depressed. She married at 15 to get away from home. She had remained with her husband ever

HYSTERIA IN CHILDREN

since, but their marriage was incompatible. She had left him on two occasions and then returned to him. At follow-up she appeared to be a depressed and discontented woman. She and her husband enjoyed none of their activities together. They fought about how to bring up the child, about their sexual life, and about their relationships to their families. Patient 3 had many problems. Her lifelong problems with her father had increased recently. Her father had been cruel, hot-tempered and subject to recurrent depression. He had attempted suicide in the past, and at the time of follow-up had been thinking of divorcing his wife. In the past six to twelve months he had turned to his daughter (the patient) for emotional support which she felt unable to give him now. The patient cried while telling of this. She had at the time of follow-up some problems with her husband. She was sexually frigid and suffered from dyspareunia. Her husband became angry with her about this and other things. He shouted at her, and this made her cry. On the other hand, the marriage had some good things in it, such as the ability to participate in and enjoy common interests. Patient 4 at the time of follow-up had several problems. She had worked for a boss, who was inquisitive, querulous, dictatorial and obsequious to higher bosses, for four years. This boss' behavior caused her to become upset and have symptoms. In spite of this she continued to work there and missed only a few days because of hysterical symptoms. When she was angry, the patient was able to talk back to her boss but she then ruminated about losing her temper and became very upset. About a year prior to follow-up, her fiance was discovered to have cancer. She accepted this news without a serious increase in symptoms. She had been living with her parents, and there was some tension in the home about the patient's wilfulness, but the home seemed to have a vein of self-critical humor in it which prevented any serious difficulties from arising.

Groups, II, III, IV, V, and VI. All Other Patients not Having Hysteria at the Time of Follow-up: The personal problems of three patients with moderately severe problems will be described.

The other 16 patients seemed to have problems of lesser severity and will not be discussed further. It was interesting to note that some patients with symptoms had few if any personal problems, and other patients with symptoms seemed to have a significant history of these problems. The two well patients in Group VI had no significant problems and will also not be discussed further. Patients 15, 20 and 11 had a significant amount of personal problems. Patients 15 began having troubles in school with a moderate amount of truancy. He entered the military services and began to drink excessively. While in the service he was hospitalized in a psychiatric ward twice, once with a faked suicidal attempt and another time with a suicidal "gesture"—cutting his wrists. He was later court-martialed because of drinking. Since his discharge from the service he suffered recurrent feelings of depression which led to alcoholic debauches lasting days. After many fights his first wife divorced him. He stated that following this his mother annoyed him with her oversolicitous attentions. At the same time, he was annoyed with his second wife for her "coldness" and lack of solicitude. Patient 20 at the time of hospitalization had a serious problem. Her father suffered from alcohol addiction and was a gloomy, pessimistic man. The patient was affected by this gloom and felt depressed. She was ashamed of her father to the extent that she did not go to school for a year. Her father's drinking made her mother nervous which the patient believed in turn contributed to her own nervousness. About two years after her hospitalization, her father stopped drinking. Since then the patient had continued to have personal problems. She described herself as a person without self-confidence. She felt that she resisted being involved intimately with anyone because of this lack of confidence. She described herself as becoming easily upset if she had to hurry, if she had to meet deadlines, and if she had to meet any novel situation. Patient 11 described herself as extremely selfconscious, chronically unhappy and subject to severe temper outbursts. She described herself as having made her mother and herself miserable. At the time of follow-up she had been married eight months and felt that she was now making her husband miserable, and as a result she felt miserable. She and her husband argued so much that they began to go out with each other with excessive frequency in order to avoid the arguments that would occur at home. He had slapped her on two occasions. On the other hand, she and her husband enjoyed themselves when they went out together and their sexual life was a source of satisfaction to both.

This brief summary makes it clear that psychologic and social maladjustments are not peculiar to patients with hysteria, nor even peculiar to patients with a diagnosable psychiatric disease. Patient 20 did not have a diagnosable psychiatric illness and Patient 11 had a non-psychiatric disease—cardiospasm. These data would suggest then that the presence of personal problems is a treacherous and fallible way to attempt to diagnose hysteria, or even to differentiate psychiatric disease from non-psychiatric disease.

The Patients Who Were Located but Not Examined. There were 14 patients located who were not examined (Table 2). The group consisted of six boys and eight girls. In four patients a diagnosis was made. No diagnosis could be made in six patients, although they had either one or two symptoms. Four patients were well (asymptomatic). It must be emphasized that these diagnoses, or absence of them, were not certain because these patients were not examined personally. The group of four patients in whom a diagnosis was made consisted of one girl with hysteria, two girls with anxiety neurosis and one girl with epilepsy. The undiagnosed group of six patients consisted of two girls and four boys. In only one of these patients was nervousness mentioned as a symptom. The other five undiagnosed patients had either one or two symptoms, such as headaches, dysmenorrhea, diarrhea or abdominal pain. However, no more than two such symptoms were present in any one patient and no diagnosis could be made. The group of four patients who were well consisted of one female and three males.

The only significant discrepancy between this group of 14

patients and the group of 23 examined patients was the excess of patients who considered themselves well, 29% versus 9%. The excess of patients who were well in the unexamined group might well be explained by these patients not reporting minor symptoms that gave no disability.

In general, then, the diagnostic status of the 14 unexamined patients at the time of follow-up rather closely follows the pattern of the 23 examined patients. The data from these unexamined patients thus does not seem to affect the interpretation of the data from the examined patients.

Over-all Prognosis of the 23 Patients Examined. One interesting finding in this series of cases was the relatively poor prognosis of a group of children in a large metropolitan children's hospital with diagnoses of hysteria, hypochondriasis or mixed psychoneurosis. Of the 23 patients examined, only two (9%) were well. Another five patients (22%) had no disability despite some symptoms. Thus, only approximately a third (31%) of the patients had no disability. Sixty-nine per cent of the patients had some disability—30% (7 patients) were severely disabled and 39% (9 patients) were mildly disabled. Patients 13 and 21 were the only patients of the whole group who received psychiatric treatment.

Discussion and Speculation

This investigation was concerned with a follow-up study of 41 hospitalized children diagnosed hysteria, hypochondriasis or mixed psychoneurosis at the time of hospitalization. Since one of the purposes of this study was to describe the clinical features of childhood hysteria, it was felt important not to exclude any possible case of childhood hysteria. For this reason the diagnostic groups of hypochondriasis and mixed psychoneurosis with manifestations suggestive of hysteria were included in the original case material. These two diagnostic groups were chosen because they seemed to the authors the ones most likely to be confused with hysteria. This lessened the chance of mistakenly excluding a case of hysteria. This assumption proved correct in that of the five cases of hysteria found at follow-up, 4 cases were originally diagnosed hysteria and one was originally diagnosed hypochondriasis. As a result, it seems that there is an excellent chance that no case of true hysteria with a psychiatric diagnosis was excluded from the follow-up study. On the other hand, if a case of hysteria had been diagnosed originally some non-psychiatric disease, then it would not have been included in the original case material. It must be emphasized that since only five patients with hysteria at follow-up were found, many of the findings of this study must be regarded as tentative. A study of a large number of cases is required to validate completely the findings of this study. Also, it must be noted, these were patients who were hospitalized for symptoms. This means they were a selected group and that they were either more severely ill than the usual patient with a psychiatric (non-psychotic) disease or that their symptoms were more dramatic or resembled an acute illness.

There were 4 cases of hysteria at follow-up, all of which were originally diagnosed hysteria, among the 23 cases examined. There was one case of hysteria at follow-up originally diagnosed hypochondriasis, among the 14 patients not examined personally. These five cases of hysteria represent an extremely small per cent (0.01%) of the over 50,000 total admissions to the hospital in the 15 year period. This small number of cases indicates either that childhood hysteria is rare or that when childhood hysteria occurs it is rarely a cause for hospitalization in children. Two other studies present data relevant to the question of hospitalization of hysteria in childhood. H. Schmidt's study presents a total of only 80 cases of hysteria diagnosed in 11 years in the medical clinic at Tubingen, and A. Tobias' study presents a total of only 46 cases in 19 years at Schritt's clinic in Heidelberg.

Some data relevant to the question of age of onset have been presented elsewhere. There it was concluded that the onset of hysteria before the age of 9 or 10 is rare. This study gives no reason for modifying this finding. In only one of the five cases did the hysteria begin before the age of nine. Hysteria in this patient began at age five. This suggests that the symptoms of hysteria do not begin in infants or very young children, and that they begin infrequently before the age of 9 or 10. These findings agree with the opinions of Cameron and Rachford.

An important question to consider is whether the criteria for hysteria used in this study excluded the diagnosis of hysteria in mild cases who only partially fulfilled the criteria. These particular criteria were developed in another study in which the clinical picture of hysteria in adults was described. The use of these criteria assures that every case diagnosed hysteria at the time of follow-up was correctly diagnosed, but may exclude mild cases of hysteria who only partially fulfill the criteria, in particular the six undiagnosed patients. It is necessary to consider whether or not some of the six undiagnosed cases in this study may be such mild cases of hysteria. Only two of the six patients were originally diagnosed hysteria at hospitalization; the other four were diagnosed hypochondriasis or mixed psychoneurosis. As has been pointed out in the Results, Patients 16, 17 and 18 fitted most nearly into the group of patients often diagnosed "tension headache." There is little question that Patients 17 and 18 do not have even mild hysteria. They have no symptoms especially characteristic of hysteria. Patient 16 has a few more symptoms than Patients 17 and 18, but most of these additional symptoms occur only with her headaches and they are not typical of hysteria. Patients 19, 20 and 21 are the most questionable cases. Of these three patients, Patient 19 comes closest to fulfilling the criteria for the diagnosis of hysteria utilized in this study. She still has aphonia three years after hospitalization, and it may be that she does have hysteria. Patient 21 presents a puzzling problem and will require a longer follow-up than the 2 years—shortest in the series—that he has had so far. Patient 20 probably does not have hysteria, although she still has infrequent abdominal pain and vomiting. It will be instructive to follow these three patients for a few more years. It is also possible that patients who were originally correctly diagnosed hysteria might have recovered between the time of hospitalization and follow-up. Since only one of these patients was well at follow-up, this consideration is not important here. Neither is the question of the influence of psychiatric treatment important, since only one of the undiagnosed patients had such treatment.

The clinical picture of hysteria in children based on the characteristics presented at hospitalization by four patients with hysteria at the time of follow-up includes the following: (1) The illness is multi-symptomatic; (2) The duration of the illness prior to hospitalization for the first time is measured in months or years and not days or weeks; (3) The "classical" pseudo-neurologic symptoms of hysteria and/or abdominal pain and vomiting are prominent symptoms; (4) Nervousness or the so-called somatic symptoms of "anxiety" (palpitation, breathing difficulty, paresthesias, dizziness, fatigue and weak feelings) are a contant feature; and, (5) The illness seems to occur only in females. It is suggested that the combination of these five findings should allow one to diagnose hysteria in children when it is present and to avoid the diagnosis when hysteria is not present.

The occurrence of many symptoms even early in the course of hysteria is consistent with an impression gained in another study. Hysteria in children as in adults is a multi-symptomatic disease. The absence of monosymptomatic hysteria in all of the patients is striking. All 16 patients originally diagnosed hysteric had more than one symptom at hospitalization. Therefore, in this study, even the possibility of monosymptomatic hysteria did not present itself. This conflicts with some of the conclusions stated in this field. This discrepancy cannot be finally explained on the basis of the data of this study. A possible explanation is that childhood hysteria that does not lead to hospitalization is monosymptomatic in some cases. However, this explanation would require a follow-up study of clinic cases for proof. There is one other study which suggests that monosymptomatic hysteria, in patients admitted to a hospital, is rare. In 21 cases, Tobias reports only one monosymptomatic case and she states this case may have not been pure hysteria, but an exaggeration of pain occurring as a result of an injury to one ankle. Another possible explanation of the occurrence of cases thought to be monosymptomatic hysteria may be that other symptoms were not asked for. A patient who complains dramatically of only one symptom may be said to have a monosymptomatic illness only if other symptoms have been asked for and denied. The absence of any study in which other symptoms were systematically investigated casts serious doubt on the concept of monosymptomatic hysteria, particularly in view of the present study and a previous study on adults. To ascertain the actual number of symptoms in a series of cases of childhood hysteria requires that the patients be asked a series of standard questions as in the follow-up in this study. This would not only be of research value but would establish clinical norms for use in everyday diagnostic work with children.

It is interesting that it was possible following the completion of this study to set up two arbitrary criteria that could have predicted correctly the presence or absence of hysteria at follow-up in 21 of the 23 cases. These criteria are a minimum of five symptoms and a minimum duration of illness of nine months at the time of hospitalization. This relatively long duration of symptoms of hysteria prior to hospitalization is open to many interpretations. Here only two will be discussed. It is possible that hysteria almost always begins insidiously and that any acute, dramatic symptoms leading to hospitalization are simply superimposed on many other less dramatic symptoms of longer duration. If this is so, it would be an important diagnostic aid in hysteria. Another possible explanation is that the parents of the child suspect an element of malingering and delay hospitalization. There is no crucial evidence for either of these possibilities, and other possible explanations exist.

The occurrence of nervousness or the so-called somatic symptoms of "anxiety" both at the time of original hospitalization and at follow-up in every one of the patients diagnosed hysteria at follow-up casts doubt on the phenomenon of "conversion" in hysteria. The concept of "conversion" and other psychodynamic concepts have not been utilized in this study. Apart from the question of their validity, these concepts are not easily applicable to clinical diagnosis by physicians who are not psychiatrists. Since this study attempts to set up criteria by means of which a pediatrician without special psychiatric training can correctly diagnose hysteria, these concepts are irrelevant to the purposes of the study.

There were no males with hysteria found at follow-up. This confirms the findings of another study in which no case of hysteria in a civilian male could be found. In this study, since there was only one undiagnosed male, even if he should prove to have hysteria, there would still be a marked preponderance of females with hysteria. It is interesting to attempt an answer to a question Kanner asks in his textbook. He is interested in what happens to boys diagnosed hysteria. In this study there were six such boys examined. The results are that at follow-up three have an anxiety neurosis, one has been diagnosed psychopathic personality, one is an alcohol addict, and one is undiagnosed.*

An analysis of the chief complaints at the time of hospitalization (Table 3) did not reveal any consistent differences between the chief complaints of the children who turned out to have hysteria in adult life and the chief complaints of those children who did not have hysteria at follow-up. This contrasts with the findings in a study of adult hysteria, where a multiple or vague and irrelevant chief complaint was characteristic of adult women with hysteria.

* "After submission of this paper for publication, two male patients of the 14 patients who had been contacted but not examined were interviewed and examined personally. Both had been diagnosed hysteria at the time of original hospitalizations, one 14 years ago and the other 13 years ago. At the time of follow-up, one patient is completely well and the other has a mild anxiety neurosis. Thus, of 8 males examined at follow-up, none had hysteria, four have anxiety neurosis, one psychopathic personality, one alcoholic addiction, one is well and one is undiagnosed.

In the present series of 23 cases examined, the use of the five clinical characteristics above noted would have diagnosed all 4 cases with hysteria correctly and (even leaving out the duration of illness prior to hospitalization, criterion 2) would have avoided an incorrect diagnosis in all of the remaining 10 cases originally diagnosed hysteria who were diagnosed something else at time of follow-up. These criteria would not have helped with the two patients undiagnosed at the time of follow-up. In summary, then, they would have probably been effective in 14 out of 16 cases (87%).

There is some suggestive evidence from this study of how *not* to diagnose hysteria in children. The occurrence of serious, disabling life stresses in the patients diagnosed hysteria at follow-up is apparent. The fact that these stresses sometimes exacerbate the symptoms is also evident, if the patient's stories are valid. But the patients who did not have hysteria at follow-up also reported these same kinds of life stresses and other symptoms in relation to them. Not only was this true in patients with anxiety neurosis, but it was also true in the patients with nonpsychiatric diseases—in the patient with cardiospasm as well as in the patient with macular degeneration. The fact that disabling life stresses cause an exacerbation of symptoms is therefore not a good diagnostic point for hysteria; it occurs in other psychiatric as well as medical diseases. Lurie has presented one case which vividly describes the pitfalls of this diagnostic approach to psychiatric disease in children. However, the absence of a history of life stresses with resulting symptoms would make questionable the diagnosis of hysteria in children or adults.

A second method of diagnosing hysteria in children that seems unreliable is the use of concepts such as, "The symptoms are too intense for the findings on physical examination" or "The symptoms and signs do not follow known anatomic or physiologic boundaries" or "The symptoms get better when the patient thinks no one is looking or when the patient is treated sympathtically." These concepts seemed to contribute to an equivocal diagnosis at the time of original hospitalization in Patients 5, 7, 10, 12, and 21.

A third method of diagnosing hysteria in children that seems unreliable is to consider the diagnosis in patients who have somatic symptoms and who seem nervous or "sensitive," without considering the total clinical picture. For example, the occurrence of nervousness plus fits in Patient 13 seemed to contribute to the diagnosis of hysteria when actually the patient has an anxiety neurosis plus idiopathic epilepsy. This kind of diagnostic approach seemed to contribute to the equivocal diagnosis of hysteria at the time of original hospitalization in Patients 6, 8 and 10, as well as in Patient 13.

No special emphasis was placed here on the presence of "hysterical" stigmata such as pharyngeal anesthesia or corneal anesthesia. Sir Arthur Hurst believed these "stigmata" did not occur spontaneously and were induced by the examiner. He was able to create new "stigmata," namely, umbilical anesthesia, nasal anesthesia, and spiraling of the visual fields outward.

No attention was paid here to one other clinical phenomenon sometimes thought to be hysteria, discussed by Creak. This phenomena is the "hysterical" prolongation of a symptom originally part of a non-psychiatric disease. This did not arise as a problem in this study and, in the opinion of the authors, this is not hysteria in the sense which it is used in this study.

From the results of this investigation, it is suggested that the diagnosis of hysteria in children might be made by following the standard method of clinical medicine; determining the facts of the chief complaint, of the present illness, of the past history, and of the physical examination. In speaking of procedures to be used in child guidance clinics, Lurie has ably stated this approach to the diagnosis and treatment of children's psychiatric diseases: "Therefore, when confronted with a child who is presenting a behavior problem . . . it is extremely important that our reaction should be that we are dealing with a child who may be sick in a purely medical sense, and our approach should be guided by that principle. This means that our approach to the problem should be the same as if the child had been brought to the clinic with the complaint of fever, or rash, or pain in the chest. To the alert physician, all sorts of possibilities present themselves immediately for differential diagnosis, necessitating careful history taking and painstaking physical examinations. The same technique should be applied to the study of . . . the problem child. The presenting symptom or chief complaint of the problem child, like the presenting physical symptom, offers a challenge in differential diagnosis. In the practice of medicine, it is manifestly unfair to the patient to make a snap diagnosis on the basis of presenting symptom alone. Similarly in child psychiatry it is also unfair to conclude from the chief complaint alone the nature of the factors involved. . . ."

In summary then, this study, by utlizing a long term follow-up, has attempted to set up criteria for the diagnosis of hysteria in children. It has not been a primarily prognostic study. All that can be said about hysteria prognostically from this study is that all four patients originally diagnosed hysteria who still had it at the time of follow-up were disabled. However, since the criteria for diagnosing hysteria at follow-up included so many symptoms, this disability might be expected. It may be added that the overall prognosis of being admitted to a children's hospital with symptoms suggestive of hysteria is not good—63% of the 19 patients who did not have hysteria at follow-up showed some disability and only 11% were completely well.

One of the chief purposes of this study was to set up a criteria for diagnosis of hysteria in children so that a follow-up study of a homogeneous clinical group could be made. Gunnarson has commented that various prognostic studies, which are reviewed in his paper, are not comparable because the various studies did "not adopt a uniform system of classification in regard to children's nervous symptoms." A uniform system of classification concerning a disease for which there is no crucial diagnostic test requires a standard procedure for obtaining clinical data that can be described in such a way that other workers of varying backgrounds can read and use the described procedure. This standardization requires not only standard questions but also addressing them to the *patient* himself whenever possible. Doctors to often accept the impressions of relatives even when the child is old enough to answer for himself. A relative is likely to describe dramatic or grossly apparent symptoms, whereas the patient himself will often describe symptoms of subjective discomfort such as palpitation or feelings of nervousness or shortness of breath, which the relative is unaware of or does not think important enough to tell the doctor.

Now that criteria for the diagnosis of hysteria in children have been set up, a primarily prognostic study could be accomplished by following for a number of years one group of children that meet these criteria and comparing them with another group of children who do not meet these criteria but who have symptoms suggestive of hysteria. It would also be possible to test the effects of treatment in such a study. It would be important to extend these studies to non-hospitalized children as well.

Conclusions

1. A nine year follow-up study of 41 hospitalized children diagnosed hysteria, hypochondriasis and mixed psychoneurosis in which 37 (90.2%) were located and 23 personally examined, revealed 5 cases of hysteria at the time of follow-up.

2. The 19 patients without hysteria of the 23 patients examined at follow-up revealed five patients with anxiety neurosis; six patients each of whom had one of the following conditions: psychopathic personality, alcohol addiction, bilateral macular degeneration, cardiospasm, idiopathic epilepsy, and a congenital orthopedic disease causing limited flexion and ex-

tension of back and hips; six patients with symptoms in whom a diagnosis could not be made; and two patients who were completely well.

3. Hospitalized children originally diagnosed hysteria in a metropolitan childen's hospital were rare—only 27 cases out of 51,311 cases admitted during the 15¼ year period considered in this study.

4. The clinical picture of childhood hysteria includes the following: (a) Many symptoms; (b) Long duration of symptoms prior to hospitalization; (c) Presence of the "classical" pseudoneurologic symptoms of hysteria and/or abdominal pain and vomiting; (d) Presence of nervousness or the so-called somatic symptoms of "anxiety"—palpitation, breathing difficulty, paresthesias, dizziness, fatigue and weak feelings. The use of these criteria would seem to help make the diagnosis of hysteria when present and to avoid the diagnosis when hysteria is not present.

5. The age of onset of hysteria in children is unusual before age 9, and seems rare below age 5.

6. Monosymptomatic hysteria did not occur in this series.

7. No male with hysteria was found at follow-up.

8. The phenomenon of "conversion" was not a diagnostic help in these patients and, in fact, was misleading, since all the patients with hysteria showed nervousness or somatic symptoms of "anxiety" both at the time of original hospitalization and at follow-up.

9. The use of such diagnostic approaches to hysteria in children as the presence of serious life stresses, the occurrence of nervousness (not further defined) and the lack of correlation between physical signs or behavior and symptoms is a fallible and unreliable way to diagnose hysteria.

10. The clinical method of diagnosis in pediatrics, that is, the use of history, examination and relevant laboratory data, seems equally applicable to the diagnosis of hysteria in children.

11. A further study of the diagnosis of hysteria in children,

with more patients, seems warranted from the results of this study.

12. A further study of prognosis in childhood hysteria utilizing the diagnostic criteria listed here seems practical and important.

CASES OF HYSTERIA IN CHILDHOOD

Marynia F. Farnham

Hysteria in children has, by the nature of its definition, been thought to be extremely rare and references to it in the literature on children are correspondingly infrequent. Hysteria involves us in the arrival at the genital phase of life and very many children's problems arise through a retardation and failure to accomplish this and many others surround the vicissitudes of the struggle to resolve the oedipal complex.

The author proposes that certain manifestations of the period surrounding the resolution of the oedipal complex, or when it might be expected that latency would have set in, are recognizable as hysterical in form. It has been found that certain children who present apparently extremely serious symptomatology with severe loss of relation to reality, accompanying very marked behavior disturbances are likely subjects of such designation. It has furthermore been noted in several cases, which will be cited later, the tendency has been for the children to produce a picture in Rorschach tests which leads the tester to the suggestion that the child is suffering from the beginnings of an early schizophrenic breakdown. In the cases to be cited here it will be observed that certain data are identical. The children are all approximately the same age; that is, they are in the oedipal stage at the point where theoretically the forces leading to latency should be operating. They all show gross disturbances of behavior and their relations to reality are grossly disordered. There are extreme manifestations of anxiety in all. They also show obviously grossly abnormal Rorschach findings and in all instances the tester was inclined to believe

CASES OF HYSTERIA IN CHILDHOOD

that one was faced with a possible schizophrenic breakdown. They were all girls. The subsequent course of their treatment and recovery demonstrated without any shadow of doubt that there was not a schizophrenic process and led one to the consideration of how such gross abnormality might come to be. This in turn has led to the consideration of the probability of a deformed or premature hysterical formation in such children.

The pseudo-hysterical structure is not widely considered in the literature. We propose to examine here and present cases of three girl children who presented similar findings. That is, they all showed characteristics on the critical side of being extremely disturbed in their behavior with an apparent departure from reality consideration and at times behavior and attitude would seem to indicate existence of a twilight state in which they seemingly were unaware of the situation around them. In these states they had an amnesia and at the same time they showed evidences of gross anxiety and abnormal behavior patterns. They were all between the age of five and eight years old. At the same time, they all had Rorschach tests which showed similar findings.

The first child was six years old at the time she was first brought to treatment because of her seeming lack of relation to reality, and because of her abnormal behavior pattern which, in her mother's opinion, indicated that there was some difficulty in the little girl's development. She was an adopted child, taken into the home at the time when there was a great deal of difficulty in the home pattern. The father was out of the home at the time that she was actually brought into it because of the war situation. Her adaptation in her earlier years had been relatively good, but as she approached her fourth year there began to be great difficulties. Her mother found it very difficult to exact obedience from her and she showed every sign of being rebellious and obstinate. There was particular difficulty in inducing her to take any self-dependent attitude and she was frequently at odds with her mother in the disciplinary setting. There was a great deal of crying and at times an apparently total withdrawal from reality, during which she would sit by herself in a seeming trance and fail to respond when spoken to. These episodes were of short duration and could be interfered with by sufficient firmness on the part of the mother.

At the time when she was brought into treatment there were no other symptoms as the mother's efforts to concede had still not been successful. On psychological examination, there were marked and interesting contrasts. While it was apparently easy to make a contact and she showed a cooperative attitude, nevertheless there were factors in the setting which made the examiner say that she believed that there was a possible schizophrenia. This was a modified consideration, but one which the tester nevertheless found to be a possibility. This child behaved like all others in this group in that she showed a marked negativism, but a surprising capacity for making contact. She entered into treatment readily and as readily began to present the material which ultimately led to her ability to master her difficulties. At many times there was a tendency to revert to the state which seemed to border on the dream or fugue, but at no time did this over-power her and she was always able to maintain her contact and return to the relationship of therapy. It was a long effort to find out the circumstances which produced the neurotic reaction. Ultimately she was able to express through her drawings the fact of her tremendous guilt and anxiety over her fantasied destructiveness toward the parental relation. Thus there had not been an adequate solution or even the beginning of a solution of the oedipal complex. This rested on the father's extreme inadequacy and the mother's attempt to take the place of the father and to assume an aggressive and commanding position in the family. Sally had little opportunity to identify with her aggressive mother who was frighteningly powerful and punishing in the little girl's fantasies. She had been forced to give up her strivings for her father and had found no compassion and help in her mother.

At a certain point in treatment masturbatory activity became of outstanding importance. This was in marked contrast to the situation prior to treatment when the mother had not observed any remarkable overt masturbatory activity. It was apparent that as treatment progressed and brought out her confusion about her own role in the parental discord she was able once more to return to the strongly repressed oedipal strivings, act them out and bring herself closer to the facts as they were.

There were times when her retreat from reality necessitated strong measures to induce her to relinquish the playing with fantasy and illusory material to a dangerous extent. It always appeared that after one of these instances the resort to masturbatory activity acted as a restorative to this child. It meant that she was able to face her guilt squarely, to face the issues that it involved, namely, her wish to undermine and intrude into the parental relationship and her feeling that her own activities actually disrupted the relationship between the parents. So she had accomplished her goal in ways which were for her intolerable and produced in her an anxiety and guilt which she was not able to handle. She was greatly given to dictating stories which were to be written by the Doctor. Most of these had to do with experiences paraphrased in the usual symbolism of animals and the extraordinary behavior of those animals, particularly those of the accepted male symbolic type. "Once upon a time I fell off a horse a long, long time ago and I didn't cry a bit. You know why, because I went too fast. That is the end of the story." Another story has to do with a little girl walking in the woods who heard something growling and then she saw that it was a lion and then it ran up a tree and "bang" she shot it and then he ran home and he was very good and went to bed and told his mommie what he did and then he had supper and said that he went up the tree and shot the lion. "Then he went to sleep. That is the end of the story. I am going to bed myself. He didn't wet his bed, he is having a nap and he woke up." Another rest in the woods—"a little rabbit came and he didn't shoot him because it was a nice rabbit." All of this had reference to the approaching birth of a brother, who was a natural child, and the discovery of this, which took place midway in treatment, activated much of her previous sexual trauma.

The next child which we will discuss has a good deal in common with the first mentioned case. She was somewhat older, being about seven at the time that treatment began, but had presented fairly serious problems for some time past. She was the older of two children, her younger sister being some four years her junior. She began to present difficulties in the form of great fears and of appearing to have enormous apprehension about physical damage and at the same time of showing a tendency to depart from reality and to present a picture of being in a trance or a fugue state. She did not show these difficulties until about her sixth year and from that time on they had grown progressively more obvious and more troublesome to the child and to the parents. The Rorschach test findings were similar to those of the previous child, with a great deal of fear and preoccupation with morbid sexual ideas appearing in the test material. She gave frequent evidence of feelings of being unable to cope with her problem and unable to manage the problems of reality. She was withdrawing greatly into fantasy. This fantasy was of no help to her but tended to make for her a private world and walled her off from reality. Her fantasy showed much more sexual concern than was usual regarding the problems of her masculinity and femininity. At the same time, she showed some difficulties in dealing with spatial concepts.

She seemed to be a very sick girl, with a probable diagnosis of schizophrenia. It was soon apparent that the first fears were not warranted as she made a fairly prompt and good contact with a tendency at first to revert back to early, much more infantile play concepts and attitudes than were consistent with her age. She repeatedly brought out evidence of having had severe sexual trauma in the sexual play, which was, perhaps, unusually common in the area in which she lived. Her intense fear of boys and her equally almost uncontrollable necessity to provoke them into a repetition of the sexual play which had proved so traumatic to her and which had apparently been the precipitating factor in her difficulties, recurred constantly in the activity of the playroom. She proceeded, after not too long a time, to act out the reassuring play of child, baby and consolidation of her feminine life. She gradually, over a period of a year, was able to gain insight into her difficulty and to establish her femininity on a fairly satisfactory and reassuring basis. She has been free of symptoms or difficulties for two years without any recurrence.

A third child was presented for treatment at the age of one month less than six years. The mother's complaints at that time were that she was enormously disturbed and from time to time seemed to present a picture of destruction which was connected with reality. She was the eldest of three children, one being two years younger than herself and the other being four years younger. She had presented her difficulties for some time, beginning approximately after the birth of the first child when she was four years old, but arising to an aggravated climax in the early months just before she was first seen. At this time she was extremely disturbed and agitated. Her relations with her mother were remarkably unsatisfactory and there seemed to be no point at which her mother could reach her or make any contact with her and that all the efforts the mother made were doomed to failure before she even started. Maisie presented a bizarre seeming psychotic picture. She was, so far as her intelligence went, superior to her age and displayed good intellectual equipment. The Rorschach test, however, showed her to have a great disturbance in the area of personal relations and particularly in the area of sexual understanding. There was a marked tendency to withdraw and become absorbed in her own inner ideas and fantasies and very limited interest in the outside world with which she had no real contact. She presented a picture of someone feeling that she was not a part of her world but one looking at it in a somewhat "split way."

The difficulties arose from the very extreme feelings of guilt which this little girl had toward her mother because of her own fantasied aggression. At this time interpersonal and emotional situations were disorganizing and disturbing. She was deeply frightened by and preoccupied with her feelings of having damaged her mother through her own fantasy relationship with her father. This was greatly aggravated by her mother's discovery and observation of her masturbatory activities and the unwise way in which this was handled. It was discovered too that there had been at about this time a sexual episode with a boy considerably older than herself. These circumstances converged and proved to be too taxing for her to handle, with the result that her defenses were breached and she was forced to the retreat of illness. Maisie behaved very much like Sally and Joan in treatment.

It was not long before it was clear that there was no occasion for the conviction that there was a prepsychotic or psychotic state. The child was actually readily accepting of contact in the therapeutic situation and entered, after a brief spell of resistance, into play activity which made use of drawing. Her drawing activities were, to a very marked extent, at first indicative of deep guilt and fear lest her forbidden sexual activities be discovered. Her first drawing was in itself interesting as it consisted of the conventional house as representative of the mother, but the house was supplied with almost innumerable windows in form of eyes and became actually a mass of eyes instead of a really formed house. It is interesting in this respect, that her tests also showed a great emphasis upon facial features in the drawing of a woman, with particular attention to the eyes. She also drew repeatedly scenes representative of the injurious situations to which she had been exposed with the guilt and anxiety which then inundated her and finally reduced her power to deal with her life problems. As with the other two children, her response was relatively rapid and when she was able to find the sources of her dificulties, she made quick use of her insight and readily relinquished her symptoms. She has been well for four years and has shown during this time no tendency to relapse. She has entered latency with no problems and is now approaching puberty.

Three cases have been presented, all of them girls, all of them show similarity in their presenting problems, even to noticeable similarity in the Rorschach tests which were applied to all of them, along with the usual battery of psychological tests. The outstanding feature of all of the tests was that there was marked anxiety which was pushing the child to the edge of her capacity to handle the situation; the anxiety had very strong guilty sexual coloration. The distortion of reality relation and the general demoralization made the probable diagnosis schizophrenia. All the children also showed the same response to treatment in a much more rapid development of good contact in therapy than would have been expected in psychotic children, and the rapid dismissal of the possible psychotic diagnosis in the early part of the treatment. They also responded promptly to the uncovering of the sexual difficulties which had precipitated their problems and have maintained their healthy condition since the termination of treatment, all three of them now being in latency and approaching puberty. It is suggested that this is a form of hysteria brought on in children at the age when the oedipal conflict is dominant. Dependent upon the sensitivity of the child, the general climate in the home, sexual traumata have induced the production of a state bordering on, or closely resembling fugue formation. The anxiety thus aroused, threatening to inundate the child, whose defenses are breached, forces the individual to a retreat from reality and the twilight state emerges. The withdrawal from reality appears most strikingly in the Rorschach and general psychological test material. The anxiety that is aroused by the suggestion of a psychotic diagnosis is very readily dismissed in the clinical setting where these children showed a remarkable ease of contact and a ready adaptation to treatment with a prompt response when the difficulties were uncovered.

THE PSYCHOANALYSIS OF A CASE OF "GRAND HYSTERIA OF CHARCOT" IN A GIRL OF FIFTEEN

Lydia G. Dawes

Many neurotic patterns, often with distinct hysterical coloring, are evident in early childhood and come into full bloom in the latter half of latency and in adolescence. We are all familiar with transient hysterical symptoms which bring children to the hospital such as fainting, vomiting and vague pains. Many of these somatic complaints clear quickly. More tenacious and difficult to treat are the cases of hysterical blindness, deafnes or paralysis that we occasionally see in early latency.

The following case of hysteria is presented to show the mental mechanisms behind the symptoms and how complex the whole matter can be. The presenting symptoms are only the end result of a long and complicated process. This process lies buried deep in the unconscious and has its origin in traumatic events in the early childhood of the patient. During the treatment the details of the unconscious mechanisms had to be first discovered and then shown to the patient so that she could function in a more healthy manner.

A Case of Conversion Hysteria

"Grand hysteria" is rarely seen today, although such cases were common enough in Charcot's clinic where Freud first observed them in the 1880's. Later, his masterly analysis of his patient "Dora" gave us the first dynamic concept of hysteria.

Sally, a fifteen year old, was referred to me when she was sent

GRAND HYSTERIA OF CHARCOT

to the Massachusetts General Hospital for study and diagnosis. She came from a remote village in the Green Mountains of Vermont. Perhaps this isolation played a part in the picture. Since the analysis was successful and her symptoms were discarded one by one as the analysis progressed, it was thought that it would be worth while to report this case in detail.

The hospital study ruled out all physical causes for her malady. All tests were negative. Physical findings were all within the normal range. A complete neurological examination with spinal puncture and electroencephalogram did not discover any pathology.

To digress a moment, this patient so interested the physicians that they were eager to see if analysis could cure her. She had a curious type of affliction—"spells" which occurred once or twice a day. Oddly enough, during the first week of each month, there appeared with clock-like regularity, an enormous increase in the number of these spells, often to 100 a day. This continued for perhaps a week and then the old pattern of 1-2 spells a day reappeared until the next month.

Each "spell" was initiated and terminated by a loud sneeze! Her gestures and pantomime behavior during these spells was arresting and thought-provoking. During her violent, 100 a day period, she showed the typical *arc de cercle*. She also had an affliction of the lower extremities. She could neither stand nor walk. If placed on her feet she collapsed immediately like a limp doll. This walking inhibition started in the hospital. All these facts were given to me before I saw the patient.

The following facts are taken from the record of the social worker. The patient was born in a small village in the mountains of Vermont. She had a sister two years older. Her father, a habitual drunkard, was often arrested for cruelty when drunk and deserted the family when Sally was three. Her mother then took her two daughters to live at the house of a friend. When Sally was six her mother died of septicemia following an abortion. The two little girls then became wards of the state and were placed in the home of the Overseer of the Poor. As was customary, they worked for their "board and keep." When Sally was 10 the Overseer died and the girls were moved again to the home of Mr. and Mrs. X. These people were poor, honest, and religious. Mrs. X had two well grown boys and since she knew the children's mother, she asked for the girls. She apparently was very kind to them. Sally lived in this home until she became ill and was sent to Boston for diagnostic study.

The social worker who brought Sally knew this family and felt that this home was a good one. She felt sorry for Sally and drove her to Boston herself. During this 5 hour drive, Sally behaved in a very "confused manner." She had one or two "spells" en route. She talked all the time in a very babyish way. When they stopped to eat she "demanded to be fed with a spoon." This social worker, thoroughly familiar with this case, was very troubled by the change in this girl, saying "she had never acted that way before." The first spell had followed an appendectomy eight months before. Sally was first brought to a home for children in Boston late in October.

The village doctor's notes sent with the patient stated that he had never seen anything like this before. He was puzzled how to diagnose it. He had known the patient since her birth and she always appeared to be healthy. There was no history of epilepsy in the family. The "spells" appeared suddenly 8 months ago, and he had attended her for the past 2 months. He had referred the patient to the nearest large hospital for study, but a difference of opinion as to the diagnosis there left him dissatisfied, and he requested that she be sent to Boston for study, diagnosis and advice as to treatment.

During the period of observation at the home for children Sally was ambulatory. She did have one or two spells per day. But after a week or so she had several hundred spells per day. This necessitated her transfer to the Massachusetts General Hospital and verified the observations of the local doctor.

At the Massachusetts General Hospital the following additional facts came to light:

Six months before admission, the patient had a mild blow

in the abdomen by a swing board in the school yard. She had a medical examination because she complained of a pain in the abdomen and then had a six hour epistaxis.

Five months before admission, the diagnosis of appendicitis was made and an appendectomy was performed at a hospital. Three weeks later, after her return home, the patient again complained of pain in the abdomen as well as headache, and had her first "spell." Following this the patient had frequent spells accompanied by vomiting and was admitted to the nearest hospital for study, All examinations, including gastrointestinal series and lumbar puncture were negative and she was discharged after three weeks in the hospital.

Patient had no more spells until the three months before admission to the Massachusetts General Hospital when she had a series of spells apparently in the first week of each month.

The patient was then admitted to the Psychiatric Service of Dr. Stanley Cobb at the Massachusetts General Hospital. Physical examination showed "a poorly nourished, small, sexually immature girl. Nascent breasts, pubic hair minimal. Blood pressure was 105/65; pulse 100-80; gag reflex was absent; there was a prominent sinus arrhythmia and moderate red flare on skin stroke. Findings were otherwise negative. Laboratory findings, including lumbar puncture and electro-encephalogram were all essentially negative."

The patient at this time was having a great number of seizures. The resident, Dr. Samuel Hunt, recorded the following description of the patient at this time. "The patient had eighty seizures per hour. In the free intervals she was cheerful, friendly and cooperative, markedly nonchalant and indifferent to her chief symptom. She laughed frequently and talked freely with considerable repartee and banter, but appeared under considerable tension. She complained only of abdominal pain and headache.

"The *spells* were initiated by a loud and typical sneeze. Immediately following this the arms were stretched stiffly over the head . . . and the legs hyperextended. The eyes rolled back, usually to the left, and the face seemed to become flushed and to assume a frown. With this there was a champing, chewing, sucking movement of the mouth, and a scraping of the lower lip against the upper incisors, frequently gasping noises, and intermittent cessation of respiration without cyanosis. The torso was frequently arched so that the weight was supported on the heels and the occiput alone. At times the right arm was brought down spasmodically with force against the face or abdomen. It was noted that touching the abdominal scar always initiated a seizure. These seizures lasted from thirty to one hundred twenty seconds. There was no clonic phase, no incontinence, moderate slowing of the pulse rate and no alteration of blood pressure in these spells. No post-convulsive neurological findings. Spells were usually followed by a brief period of semi-confusion but at times the patient was immediately lucid. On attempt to walk patient had repeated seizures and fell toward the bed. Three days following admission there were two to ten brief, milder spells per hour. Abdominal pain initiated each spell. At times these spells were initiated or terminated by a sneeze but not always."

After two weeks of hospitalization the spells occurred two to five times during an hour interview and less frequently at other times. These spells involved only the arms and head. The analyst was contacted at this time because it was felt that all findings were negative and both physical and neurological studies had produced no clue to this illness. A psychological test had been given in which Sally rated in the dull normal group. Dr. Cobb thought it would be interesting to see if this case were suitable for analysis. Diagnosis was made at this time of "grand hysteria."

Period of Observation in the Hospital (Analyst's Notes)

The first visit of the analyst to the hospital took place at this time. The patient was a pathetic looking young girl, who did not look her fifteen years. She was very unsophisticated in appearance. Her complexion was sallow, hair and eyes were brown; she wore glasses which were small and old-fashioned, and her body was slender and immature. The old-fashioned glasses gave her face a quizzical expression. She wore pajamas and a bathrobe and was tied in a wheel chair by a heavy strip of cloth passing around her waist. A blanket covered her legs and a pillow was tucked behind her. She did not look particularly ill, but one might say rather thin, undernourished and bewildered. Immediately after being introduced she sneezed, twisted her body to the left, thrust both arms out in front of her with fingers widespread. She rolled her eyes to the left as though looking for something. She seemed to raise her pelvis and although her legs were rigidly held there was a noticeable trembling. She was out of contact, apparently did not hear the examiner when spoken to, but made peculiar noises with her mouth part of the time chewing loudly and clucking with her lips and tongue. After a few seconds, she sneezed again, looked directly at the analyst and became quiet and appeared to be interested and lucid. She was then easy to contact, and the following material came in a hesitant manner with many pauses:—

"These spells come often and that's the reason why I'm in Boston. They started after the operation (appendectomy). I was sent to the hospital in the city of ——, and there the doctors used to slap my face when I got in such a state."

She emphasized the following: "These spells get worse around the first of the month. The doctors there said that if I had my period that this would all go away. I'm worried because I'm fifteen and I still have not menstruated but my sister had her period since she was thirteen. What do you think of all this?" To this the analyst responded, "I would like to hear more about what you think about it all and how you like Boston." The patient then began to talk about the children's home from which she was transferred, and enthused about the babies there.

Sneezing suddenly, she had another spell and after a few seconds it was over. Sally continued the conversation as if nothing had happened, and added, "There was a baby there with something the matter with his leg and I felt very sorry for him."

After the above conversation the patient returned to the subject of her "seizures" saying, "I wish these spells would stop because I have an awful pain in my stomach. It's worse before they start and it's there when they finish. I know when they are coming because it is sharp, like a knife." She localized the pain by placing her hand on her lower abdomen, then continued saying, "My hands get numb, and I am awfully frightened."

She then, at my request, gave me a sketch of her home, which was, from her description, a very simple one, typical of the poorer type in any country village. She said also, "My mother died when I was between five and six. She was lame and walked on her ankle. My foster mother, Mrs. X, told me that my mother's mother threw her against the wall when she was a baby and hurt her leg so that she was always lame."

"After my mother's death, my sister and I lived with the Overseer of the Poor. He was a very mean man. He beat us with a horse-whip whenever we did anything we shouldn't have. We stayed in his house until he died. I think I was about ten years old then when we moved to Mrs. X's. (Her present foster mother.)

In subsequent interviews many months later the patient mentioned that she felt her foster mother, Mrs. X, had rescued her from a very unhappy fate and stressed that this foster mother and her own mother had been friends. Mr. X was the village carpenter, active in small-town politics, and he was also the sexton and buried the town dead. Mrs. X did the washing for the neighbors. Mr. and Mrs. X had two sons who at the time of the patient's admission to the hospital were twenty-two and seventeen. The foster parents usually made a yearly trip to the near-by state capital when the legislature was in session because Mr. X was the janitor for the state house and was on duty there during this time. The foster parents were always absent from the home for several weeks, leaving all the children at home to time after this asking me for a definite appointment, as she was eager to begin analysis.

Several details held us up. Living quarters in a suitable foster home had to be found when she was transferred from the hospital. She was now unable to walk which further complicated matters. Also, since she was a state ward there was no money available for analytical fees, which later made difficulties in the transference. There was great difficulty in obtaining money for foster home care and transportation. Finally enough money was advanced to pay for her living expenses for one year, with the provision that she would be returned home unless she showed definite improvement. When these details were settled another hurdle appeared. No available foster home was suitable, so finally one was located in a distant Boston suburb which necessitated transportation by taxi. Not being able to walk meant that the patient had to be carried in and out of the analyst's office and up and down in the elevator by the taxi man.

Arrangements were completed and Sally was transferred to the foster home during the first week of January. Of course she had a series of "big spells." The foster mother was unknown to the analyst. Before contacting the analyst she became involved in treating the patient for "epilepsy." This foster mother, over sixty years old, had been a teacher for feeble minded children and also had cared for an "epileptic" relative for years. So she, being a determined person, began to give the patient medication which had been prescribed for her relative. It was only with the greatest difficulty that she was persuaded to discontinue her activities and leave the patient to the analyst. After this initial bad start, this foster mother cooperated well. The patient, however, remained away from analysis for the first week of every month.

First Phase of the Analysis

The patient's behavior in the first hour is worth recording. Sally was carried into the office. She was inert weight, rigid and heavy in the arms of the burly cab driver. He laid her on the couch and she promptly rolled like a log to the floor. Then she became angry, said that she had hurt herself, and refused to go back on the couch. She stayed on the floor during the entire first hour, talking in a loud strident tone, revealing her ambivalence toward the analyst. At the end of the hour she was carried out, silent, stiff and unlifelike. This was the beginning of a phase of "acting out" which lasted for several months. During this period the patient remained on the floor where she was made comfortable. She sneezed and postured frequently but it was noted that the seizures became less frequent as her aggressiveness increased. The aggressive attacks were directed at the analyst. Although the rules had been made clear to her she broke all of them. Not only did she refuse to lie on the couch, but she stared at the analyst continually, twisting herself on the floor to manage this. After the first few hours she became extremely abusive. She pelted the analyst with scurrilous names, glared with hatred as she spat them out. Her contempt for women doctors in general was poured out and concentrated on the analyst in particular. When she received no response she began to threaten physical harm. She boasted of her own strength. She often spoke softly of her beloved intern. She felt that there was no doctor as good as he. One had the impression that she felt as if she had been taken away from him by the analyst. Interspersed with the aggressive verbal attacks were fragments of her past life, partial memories with no integrated connection. Finally, after an especially frenzied and angry vituperation, she crawled over the rug on her hands and knees and struck the analyst a blow on the leg. The next day a table was placed in front of the analyst's chair and when Sally saw this barrier she became very contrite and very unhappy. As a compensation for the analyst's attitude of forbearance she gave the first piece of material which explained her behavior. She described the house of the Overseer of the Poor, in which she spent so many years of misery. There was a room in this house that she hated. It was in the attic and she said it was the size and shape of the analyst's office. The memory of frequent whippings and violent scenes that had taken place in this room flooded back into consciousness. Mr. C. had horsewhipped her and after he did this he locked her in this room for an hour. All the time that he beat her he yelled and cursed and forced her to look at him, always in the eye. (Old records show that when Sally came away from the C. home she was covered with bruises from beatings she had received from this man). She had felt terror-stricken and helpless and had minded being alone and locked in more than she had the beating. She expressed also her terror and fear of the unknown room and the analytic treatment. The patient was given the first interpretation at this time. She was shown how her behavior had been understood by the analyst and why the analyst had remained passive. The analyst told her that we had learned, first of all, that when she became afraid of an old memory becoming conscious she became aggressive. Secondly, that what she tried to push out of consciousness were ideas that had begun to crowd forward when she noticed the shape of the office. Third, she then lived out actively what she had endured passively in the room of Mr. C.'s house. Fourth, she became aggressive, striking the analyst as she had been struck when she was beaten. It was necessary for her to verbalize this all, after acting it out, before she really understood it. Sally was impressed that the analyst did not retaliate or punish her for her behavior. As a present to the analyst for her forbearance, Sally said, "Tomorrow I will go on the couch," or, in other words, now I will show you that I can be a good child.

The next day she was laid on the couch but rolled off again. This time she landed on her wrist, and since she complained that it was painful she was sent to the hospital to have an x-ray taken. Her wrist was slightly sprained, but there was no fracture. Her beloved intern was not on duty. It was a great disappointment to her, but that was probably the real issue—she wanted to get hurt and go back to see her doctor.

For the next six months the patient refused to go near the

couch. She was made comfortable on the floor on a thick quilt, and the analysis continued. During these months Sally brought out, for the first time, memories of her own father. He was a very violent, cruel man, who drank heavily and was often arrested for abusing his wife and children. She remembered the frequent visits of the police who came to lock him up. He deserted them when Sally was three. Sally, her sister and her mother came to her mother's foster mother's home. Sally's mother had been reared by this woman, Mrs. D. whose own son, Harry D., lived there also. Sally thought for a long time that Harry D. was her Daddy, and did not learn until years later that her mother and he were not married. The descriptions she gave of the D. home were vivid. It was squalid and overcrowded. Sometimes she, her sister, or some other child slept in the bathtub. She often slept on a cot in her mother's bedroom and remembered how Harry D. forced himself on her mother. There were frequent and violent fights between her mother and Harry. Each time after one of these upheavals, the mother took the two girls and returned to her own house on the edge of town. Sally said that everyone knew that her mother entertained men there, but she excused her mother's promiscuity by saying, "I was to blame for what my mother did. I cried all the time because we were so hungry. I used to go with my mother along the roads. We picked up apples and ate them. Even if they were rotten we ate them, we were so hungry. There was nothing in the house to eat. My mother would come home after we were hunting for something to eat and would scream and cry and tear her hair." (It is to be noted that she depicted in her spells these hunger experiences by clucking and sucking noises. In addition she also expressed in the spells anger and despair of her mother.)

Sally said, "Mother finally had to take men for money so we could eat." Her mother spent a great deal of time off and on in her own house. The rooms that her mother occupied were on the ground floor, so that Sally said she saw men frequently slipping in and out of the bedroom windows. (These facts reported by the patient have been checked through police and social service records which show the brutality, poverty and sexual degradation surrounding this girl in her early years.)

Harry D. discovered that her mother was frequently absent and he found out about the men. He wanted to know how many men came and was very jealous. He paid Sally to spy on her mother. Sometimes, Sally said, her mother took men upstairs and then she would either send the children out into the fields or send them on an errand or would pretend to be sick. Usually the mother claimed faintness and the man who had come would carry her upstairs into the bedroom and place her on the bed! (Compare the taxi man who carried Sally into the analyst's office and placed her on the couch.) The windows were covered and remained so and her mother would not answer when she called. (Sally kept her eyes covered with her arm.) But she and her sister would slip in barefooted and look through the keyhole. Sally gave vivid description of all the sordid details of prostitute practices. They seemed to be etched on her memory. Curiously enough she had the most difficult time telling about the men fondling her mother's naked breasts. This seemed especially shameful and abhorrent to her. (Sally did her best to conceal her breasts and expressed a hatred of her shape. She wanted to remain flat and childlike.) As she verbalized this material she punctuated her remarks with many sneezes and the oft-repeated phrase "It's all my fault, it's all my fault. I'm afraid I'm going to die" recurred over and over again with curious regularity. She was unaware of what she meant, repeated this statement to the analyst and asked her to explain it.

As the transference grew steadily more positive and as Sally began to understand that the analyst did not react the way people usually did after they became aware of her mother's sordid life, she said, "I love you, and I will go on the couch now, if only you will put a big chair next to it so that I won't fall off." The new position of the patient made it possible to understand that oft-repeated phrase "I'm afraid I'm going to die." The first idea that emerged was that "the couch is shaped like a coffin and I am afraid." Each day when she was placed upon the couch she would sneeze and roll to the edge, where, of course, the big chair stopped her. She would remain quiet and apparently out of contact until the second sneeze came, and then she would roll back toward the wall and would exclaim, "I'm afraid, I'm afraid I'm going to die!" She held her body rigid, her voice was thin, high and childlike, as if she was terrified. Her mind seemed to be filled with dread. Very little was said during these hours. She was fighting a paralyzing fear. She lay stiffly hour after hour, avoiding, as she finally admitted, the thoughts that came up, "by sneezing and going away." She kept this up for many days. But the thoughts she tried so hard to elude finally burst through in speech. She began to talk.

There was a picture that seemed to recur again and again in her mind's eye. She saw her mother lying dead in her coffin. All the terror attached to this memory returned too. She trembled and became pale, but she used her usual defense mechanism to deal with her anxiety. She warded it off by abusive shouting, "I hate this couch, I hate this analysis. I hate you. It is all silly, I am no better, I still have my spells, " and so on. When she quieted down, she slowly accepted the interpretation that she was using her characteristic method—aggressive attack—to escape from the anxiety which was connected with old memories and thoughts that she did not want to think about or remember.

Slowly and suspiciously, as a child whose experiences have taught it to distrust adults, she began to test the validity of this idea. She decided to try to discard her old method of dealing with her fear. Haltingly she told about the "half-awakening, half-sleeping terror" that she had experienced every night. "My bed with the high sideboards seems to turn into a coffin. I wake up, everybody in the house hears me screaming." From the time she came from the hospital, her foster mother had placed sideboards on her bed every night. The foster mother reported that Sally had nightmares and woke up everyone.

Sally had very vivid, recurring and frightening dreams at this time and these intesified her anxiety. When she dropped off to sleep she would dream "that my dead mother appeared and beckoned to me" or she would dream "I ran after my mother who always disappeared in the distance." She would awaken, crying and sobbing.

These dreams gave a wealth of material, and analysis of them resulted in better sleep for Sally. Her associations centered around her early relationship to her mother. "When I was little I adored my mother. I wanted to be like her in every way. Then I learned about what she did with the men and I tried to get rid of everything in myself that reminded me of my mother." (Here the ambivalent attitude of the patient is clearly visible. There is denial of love and at the same time longing for the mother. The early love repressed was expressed consciously in the opposite defensive hatred and rejection of everything connected with her early memories of her mother. The anxiety and the dreaded dreams concealed also the unconscious longing of the patient to join her mother.) Sally was especially grateful when the analyst explained that if women like her mother had had help, as she was having it, when they were young, that they might never have chosen such a way to solve their difficulties. She caught eagerly at this and said in a warm tone, "My mother was not bad, she was nice."

After six months of analysis the patient began to try not to remain away from the analysis for the first week of every month. She finally stayed out for three days when the seizures were such that she couldn't be brought in. The foster mother reported at this time that the seizures were no longer as violent as they had been at first. The patient could now stay in bed without the sideboards, and was attempting to move about the room, supporting herself by holding on to a chair or pushing it in front of her. Sometimes she crawled on all fours to the stairs, and sometimes she came down the stairs like a small child by hitching herself from one step to another on her buttocks. The sneezing continued. She talked baby talk and wanted to be fed by the foster mother during the three day absences and even wet her bed, though she had not done this in the hospital. She became compliant and loving toward the foster mother at this time and seemed to crave affection.

Finally Sally was willing to bring into the analysis her fears and thoughts concerning these strange and regular absences of hers. She understood that she was "acting out" something and that it was to her interest to find out what it was that she was avoiding. Cooperation began to supplant her earlier resistant attitude.

One day she began to tell me about her "big spells." "I know nothing for three days. I am as if dead—like my mother. She was dead for three days and in the coffin. I was afraid of her, she was so cold and still." Fragments and ideas surrounding this whole theme of the death of her mother emerged in a crystallized form. Sally feared her dead mother who had become for her a punishing, powerful figure. Sally felt that her disloyalty and rejection of her mother were known and that her mother was coming from the grave to get her as she did in Sally's recurring dreams. Sally said, "I am to blame for her death." She also confessed in a childlike voice, "I have to suffer for the sins of others. Christ suffered for the sins of others and He had to die. These spells are my punishment. My mother was dead in the house for three days. I am dead too for three days. Then I am like reborn after three days. Christ was reborn too."

Why did the patient blame herself? Why did she have to be punished by these "big spells"? These questions were put directly to the patient.

From her free associations one determinant connected with what Sally called "the three-day spells" became clear. Sally had quarrelled violently with her mother. She actually wished her mother would die. About this time her mother became critically ill and died. In the "big spells" Sally acted out symbolically the punishment that she feared. To quote Sally, "For my bad wishes my mother will kill me. She will kill me as I wished to kill her." The analyst continued, "You have to protect yourself so you die and remain dead for three days. So you are absolved." Sally answered, "Yes. I'm reborn like Christ was, and I can live again as a baby."

We went over this many times. When the patient understood what she had been doing, she said over and over, as if to make a point clear: "My mother died in the hospital after an operation." There were many little spells initiated by a sneeze during this time. It will be recalled that the patient's first seizure came after her hospitalization for appendectomy. So the linkage between the mother's death in the hospital and Sally's own fear of the same fate became clear and was understood by the patient. The violence of the big seizures subsided as she worked through her fear of the dead, avenging mother.

So far it was unclear why the "big seizures" came so regularly the first week of each month, and why Sally absented herself for three days from analysis at that time. The regularity was understood by the patient as an equivalent for menstruation. Up to this time Sally had not menstruated. She said she was jealous of her sister because her sister had menstruated at thirteen and had her "period regularly the first of each month." (Here she stopped—the anxiety was too great.) She said she could not even try to come to her hour in these three days.

The association chains now branched toward the chair which still stood next to the couch and prevented her from falling when she had the spells. She continued to have several per hour. She would sneeze, be out of contact, sneeze again a few seconds later and continue speaking where she had broken off. The chair made her think of the time she had pneumonia. She was about three years old, and night after night her mother sat in a chair next to her bed. She recalled that she was so ill that she thought she would die and that she clung to her mother. Her mother was always there. As this memory became conscious, the menacing, revengeful mother was displaced by a kindly, protecting figure. The transference was analyzed. The loving mother and the analyst became one. She accepted the analyst as a protecting figure. The chair was removed and the patient no longer rolled from side to side during her spells but remained in the middle of the couch.

The sneezing continued and the small spells interrupted our work constantly. She talked calmly about her mother's death. As she approached the next dangerous material the spells increased.

She said that her mother had lived with Harry D. and had grown very fat before she got sick. Sally knew her mother was expecting a baby. One day she came home from school and found her mother very ill, with a high fever. She was delirious and unable to recognize anyone. She screamed and yelled violently. The doctor removed her mother in an ambulance to the hospital and there her mother died. Sally went on to say that after her mother was taken to the hospital she went into her mother's room and found a bloody wire on the floor. She remembered how she carried this wire to somebody in the house. The furtive, disgusted attitude of the adult as the wire was snatched away caused Sally to retain an impression that something awful had happened. Much later Sally said, "I overheard conversations about Harry and my mother.'" Here apparently she was referring to the sexual act that her mother had committed with Harry, and the pregnancy and abortion that followed. Sally also accused Harry of murdering her mother. She had also overheard that he was the father of the expected child and he put the wire into her mother. She said that the baby was born before its time and was buried in a box in the garden. (The mother's baby actually was buried on the property of Harry D. The old doctor who took care of Sally's mother during her last illness confirmed this fact and accused Harry of being a murderer. The doctor did not prosecute the man because he felt that the two girls Sally and her sister needed protection and this scandal would damage them more. Several years later Harry D. was prosecuted for an incestuous relationship with his own daughter who was pregnant by him.)

Again Sally said, "It was all my fault, because my mother had to do things because of me." At this time she showed a thorough knowledge connected with the abortion. She linked her own severe bleeding from the nose, which occurred six months before her admission to the Massachusetts General Hospital, and her confusion about her retarded menstruation with the fear of a bloody death from menstruation. Here there was undoubtedly a displacement in which the nose became eroticized, and the bleeding nose, which was packed after a six hour epistaxis, became symbolically a bleeding genital. The patient understood how she had identified with her dead mother, so that the hospitalization which followed her severe nosebleed was a confirmation that she was going to die too the way her mother had. The anxiety had been displaced from the genital to the head. When this material was worked through and analyzed, it brought to an end the big seizures and the menses were established a year after the patient was first seen. This was the first menstrual period that the patient had, and the menses continued regularly after this.

During the next six months, the patient behaved in the analysis as she had when she was on the floor. She was highly abusive and aggressive most of the time. The name-calling kept on. When she was most anxious she shouted, "Dope, fool, you are like all the rest. You tell everything. Shut up, shut up. Stop that mush, mush. I hate you. I wish you'd get out of here." She was taunting and provocative, tried to pick fights with the analyst and the silence of the analyst seemed to provoke her more. Finally she turned on the couch and verbally ripped the analyst to shreds. She criticized the analyst's voice, her person and her appearance. She jeered, laughed, sang, made fun of analysis and played dumb for hours, sneezing occasionally. Finally she accused the analyst of not helping her.

What she referred to were the small "spells" that continued in the hour and at home. These were different from those described earlier, but were nevertheless very annoying to the patient. A sneeze introduced and terminated a "spell" lasting a few seconds. During this "spell" she lay inert, quiet and motionless on the couch, out of contact. It seemed as if she had dozed off. During her abusive verbal attacks these spells mounted to 6-8 an hour. After coming out of such a quiet period she would take up her conversation where she left off.

Hours of provocative behavior, which became almost unbearable, finally stopped. Formerly attempts to analyze the sneezing were of no avail. Now analysis became possible, because Sally, contrite and appreciative of the analyst's forbearance, began to work on this problem.

We learned that the "sneeze" was a magical gesture with two valences. First it meant "I wish you (the analyst) would disappear" i.e. die. When Sally recognized this thought consciously, she became frightened. She sneezed and lost consciousness for a few seconds, thereby experiencing a "little death" herself. Having atoned for her death wish toward the analyst, she sneezed again and consciously denied such a wish, saying, "I do not want you to die."

When the patient worked through her anxiety in the hour and learned that her wishes did not harm the analyst, she was able to speak freely about her belief that her death wishes had killed her mother. By analyzing the transference and linking her behavior in the hour to the symbolic three day death in the big seizures, Sally finally understood and mastered her infantile fear of the death wish. Then the sneezing and the "little spells" in the hour also disappeared.

The analyst had become alternately the loved and hated mother, whom she had killed by her bad wishes. But the foster mother reported that the sneezing occurred occasionally at home when Sally quarrelled with her. Shortly after this Sally became more active at home and took an interest in the housework. She began to sew and to move around her room. The sneezing at home then disappeared. She still held onto things in her room and refused to try to stand or walk alone. She told the analyst all about her trouble with her present foster mother and her fear of walking, and said, in a timid voice, "I'm awfully ashamed of myself, the way I've acted." Her expression of shame was genuine. Then she voiced her love for the analyst but confessed, "I am awfully afraid of you, you have a power over me." The transference situation was analyzed further. Sally understood that it was something in herself that she feared. She became eager now to find out what that was. She also became much more like a girl of her age from this point on, and began to bring in her daydreams to be analyzed. She had many day dreams:—about her future husband, about the number of children she was going to have, about the life she was going to lead later on when she got well. Two typical examples are: "My dream as I would like my life to turn out is this. First I want to get well, and by that time I will be seventeen, a young lady. Then I will finish high school, and then I am planning to become a teacher for small children. After I am twenty-two I would like to be married, and here is a sort of fairy picture of my future husband. His name is Roland and he will be about five feet, six and a half inches tall, not handsome but good-looking, so I won't have to be jealous of him. I want him to be a year or two older than I am, and here is what I want my house to be like,—a little white cottage by some little grove on a lake, a little white house with pea green trimmings and I will call it my house of dreams. I want two little babies, a baby boy and a little girl. I would like them to be twins. I would like the little boy to be golden-haired and have blue eyes, like his Daddy; and the little girl I would like to have dark eyes as my sister has. I would wait for picking out their names until I saw what my husband liked. I could see my babies grow up together and take care of one another in sickness or in health, and teach them to stand up for one another when they are older. They will be fine children. And there will be grandchildren, and I will be able to love their children as I did my own when they were little."

The second daydream, which also appeared in various forms, was "When I am rich, I will repay you and I will plant my mother's grave with pansies too." She expressed that pansies meant thoughts. "I will become a doctor and I will help people like myself."

During these months, when the most abusive attacks took place in analysis, I learned that she was also hiding something about which she was very guilty. She had been very busy writing to her former foster mother. The present foster mother found several of these letters and brought them to the attention of the analyst. The former foster mother had been a great hindrance all along to the analysis. She no longer received the weekly stipend from the State because Sally was now in Boston. She wrote to the girl, begging her to give up the treatment and telling her that it was no good. She cautioned her not to tell the analyst anything about her mother or her early life. She also wrote that Sally should not believe the analyst and that she could not be cured by talking. The former foster mother wanted Sally to come back to her and have the chiropractor in the village give her treatments. Finally Sally brought all this to the analyst and told her that she was sorry for what she had done. So we see that the girl tried to serve two masters. From that came the conflict and aggression which I have recorded.

A few words might be said here about the present foster mother in Boston. She had a very hard time for a good many months because, as in child analysis, the patient acted against the foster mother when she was in a positive relationship to the analyst. But when she was in a negative relationship to the analyst, the present foster mother took over the analyst's role actually, and received confidences from Sally and gave advice. This, of course, added to the patient's confusion and resistance. This well meaning interference was very difficult to handle. The patient's own part in creating the situation had to be worked out so that she understood how she was holding up the analytical work. Sally usually confessed what she had done. The relationship on the surface would be positive to the analyst for a short time after such a confession. But the competition on the part of the present foster mother, created a very serious difficulty. Finally the patient refused to allow the analyst to have any contact with the Boston foster mother, so that it was impossible to find out what went on at home for a good many months.

At this time also the patient's sister, who wrote regularly to Sally, became very intimate with her boy-friend whose name was Harry. As soon as Sally found out that her sister, Elsie was in love with Harry, she began to correspond feverishly with Harry, in an endeavor to sever this relationship and get Harry for herself. Here she showed her identification with her mother as well as her competition with her mother. These two figures, Harry and Elsie, had the same names as the original pair in the past. (Sally's mother's name was also Elsie, and it will be recalled that Harry D. was her mother's lover.) The same names facilitated the acting out of the old oedipal situation. Analysis of this material brought an end to the letter writing and deepened the patient's insight and understanding.

The shadows of the past now moved towards the taxi driver, who became increasingly important in the analysis. At first Sally was only an inert, unresponsive weight in his arms as he carried her from his cab, but as the analysis progressed a subtle change began to take place. She behaved as if she were attempting to seduce him, especially during the time that she was so busy writing letters to Elsie's boy friend. For Sally became very soft and pliable and snuggled in the man's arms when she was carried in and out of the office. She told the man suggestive stories, giggled in an excited manner, and several times maneuvered to leave the elevator door partly open so that she was trapped in the elevator with him for some time. Sitting on this man's knee gave her a lot of satisfaction. He, then, began to react to her. He began to take her on detours, buy her ice cream and candy, give her money for stamps and mail her letters. Many of these letters, as I learned later, were full of complaints about the analyst. Apparently she had voiced her love of the analyst as a protective measure. It was about this time that Sally requested that there should be no further communication between the analyst and her foster mother, but the foster mother, acting on her own, reported by telephone that the taxi man had complained about the patient's flirtious behavior. The foster mother, too, was worried about the patient's behavior. A neighbor of the analyst also complained about the noise that the patient and the taxi man made in the elevator. The patient's behavior was brought to her attention by the analyst. Sally first reacted with an outburst of rage, but then became very ashamed, and was shocked at what she had been doing. She cried bitterly for quite a while and said, "I do not want to be like my mother. But I am like my mother." And in broken sentences she brought out, "The taxi driver is just like Tom." She recalled that her mother had had an affair with a man called Tom, and that Tom looked like this taxi driver. Tom was the man who always carried her mother upstairs to the room, and he was the man with whom her mother pretended to faint. In this way, by pretending illness and faintness, she got rid of her children. Tom was a big man, and he always turned and explained to Sally that her mother was sick and then he would pick her mother up, carry her into the room and close the door. Now again we can see how the patient acted out in plastic form her identification with her mother in relation to the taxi driver. As was characteristic of this patient, the old memory was acted out before the verbal level was reached. The taxi driver became Tom, and day by day as he carried her in his arms and laid her on the couch in the office, she was in fantasy, her mother. The laughing, fooling and uncontrolled behavior of the patient was understood by us now as an unconscious equivalent of the rejected and repressed wish to act like the sexual mother. When this material was interpreted and worked through the patient became discreet and quiet, insisted on wearing slacks, and would never allow the chauffeur to touch the skin on her legs. Before this she had worn a dress. She was ashamed of her former seductive behavior and tried in every way to appear lady-like. The analysis seemed to progress normally into the next phase.

Second Phase of the Analysis

Since Sally had matured physically she was happier, and since she no longer feared the "big spells" which had completely disappeared now she continued to gain weight and her body took on the rounded contours of a young girl. She had changed characterologically too. She was working well in analysis, having gained enough insight to realize that the traumatic happenings in her early childhood which she had tried so hard to forget and ignore were connected directly with her symptoms. But there was still another symptom which troubled her very much—she was unable to walk. She admitted now that she was very worried about this. She had not walked for many months and feared that something had happened to her legs. She thought that she had actually damaged herself by her stubborn refusal to try to walk. She began to verbalize all her anxiety about walking. "Perhaps I am really paralyzed" or "The doctors had missed it while I was in the hospital." Her associations revolved around this central fear. After several weeks she could no longer push this anxiety aside. She decided, with the help of analysis, to get an objective viewpoint about her physical condition, and to meet her anxiety concerning paralysis by returning to the hospital for a neurological examination. She had a great deal of confidence in Dr. Cobb and it was arranged that he would examine her at this time. She verbalized her anxiety to Dr. Cobb, whose note follows:

"Examined by me in my office. On my entering the room she immediately sneezed three times and went into a moderate extensor spasm with her legs crossed and her hands over her face, which was turned toward the right. She then looked up at me and smiled. In the interview, she reported that she had lost almost all of her symptoms and that she was not much worried by the sneezing and the short spells of unconsciousness; that the real trouble now was that she was unable to walk without having sneezing, that as soon as she sneezed she would lose contact for a moment and her legs would go out from under her, therefore she did not dare to try walking, but dragged herself around on her rump like a child. My neurological examination was entirely negative. The legs have rather small muscles but they are perfectly adequate. I told her that Dr. Dawes had done a remarkable piece of work in removing her other symptoms and I had no doubt that she would also remove this, that the legs would be able to carry her as soon as she worked out the psychological obstruction to walking. She asked my advice about eyes and having headaches, and about her teeth. These were incidental but should be looked into. I advised her to go to summer camp and said that I thought that with everything going as it is, she ought to be able to walk by then and really enjoy the camp."

After this examination Sally was able to breathe easier. As she talked freely about her fear of paralysis she brought out the anxiety that she had hidden so far from the analyst about her earlier hospital experiences. Of course, the visit to the hospital mobilized this material. Her new impressions caused her to compare and reminisce about her feelings then and now. She was not in resistance, and the relief after the examination made her eager to go on. It will be noted that Dr. Cobb states that she had a recurrence of the type of spell which she had when in the hospital!

Sally's next associations connected her anxiety with the terror she felt when the electroencephalogram was done in the hospital before she came to analysis. She said, "The night before it was taken I had the following dream. I was alone in a large building, there were no doors and no windows. There was no way out, and I was very frightened." But the next morning Sally related, "I laughed and joked with the nurse and the intern on the way to the laboratory. I thought they were completely fooled by me, because they praised me and said, 'Isn't it wonderful that she isn't scared'?" However, when the wires were placed on Sally's head she became so frightened that she had no memory of what happened subsequently. (She had a "spell" during the recording, but the electroencephalogram showed no abnormal waves.)

Sally began then to puzzle why she had had a spell just at this time, since she consciously was not afraid of what was going on! Through free association two trains of thought were connected with this procedure. The first linkage had to do with placing the wires on her head. The whole story of finding the bloody wire, and the mother's abortion and death was again repeated along with the details of her severe nosebleeds which had occurred when she was still in the village and shortly after she had had a blow on her abdomen in the school yard. Finally the unconscious meaning became clear. The blow in the abdomen certainly had the unconscious meaning of an unexpected sexual asault. No more ideas came at this point. The second train of thoughts began again with the wires. The intern had placed them there. This intern was much beloved by the patient and in her fantasy he again and again became her lover. So it came out that when these wires were placed upon her head they had a symbolic meaning to the patient. The patient said that her mother's lover, Harry D. "put a wire into her to get rid of the baby." Here we see the mechanism of displacement at work. The male intern put wires on her head! Apparently the anxiety attached to the genital had been displaced to the head. Again the patient's identification with the mother was clear. She felt she was in the same position as her mother. Something was done to her with wires, and it was something sexual by a man. The anxiety, that she was in the same predicament as her mother, was so overpowering that she was unable to do anything but have a momentary lapse from consciousness. Hence the spell during the electroencephalogram procedure! The unconscious linkage of wire—bleeding—hospital—death, now was understood.

There was a great deal of mystery surrounding the time that the patient fell ill. So far all that was known was given to the analyst by the patient, that is—accident in the school yard, appendectomy, nose bleeds, spells, illness, and hospitalization.

Sally avoided all discussion of the circumstances surrounding the accident.

She veered away from this and started on a second group of ideas about the electroencephalograph machine. "It was a lie detector" and she feared that her secret would be found out (i.e., masturbation).

She also connected this topic of masturbation with the fear she had when the interns came and stroked the scar on her abdomen. She came to dread the time when they came, why she did not know. She protested that the stroking had been pleasurable. This is another instance of displacement—the scar was equivalent to her genitalia. She brushed aside this interpretation, but began to free associate, "Why did the stroking of the scar always frighten her so?" It had always initiated a spell. The puzzling phenomenon was finally clarified. She haltingly recalled that during the time between three and four years, when she had pneumonia, her mother had sat with her and never left her side until she was out of danger. Then she added something to this memory, and apparently was able to do so because the analyst had been accepted as a protecting mother figure. She told of a memory that she felt was very shameful. She kept her eyes covered, blushed and was very, very miserable as she brought it out. She began in a halting voice to describe in detail the room where she had been in bed at this time. Then she said, "One day when I was better mother left me for a little while. I was still so weak, having been in bed so long, that I was unable to sit up alone. So mother *tied me in my chair* and went out on an errand. While she was gone Harry D. came to see me, and found me alone in the house. He put his hand between my legs and did 'it' to me." She found that all the shameful misery, that was connected with this memory, seemed to evaporate when the analyst did not condemn her. Again, as a present to the analyst, she gave up tying herself in the chair at home. She talked freely now about how she had been accustomed all these months to winding a clothes-line around her waist and tying herself securely to her chair, as she had also made the nurses tie her into the chair in the hopsital. Her foster mother had reported that whenever she had tried to get Sally to desist from this, that the patient became extremely anxious. This restraint was not removed until the patient ventilated this old memory and no longer feared it. Then she no longer needed the rope.

When the rope was discarded Sally felt very encouraged. She could stay in the chair without falling and decided to try now to find out why she had been so frightened about undressing for a physical examination. It might be remarked here that she still refused to remove her hat and coat when she came to the office. When the doctor had tried to examine her in the hospital she had a spell each time. She felt this had something to do with "a love scene." Later analysis clarified this equivalent also. She had consciously felt so anxious that she absented herself in a spell, but unconsciously the wish was very clear that she wanted to be like mother who in this way made herself ready for the man in the first part of the love scenes that Sally had witnessed as a child.

She felt more relaxed now, verbalized how glad she was that the analyst did not criticize her, and again voiced her love for the analyst. Her associations next linked the doctors in the hospital with cruel practices. She accused her beloved intern especially of being cruel. He had repeatedly stood her upon her feet. She had "blacked out" each time. She said when this happened she had fallen toward the bed. Sometimes she was unable to get to the bed and had hurt herself by falling to the floor. Now the reason she gave for not trying to walk at home was that "Every time I try it everything gets black in front of me, and I feel as if I was pushed from behind." She persisted in trying to stand, however. Usually somebody was in the room with her. She never actually fell, from any reports I had, but her extreme anxiety of falling held her prisoner.

After some days she brought out another memory of the time when she was convalescing from pneumonia between three and four years of age. Again she was alone in the house when Tom came in. He sat her upon his knee, and put his finger into her vagina. She tried to run away from him but everything got black and she fainted. Her mother returned and found her on the floor in a faint. (The scene in the elevator with the taxi driver will be recalled. He was linked with Tom in the patient's mind. She always sat upon his knee, giggling and laughing. The flirtatious behavior that occurred at that time apparently was a sexual equivalent for this unconscious memory which the patient had repressed and rejected.)

She tried now to stand on her feet. She no longer had any trouble about fainting, but her feet were extremely painful. She soon desisted and using the pain in her feet as an excuse, her aggression turned to target the doctors. She was very ambivalent toward all of them, principally because she had had the fantasy that doctors always made love to their patients. She substantiated this fantasy with citations from her own experiences. The first one she gave was that the old doctor in the village who sent her to Boston had petted her, kissed her, and sat up all night with her when her "spells" began. He was also the doctor who had attended her mother during her last illness. Sally overheard this doctor tell her former foster mother that she was very ill, and that he could do nothing for her. She embroidered this fragment of conversation further and said, "He thought I was going to die like my mother did, and he sent me to the hospital to die the way she did, because of those sexual things that I did with those men."

She spoke of other daydreams about interns kissing their patients. One intern, after she had had her appendectomy, had always kissed her goodnight. She continued "Everyone on the psychiatric ward knew what doctors did with those women patients behind a closed door in their offices." Sally never would go to see the intern alone in his office. He had told her that unless *she walked to his office* he would refuse to see her except on the ward. (It will be remembered that Sally was able to walk al Children's Home in Boston before she came to the Massachusetts General Hospital.) Therefore, her walking inhibition started in the hospital and protected her from seeing the intern behind a closed door—a situation she felt was dangerous. All sorts of exciting sexual stories began to appear at this point in the analysis. Her early spying activities had been extensive. One fantasy which had appeared earlier in the analysis, e.g. "a girl was tied to a tree and raped by Tom" now was said to have actually happened. Sally had seen this as she walked through the woods with her sister! Many other sadistic fantasies appeared before she finally told the facts surrounding the accident in the school yard. She had been greatly shocked just before the swing board hit her. She had come upon her adored foster mother, whom she had come to regard as a very pure mother type, embracing and kissing a man. She had run away and had been disgusted. A few nights after this, and shortly before she became ill and was sent to the hospital, she had been sweeping out the school house. "I finished sweeping and I was coming across the school yard. I saw Harry D.'s car parked and I went over. My sister and Harry were having intercourse in the back seat and they never even heard me. I saw everything." The story that she had told the intern about being hit in the abdomen by a swing board in the schoolyard was true, but it was simply a substitution to avoid talking about what she actually had seen because of the intense excitement that was generated by witnessing this sexual pair. All the sadistic sexual fantasies emerged before she was able to verbalize these ideas which had been apparently perfectly conscious during the whole analysis.

The patient's associations then veered sharply away from this whole topic. Nothing further emerged about the swing board hitting her in the abdomen. Many subsequent hours were spent testing the analyst, trying to find out what the reactions of the analyst were to her. She began a theoretical discussion of love versus infatuation. She reported that she had overheard a conversation between her former foster mother and a neighbor. These women were talking in low voices about girls touching each other and her foster mother wondered if she should allow the patient and her sister to sleep in the same bed. Sally pretended now to be very naive and said, "What did they mean? What could they have meant?" As she realized that the analyst was not shocked by her hints, she talked freely about masturbation. Before this confession Sally behaved as many children do in analysis. She became very aggressive toward the analyst, and acted toward the analyst as she expected the analyst to treat her. She kept her eyes covered with her arm, also, because she was afraid, as she told me later, that I would read her secrets in her eyes. She still continued to wear her coat, hat, and gloves and refused to remove them. After she did not get the expected punishing, aggressive response, she became very silly and had a foolish expression on her face. She often appeared in the doorway, as the taxi man carried her into the office, with her finger in her mouth, acting and looking like a feeble-minded person. This was brought to her attention and she clarified it, after some time, by confession that she had believed her former foster mother and her foster father too, who had tried to help her fight her rather excessive masturbation by threatening her with the consequences that would follow such an activity if she persisted. That is, she would become crazy or foolish, like the women in a nearby mental hospital, whom they were convinced had become inmates there because of this practice. As usual, Sally acted out what she feared. It is probable that this confession of masturbation came just at this time because of pressure her former foster mother exerted on the patient. The social worker received a letter from this foster mother at this time in which she stated that she was convinced that this practice was connected with the patient's illness, and she felt sure that Sally had hidden all knowledge of this practice from the analyst, and she felt it was her duty to see that this information was given to the analyst. It seems that Sally's sister had tattled to the former foster mother about Sally's masturbatory practices. Sally found this out and for days and weeks she was occupied with ideas of revenge. All the former love that she had had for her sister turned to hatred and she directed all sorts of death wishes toward her sister and her foster mother. When this explosion of affects had spent itself Sally began, then, to tattle to the analyst just as her sister had tattled about her. Sally described in detail her sister's numerous sexual escapades, and was especially bitter because she knew all about these things, had spied upon her sister, and had never told the foster mother. Not only had her sister had a sexual relationship with Harry, but also with a boy named Arthur. She also had a long affair with the elder son of this former foster mother when the foster father was away from home, acting as janitor of the state building. There were other boys, quite a number of them, in the village, whom she had entertained also. Of course the foster mother knew nothing about this. The patient had always been extremely jealous of her sister's good relationship with the foster mother, and now she was very angry because she felt that her sister had tattled on her and that she also had betrayed her. She said that for years her sister and she had slept in the same bed, and that they had masturbated each other until the foster mother finally separated them.

It is remarkable that each sister had found a different solution in puberty for the traumatic experiences which they had shared in childhood. Our patient had become ill with a severe neurosis, but her sister who was only a year and a half older had found her solution in free and uninhibited sexual promiscuity. Sally was angry and revolted by her sister's behavior, for she linked it with her mother's own disgraceful life. She was especially bitter because the former foster mother's criticism had been turned on her and, in this way, her sister had hidden her own disgraceful conduct. She screamed hour after hour, "I hope my sister gets a baby. Then she will be disgraced for her whole life." Sally noticed how often she said this and she began to wonder why she wanted her sister to go through a pregnancy. After she had overcome her strong guilty feelings about discussing her own masturbation, it came out that she felt that this practice resulted in disgrace before the world, that is, if one kept it up one got a baby. She also believed that if a girl masturbated excessively she ruined the genital so that no baby could be produced. (Again we have two diametrically opposed notions about the same thing. Might this also be another reason why at the beginning of the analysis the patient did not have her menstrual period?)

As the fears about masturbation crystallized and were worked out, Sally again tried to exercise her legs at home. She talked to the analyst about her legs and asked advice how best to exercise them. After crawling to the bathroom and around her own room for weeks and exercising her legs, she stood up and tried to walk about her room, holding on to things. She could not go without support and her legs were badly swollen. If she tried to let go of the support she sneezed and felt as "if I'm pushed from behind." Her present foster mother watched the patient and reported that Sally was trying to do as I asked, but gave up easily. She managed to crawl to the kitchen and helped with the dishes. There was no recurrence of the "spells" that the patient had had earlier. The analyst realized that the patient was getting a great deal of enjoyment out of this role of a sick girl, as the foster mother fussed over her a great deal still and babied her. Sally loved the daily rides into Boston and the contact with the taxi man who still carried her into the room. This state of affairs could have continued indefinitely. The patient really had no incentive to lose her helplessness, which she was able to rationalize by saying that she could not stand. She steadily refused to try to stand alone in the analyst's office.

The secondary gains were enormous and it seems as if the unconscious meaning of the symptom, that is the walking inhibition, would remain hidden for some time unless something happened to disturb this pleasant life she enjoyed. Fortunately for the analysis, a sudden change in the reality situation did occur. Her present foster father died suddenly of a heart attack and her foster mother was compelled to give up her home because of lack of funds to run it. The patient was given notice to leave within a week after the death of the foster father. At the same time, fortunately for the progress of the analysis, the funds for the taxi, which had been supplied by a private indiidual, ran out and Sally was confronted with the necessity of making the initiative if she was to continue her analytical treatment. The foster mother was so overwrought by the tragedy in her own life that she was unable to help the patient in any way to solve this dilemma.

The summer vacation was approaching. One day the patient saw the analyst's baby daughter as she was coming to her hour. Sally expressed conscious pleasure and praised the analyst's baby, but repressed her negative feelings. Her negative reactions began to target the former foster mother. Sally complained of the foster mother's preference for her sister and said she did not want to go home to the country for the summer.

For the first time, Sally turned whole-heartedly to the analysis, which she felt offered her her only chance to get well. She felt that the analyst was the only friend she had in the world. Crutches had been suggested a month earlier, after her visit to the hospital, but she had stubbornly refused them. She used the crutches now and accompanied by her social worker came to her hour by subway.

The death of her present foster father precipitated many more memories relative to her mother's death. She wept bitterly and with great abandon for several hours and all the associations between her sobs were concerned with her love of her mother and her feeling of loss, which I think was supported by the fact that the two foster mothers had both withdrawn their support and vacation was approaching. Sally was bewildered and angry at her own mother and, as usual, ignored her feeling of frustration in relation to her present foster mother. She behaved like a little child, was very unreasonable and lost. She left a note on the couch one day which read, "I was only a baby when I lost my mother. I hated to think what she did, but I also loved her; but I was bewildered and hurt when she forgot to say good night dear when the time came. I trusted her and adored her with my whole heart, but she hurt me and that is why I don't believe in any other person. You can't count on people."

Sally recalled that she and her sister had gone to the hospital when her mother was dying and the doctor had left them outside in his car. She was ashamed to say that she blew the horn so much that the nurse had to come out and reprimanded her for the disturbance. Reproaches now centered on herself; she cried and cried and wished that she had not done this. She said that she had been unable to cry when her mother had died. She spoke of her fear when she found that she had been unable to make her mother recognize her when she lay dying. She also described how her mother's eyes stared and how she had spoken incoherently and acted in a crazy way. This had frightened both the children. All the real longing and grief that she had felt for her mother's death and all the misery that she had borne because of her mother's life, came to the surface now and spent itself.

The transference was analyzed and the analyst's departure on vacation was linked to her mother's death. The patient brushed this aside and spent the remaining hours before vacation sullen or petulant because she had been returned to the Children's Home for the summer. She again began to vent her resentment by writing letters to her former foster mother, whom she professed to hate, complaining about the home and the analysis.

Without consulting the analyst, the patient completed plans with the social worker for a visit to the home of her former foster mother at the end of the summer. She was going back to the village in the role of a little crippled girl. It was evident that this foster mother agreed with the patient that analysis was worthless and urged Sally again to try the local chiropractor. It was clear that Sally turned to this foster mother because all her infantile desires which had been brought in transference in relation to the analyst could not be satisfied but were now to be indulged by this foster mother. (During the first part of Sally's illness this foster mother had treated the patient as a helpless baby and even taken her into her own bed, cuddled her, petted her and kissed her.) Naturally when the patient lost her present foster mother, and was frustrated by the analyst, she turned back to her former foster mother in her disappointment.

On the first day of analysis in the fall, the analyst received a phone call from the Boston social worker who said that the patient had been put on a train for the country for a two weeks' vacation with her foster mother. The social worker had understood from Sally that these plans had been discussed with the analyst. Sally had maneuvered it so that her stay was thought by the former foster mother to be indefinite. Of course the patient was acting out her transference resistance. When the two weeks stretched into two months there was a very serious danger that the patient would not return at all, thereby spoiling the results achieved so far. The analyst at this point stepped into the reality situation and requested the return of the patient. Sally's legal guardian was contacted and she was sent back to Boston. The return of the patient and the acting out that followed this move on the part of the analyst made the analyst regret many times that she stepped out of her analytical role. Not only did the patient return to analysis in poor physical condition, but she was hostile and uncommunicative. She sneezed frequently. At the Home she fell down whenever she attempted to stand without the support of her crutches. She had definitely worsened during these two months. Spite reactions were coming to the surface so that a foster home would have been inadvisable for the patient at this time. A group placement was chosen because it was thought that Sally's strong wish to satisfy her infantile longings with a foster mother, which had created so much danger in this analysis, would be lessened.

The patient was placed in E. House, a home for girls, and plans were made for her to enroll in a nearby trade school to learn to become a seamstress. This was the type of work in which Sally had shown interest. She had done a lot of needlework and wished to learn to make her clothes.

Unfortunately the school would not accept her school credentials but required a ninth grade certificate. So a tutor was found to help her fulfill the requirements. This external blocking of her desire to become a dressmaker offered fresh fuel for her resentment and increased her aggressive outbursts in the hour.

Her sullen silences became a thing of the past. Loud, strident shouting, "You brought me back to Boston but I intend to wreck the analysis" could be heard outside the office. She cursed the analyst, used vile terms or yelled, "You got to be bumped off. You know too much, you heel. You tell everything." She was tough, behaving at this point like a gangster's moll. She was an ardent radio fan, listening to all the gangster stories and reproducing the intonations and expressions which she had heard. Many times she reiterated, "No matter what you do, wise guy, you'll never get me well. I'll make you the laughingstock of everyone. I'm going out to tell everyone how silly the analysis is," etc. Although she was in a negative phase of analysis she made a fair adjustment to the group in the home, but usually chose as her companions the dull girls who dwelt on their sexual experiences and told risqué stories. She was a champion of the younger children, who were frequently punished by the matrons. She divided the matrons in the home into "good" and "bad" ones. The analyst was put in the latter category. Sally quoted her father often at this time. She complained that he had never had a chance, that everyone was against him and that he was right in saying, "You should get all you can out of every one." She would then add, "He was no good. He was a drunkard and a bum and I'm no good either, and no matter what you do you can't change me." She described his drunken behavior and then would tell how kindly he was, when he was not drinking. An attempt to analyze this material resulted only in a further outburst of aggression. She was acting like her father at this time, and her walk with her crutches reminded one of the rolling walk of a drunkard.

On one of the days that she was less resistant, she repeated a story about her dog, which she had told the analyst while she was still on the hospital ward. The story was as follows:—"My dog ate some poisoned grain. He found it accidentally under the woodpile. It was rat poison. He got awfully sick and limp from it. He couldn't walk. He nearly died. The old doctor [who cared for her and sent her to Boston] took care of him." It was not until a year later, when she repeated this story again, that the reason for its repetition became understandable. Her associations showed that she apparently identified herself with the sick dog who had eaten something poisonous. It became clear that this story connected directly with more old forgotten material. *The sucking movements of her mouth* that had been noted in the hospital during the "spells" were repeated as she told the story. She recalled that when her father was drunk, he quarreled violently with her mother. She and her sister were very tiny and frightened. She would cry and then he would come into the room and force Sally to take his penis into her mouth. She was very much disturbed as she brought out these memories. She wept, ashamed and miserable. She pathetically asked, "What made all this happen to me? Is anyone in the whole world decent?"

There was the usual pause in her hostile attitude with an outpouring of her gratitude and love for the analyst but it was short lived.

She once again became resistant and difficult. Often coming late to her hour, she chatted about inconsequential matters. She spoke in a high irritating tone, adroitly avoiding any mention of her inner thoughts or activities in reality. She finally told of her annoyance with people whom she met by chance in the subway, and their questions about her "crippled state."

In spite of her vigorous protests, she thoroughly enjoyed talking with strangers, especially about how she had become crippled. To some people she told a beautiful story about an operation on her legs, to others she gave the idea that she had had infantile paralysis. In fact, she was so convincing in her ability to tell a good story that the social worker who had charge of her believed that Sally was unable to walk alone on the street. For months and months, this worker would meet her before and after the hour and walk arm in arm with her down the street. Another time a woman who was connected with the Orthopedic Department of the Massachusetts General Hospital visited the analyst to offer assistance to the patient. She had been given the analyst's address by the patient. Sally's pathetic plight had so touched this woman, that she wished to provide her with crutches which were the proper height, remonstrating that those the patient were using were too short for her! There were also many telephone calls from Sally's numerous friends who championed her cause, telling the analyst of Sally's unhappiness.

When these facts were brought to Sally's attention, she was contrite and continued to reiterate: "I am just like my father, he was an awful liar. I am no good, he was no good either. Why don't you give me up?"

Third Phase of the Analysis

The third phase of the analysis began with the anxiety attaching itself to "being alone in the street." Sally mentioned this but did not elaborate. She avoided talking about it, but maneuvered very cleverly to get her young Boston social worker to escort her to and from the analyst's office. As usual, Sally's ambivalence targeted this worker. She confided to the analyst that she hated to have someone hang onto her arm and watch out for her as if she was a baby. When it was clear to Sally that she had tried to avoid the thoughts that were crowding into consciousness, she agreed to come alone and bring the thoughts to the analysis.

For several days she had a very hard time. The anxiety broke through when she came alone and all the fear of living out her sexual fantasies was clearly behind her anxiety.

This problem had to be worked out. She began to be occupied with two boy friends, "Curly" and "Joe", both of whom were in love with her and were following her and meeting her in the subway. Joe was the brother of her old rival in the ward of the Massachusetts General Hospital. This young woman ally thought, was favored by her beloved intern. "Curly" undoubtedly was a fantasied lover. (Months earlier Sally left a closely written paper on the couch. It bore the title "A Young Girl's Dream." "When I am 20, I would like to meet a very nice young man and fall in love with him. I will describe him. I want him to be tall and strong, with *curly hair* and gray eyes and if I marry him I want to understand and guide our married life. I want him to be able to take me in his arms and say, Darling, I'm so glad to see you' and really mean it.")

All "Curly's" letters were neatly typewritten. (Sally had been given a typewriter). She brought two letters daily. They were very sentimental, full of terms of endearment and of plans for the future. Along with these letters Sally brought two stories she had written. These were rough drafts of romantic adolescent daydreams, in which she was the thinly disguised heroine. The scene of the stories was laid in a hospital. A surgeon, an austere, forbidding man, with "curly" hair and blue eyes (her beloved intern) fought off his love for his patient. In one story this woman was having a child, in the other she had sustained a desperate injury. In both cases the surgeon's skill saved the patient. In another story she became a nurse who assisted him and in the other his wife who helped him to carry on his too heavy practice.

Then Sally began to elaborate on the "Curly" story. "Curly's" father had been a doctor. He was now in Boston to have an operation performed on his crippled hand, which he had injured in a machine. He was supposed to be in a Boston Hospital waiting for this operation. From the hospital he wrote Sally!

As for Joe—he was meeting Sally daily in the subway. One day she came to her hour. Her left hand was bandaged. She said she had fallen on the subway steps and cut it. The hand began to swell. The Home, at the analyst's request, had a surgical consultation and X-ray. Nothing but a superficial injury was diagnosed. But there was an enormous swelling of the soft tissues of the hand. There was no fever. Finally an orthopedist was consulted and the patient was hospitalized.

Sally did not like it at the hospital. The report to the analyst stated that Sally had been very uncooperative, refused to follow directions about soaking the hand, had removed it from the sling and had hung her arm over the edge of the bed and in every possible way delayed her recovery. Finally the wound on the back of the hand opened. Since this occurred immediately after the hand had been dressed and the nurse reported that the patient was observed tampering with the cut, she was peremptorally dismissed from the hospital as a malingerer. The orthopedist was extremely irritated at the patient and severely reprimanded Sally.

Sally returned to analysis subdued. The cut healed but the hand and arm remained very swollen. There was no pain. The associations soon clearly linked the unconscious meaning of the swollen hand and arm with the erect penis. She envied the men. She wished she had a penis instead of her female genitalia. She reiterated, "I'd rather be a man because women die having babies!"

Reality was brought clearly to the patient's attention and the wish for and envy of the male organ was analyzed and discarded by the patient. Many questions about the female body were asked and answered. The swelling of the hand and arm subsided as quickly as it had occurred as this material was worked through.

But soon she managed to cut her right hand. This hand she said was her "bad" hand. She was very superstitious and remarked that the injury was a punishment for masturbation.

She again discussed her exciting thoughts. Every type of masochistic fantasy came tumbling out. Finally she reiterated the story of the "girl who was tied to a tree and attacked sexually by Tom." (This story now fell into its proper place and we see that it belonged to the period when she tied herself up in the chair and warded off the fantasied aggressor with outstretched arms and widespread fingers. At the same time her legs moved in a very suggestive way!)

These ideas clarified the pantomime gestures depicted in the "spells." Because the ideas were rejected and had become unconscious they were out of reach. Sally was working hard at this stage of her analysis. She was greatly relieved to unload these shameful thoughts. She poured out many stories centering around the whipping or beating and sexual maltreatment of a woman by a man. (These sadomasochistic fantasies explained also the maltreatment of the analyst in transference. She was the cruel sexual male.)

When this interpretation was made, the patient confessed that she had been flirting with Joe for months. She had been meeting him and seeing him regularly in the subway. She had led him along and the affair had progressed to the handling stage. She became frightened, pushed him off, but he met her again in the subway and tried to become familiar. She shoved him away and tried to get down the stairs but he tripped her. She lost her balance, and she and her crutches tumbled to the bottom of the stairs. She cut her hand on the iron steps. This was the story of the injury that resulted in hospitalization. The old theme was repeated: sexual sin—injury (punishment)—hospital.

She began to tell more stories about "Curly". His hand was not cured by the operation. He contracted pneumonia while waiting in the rain for her. He was again in the hospital and he was slowly dying. As he neared death, he entrusted his two children, a girl and a boy, to her and she planned to adopt them legally! Then a long, involved and incredible story about visiting a judge and filling out papers for adoption came next. About this time, the story was too much for Sally and so "Curly" died! The analyst showed scepticism and pointed out that "Curly" was anything but a masculine character and it was a curious coincidence that he had so many troubles similar to her own. The crippled, damaged hand of the fantasy lover was linked with the damaged genital, caused by masturbation, that Sally herself was so worried about.

Before each menstrual period, Sally now became increasingly aggressive and verbally abusive, literally pounding the analyst with scurrilous words. She began to flirt with men on the street, flaunting her escapades and saying that many men were interested in her. She masturbated frequently and boasted about it. (The interpretation was given that she seemed to be trying to master her fear that she was like her hated sexual mother by behaving like her.)

The interpretation resulted in a penitent, tearful Sally. She had received understanding instead of punishment. She then gave up another secret: "My sister used to entertain boys in the living room—you know what I mean—while my foster mother and father were out of town. We used to be left alone with the boys for several weeks. Just before I got sick my foster parents were away and my mother and I used to go upstairs. She and the younger son of her foster parents had indulged in a lot of sexual play. He had tried to insert his penis into her vagina. This happened just before the onset of her illness. After this attempt he became more and more insistent. She became very afraid that she would become pregnant if she allowed this. One day when they thought they were alone in the house, her sister came upon them, surprising them in the act. From then on her sister had the upper hand over Sally. For years Sally had known about her sister's sexual looseness and had threatened to expose her to the foster mother. Now her sister had the added advantage of being the preferred foster child and was more adept at deceiving the foster parents, thus she could easily throw suspicion on our patient. So it became understandable why Sally, earlier in her analysis, was so full of resentment toward her sister. Her sister had told about Sally's masturbation but had not told about the affair with the boy; this she held over the patient's head as a constant threat—enjoying the place of the favored child at home.

Sally had never been the favorite with the foster parents who caught her masturbating and had warned her that she would "Go potty doing that." They had tried to break her rather excessive masturbation by pointing to the sad examples of insane women in the nearby hospital, all of whom they described as being there "because of that."

Sally said in addition that before she became ill she had become "more and more worried about doing it," and also about the secret sex play with the boy. She was afraid she would be found out. She was convinced that she had injured herself by these practices. When her menses were not established by the time she was 15, she was sure of it. Then the "spells" came and her sister told about the masturbation with the result that her foster mother rejected her almost completely.

As the boy became more demanding, even after her foster parents returned home, her days and nights became fraught with anxiety. "I'm like my mother and I will follow in her footsteps." This overwhelming fear of promiscuity forced Sally to seek a means of escape from an unbearable situation. Apparently the conversion symptoms that followed the appendectomy furnished the way out! Here we see this girl's ego pushed from within by unbearable tension and threatened from without by a dangerous reality situation. The repressed unconscious fears and fantasies (which had been unearthed in analysis), pushed forward for expression. The upsurge of the sexual tensions in puberty almost tipped the balance in favor of promiscuity. Fear of death acted as a counterweight. The conversion symptoms with the unconscious linkage: (promiscuity—baby—bloody abortion—hospital—death) provided a partial expression of forbidden wishes and punishment for them.

Fourth Phase of the Analysis

The fourth and last phase was concerned with Sally's inability to walk. The hysterical paralysis of both legs continued, and she had given up her exercises and was content to swing along on her crutches.

Whenever an attempt was made to call her attention to this symptom, she shouted, "They can't make me give it up" over and over again. When an attempt was made to analyze this phrasing and to show the patient that "it" probably had another meaning, every abusive term that the patient could think of was hurled at the analyst. Again, this provocation, hostile behavior continued for weeks. The analyst was unable to penetrate the wall of aggression. There was nothing to do but wait.

One day Sally was silent at the beginning of the hour. An interpretation was again attempted. The patient was asked to consider the phrase which she repeated so often: "They can't make me give it up" and was told that "it" did not refer to walking, as she would like to make the analyst believe, but to masturbating, and that until she was able to work out that problem with the analyst, the puzzle of her inability to walk could not be solved. With great difficulty the material slowly emerged, interspersed again with hours of aggressive behavior. Sally had masturbated actively for years many times a day and always before she went to sleep. This she did in the hospital too. She would usually put her finger in her vagina. As she masturbated, she had fantasies about the finger being a penis and that she might have a baby. She refrained from speaking about masturbation, not only because she feared she would lose the love of the analyst, but also because whenever she talked about it, memories of her mother in sexual activity with Harry D. and other men came vividly before her eyes. She wanted to be rid of these ideas. So the interpretation was given that her way of evading them was to scream, yell or shout at the analyst whom she held responsible for reactivating them. She understood this and agreed. Then she yelled in a fresh attack of anger, "There's something I'll never tell you and that is something about you." This statement was reiterated many times and the analysis was nearly completed before its meaning became understandable.

Reality interrupted us at this point. It was necessary to find a new place for Sally to live. Complications at the girl's home, which had nothing to do with the patient, led to the termination of her stay there. Before she left, the matron sent the analyst a report stating that Sally had changed greatly during her stay. She had become a very likeable person adjusting well in the home and had lost many of her unpleasant mannerisms. In addition she had passed the ninth grade and had dropped all her old acquaintances. She was placed in a foster home again, this time with a very warm, well-balanced foster mother, who took a tolerant, objective view of the patient's peculiarities. The reports from this foster mother indicated that the patient was happy and seemed to be adjusting nicely.

The social worker who placed Sally in this new home was a great hindrance at this stage. She, for reasons of her own, was unable to cooperate with the analyst. She indulged the patient and the patient clung to her tenaciously. Sally talked freely with this worker, sharing her secrets as she came to her analytical hour accompanied by the worker, who patiently guided her on the street!

Needless to say, Sally was very guilty about her part in this. Very little progress was being made in analysis. Sally again seemed to act as she had months before, aggressively and abusively. Any attempt on the analyst's part to call her attention to the fact that she was guilty and avoiding something led to a loud "Shut up!" from the patient.

After an especially trying hour, the interpretation was again given to the patient that her behavior in the hour seemed to be an identification with her brutual, abusive father and her violent treatment of the analyst was a reflection of this identification. (The patient's father was in jail at this time, for beating a horse to death.) Since she was using the hour to gratify her cruel fantasies and was unable to cooperate any more or try to work out in the analytical way, it was felt that it would be wise to stop the treatment! *A definite termination for the analysis was set at this time, for, as the analyst informed the patient, no progress was being made as a result of her attitude, and so the analyst did not feel that she had anything further to contribute.* The social worker was contacted and arrangements were made to stop the analysis in three weeks.

The day after this happened, the patient came to her hour

very unhappy and seemed a changed human being. For the first time in many months, she removed her hat and coat. She realized that the analyst was in earnest and that the analysis was to be interrupted and so she gave the piece of material which she had been withholding all these months. She confessed that for weeks and weeks she had had florid mastubatory fantasies about handling the analyst in the genital region and having intercourse with her. She was afraid to tell these fantasies because she thought the analyst would immediately "throw her out" if she knew them. This was what she had referred to previously when she reiterated, "There's something I'll never tell you and it's about you." She verbalized this material with great relief now that she felt there was nothing to be gained by withholding it. Following her confession, she became very earnest and exclaimed, "I do not want the analysis to fail because you are the only one, really, who has always been kind to me and I really love you." Then there was a pause. "I was afraid that you would not love me if you knew what filthy ideas I had about you." This last material was analyzed and understood as the last fragment of the primal scene material in which the child had identified with the brutal, sexual father. The patient, in her sexual fantasies about the analyst, was the active man. This explained her reactions in the transference situation.

The patient realized that the analyst, even after hearing this most feared group of ideas, remained objective in her attitude toward her, understood and analyzed this material. With this realization a remarkable change came over the patient. It was as if she were suddenly released from a terrible fear. She became quite docile, was friendly, lovable and cooperative. She reiterated that she wanted to make the analysis a success in order to demonstrate to others that children like herself could be helped. Then she asked what she could do first in the time that remained to regain the use of her feet. At the end of this hour, instead of taking her crutches as she arose from the couch, she stood upright without support and walked across the room! Then she reached suddenly for her crutches and said that her feet hurt her terribly. She admitted that she lied to the analyst and that she had been trying to stand up and walk for a long time. She felt that the masturbation had, in some way, permanently injured her legs and her feet. However, since analysis had cured her other symptoms, she wanted to try to walk.

The next few hours she was very bitter about her former foster mother. In her positive relationship to the analyst, her aggression turned toward this foster mother and then toward all other women who threatened children about masturbation (revealing, of course, that she had been convinced that her foster mother was right, i.e., that sexual crimes had caused her sickness). She had been angry at the analyst all these months *for not stopping her masturbatory practices,* but now she wanted to go out into the world and demonstrate that she was cured of her illness. She outlined what she wanted to do. "I want to get a job and get to work. Will you help me? What shall I do about my feet? They are so swollen and they hurt so when I try to use them." Sally was referred to an Orthopedic Clinic. There her feet were strapped, and she was given instructions to use her feet and legs and advised to drop the crutches.

On her last analytical hour she was walking part of the time with crutches, part of the time without them. She told the analyst that she would make a visit to her office within three months and that she would then be walking without the aid of crutches.

A month after Sally stopped, she rang up the analyst and asked for an appointment. She walked into the room leaning on her crutches, put them against the wall and began to walk around the room unaided, laughing and saying, "I just did it for a surprise. I cannot understand how I could have been so silly for so long. I have a job in a factory, sorting screws and bolts and earning real money. I want to visit Dr. Cobb and show him I'm well." This day she made plans to visit the Chief of the Children's Home in order to return her crutches. The analyst learned later that she not only delivered her crutches but also thanked the chief for his help in making it possible for her to have an analysis. She said to him, "Analysis is a fifty-fifty proposition—the analyst did her 50% and now, although it's taken me a long time to do my 50%, I'm going to finish it up." Next she went back to the village in the country, visited her guardian, her friends and her former foster mother to show them that she was really well and also to prove to herself that she had overcome the influence which she felt this former foster mother had over her. She returned to Boston, relieved and reassured at the time of her next visit to the analyst. She reported that everything had been very comfortable at home and that her foster mother had treated her like an adult. She had gained weight and looked happy and healthy.

A few months later, she secured a better job in a box factory. A year later she returned for a visit, was well nourished and well developed, appeared to be entirely normal physically, walked without difficulty and seemed happy and well-adjusted. She had a Sunday School class and had joined the Church. It seemed as if the unpleasant past no longer marred present or future. Sally was looking forward, at the age of eighteen, to marriage and motherhood, and had very definite ideas concerning the rearing of children. She had several boy friends but unlike her sister, was circumspect in her behavior with all of them. She was like any other girl of her age, busy with her work and social activities.

About three years after the close of this analysis, which ran roughly over a period of three years, about 600 hours, Sally wrote to the analyst asking for an appointment. She came looking well but older with a little baby girl in her arms. She had given birth to her daughter four months earlier. The father of her child was a service man who was married and who had mislead her (according to her story) into thinking he would marry her. His unit had gone overseas and when she notified him of her pregnancy he wrote her that he was already married. She was frightfully upset and wanted to come back to me but feared that I would condemn her as she condemned herself. She kept her baby and was very proud of it. She had a job and was engaged to a young man who was going to marry her and who loved the baby as well.

She wrote once or twice after this, enclosing pictures of the baby. She apparently kept well and had no return of her old illness.

Conclusion

This typical conversion hysteria demonstrates what actually takes place during the course of a psychoanalytic treatment. The decoding of the unconscious meaning of the symptoms through interpretations brought about alterations in the transference and symptomatology. The correctness of the interpretations resulted in the steady progress of the analysis. The historical and genetic reconstructions were made by utilizing the fragments which appeared in dreams and free associations of the patient.

When the analysis was completed the patient had matured physically, had changed characterologically and was able to stand and walk about freely not only in a literal sense but also in a symbolic sense as well. She appeared, in behavior and attitude, to be well within the norm for her age group.

ANXIETY IN CHILDREN CONVALESCING FROM RHEUMATIC FEVER

Irene M. Josselyn, M.D., Albert J. Simon, M.D., and Eleanor Eells

Evidence of anxiety in children convalescing from rheumatic fever is not uncommon. This anxiety may become evident in the verbalization of the child or in his questions about the results of various examinations to which he is submitted. The child may appear frightened without being able to describe his feelings or his fears. In some cases the anxiety expresses itself in inhibited behavior. The child is more inactive than his past history would indicate was his normal pattern. He curbs his activity more than the physician indicates is necessary and more than would be commensurate with his own returning strength. In such cases a cursory observation of the child suggests he is depressed and only closer study reveals the underlying anxiety. In contrast the anxiety may be masked by behavior characterized by excessive activity, a verbal denial of the illness, and a refusal to accept the necessary limitations. In some cases severe nightmares are the only manifestation of the child's chronically anxious state.

Anxiety is a psychological response to which there is a physiological reaction. Physiologically in anxiety states there is a modification in glandular secretion and an increase in vasomotor tonus. The heart rate increases; changes may occur in the electrocardiogram. A transient response of fear is undoubtedly not as significant as chronic anxiety may be. In the former the physiologic changes are transient, while in the latter they also take on a chronic nature.

It would seem likely that the physiologic effect of chronic anxiety may be especially significant when the heart already is crippled by disease. If this assumption is correct, a significant aspect of a child's convalescence following an acute rheumatic fever episode would be to attempt to alleviate chronic anxiety in those cases in which it is recognized, and to avoid where possible the creation of anxiety in children where it appears to be absent. Because this hypothesis has appeared valid, the staff at Herrick House, a convalescent home for children recovering from rheumatic fever, has concentrated considerable attention in the last eight years on the over-all problem of the anxious child among the patients at the institution.

Even a superficial study of this subject gives many explanations as to why the child may be anxious. The child has been away from home for a long time and is fearful because of the separation from his primary source of security, his parents and the home. The hospital experience itself has often been frightening over and above the separation from the parents. To begin with, the child enters the hospital seriously ill. He often experiences considerable pain accompanied by symptoms or toxicity. Even after the acute condition subsides, his anxiety is not completely relieved because he fears a recurrence, having been told realistically of the possibility of and the dangers in a recurrence. Any mild joint pain that another child might ignore may cause alarm, because of its similarity to the prodromal symptoms experienced at the onset of the acute rheumatic fever.

Many children experience another anxiety-stimulating situation which is unavoidable. Even after the child is consciously free of symptoms, he is not allowed to get out of bed and participate in activities he feels capable of doing because of the medical necessity of a period of bed rest even in the absence of pain. He thus comes to know that the disease is not limited to the period of actual physical discomfort. There is something mysterious going on that does not give symptoms discernible to him, but which, as indicated by the general regime, is significant to others. Many of the children have been aware of the death of friends, friends they have found in the hospital, at the clinic or in the special school for cardiacs. The child becomes aware of the possible ultimate fatal outcome of the disease.

In teaching hospitals, the child faces another source of anxiety. On ward rounds he overhears discussions of rheumatic fever, of complications, of the possibility that the disease will finally prove fatal. Under some circumstances he may actually hear a discussion of his own case from which he may glean only the negatives and not be aware that possibly in the discussion positives are also apparent.

Parents undoubtedly often increase the anxiety of the child. The doctor has perhaps unwittingly given them an unjustifiedly pessimistic picture of the situation because of his eagerness to have the acute phase handled optimumly. Publicity in regard to rheumatic fever unfortunately has tended in some instances to alarm parents unduly. While the disease is the major cause of death in the young from the ages of 6 to 24 years, parents are unable to evaluate what that means. They interpret the statement as indicative of the probability that the disease will prove fatal to their child. This parental anxiety has been then either directly verbalized to the child, or because of the child's sensitivity to parental feelings has been more indirectly transmitted. It is not surprising that as a result of these multiple factors, many children who come to Herrick House show signs of unwarranted anxiety in regard to their heart.

In order to counteract the effect of these unavoidable situations and still assure the cooperation of the child during the period of convalescence, the initial relationship with the attending doctor at the institution becomes extremely significant. After carefully and thoroughly determining the child's current physical status, the doctor explains to the child that he has been ill, that it will be a while before he can be as active as the other children. He will return to activity by stages. He will finally be able to be active more nearly as other children are. He answers any questions the child may raise. With many children this is sufficient. They depend upon him to determine how much they can do and apparently feel safe under his guidance and that of the other members of the staff. If there is obvious anxiety shown either directly to the doctor or reported to him by other staff people, he will often give a more complete explanation of the disease and the effect it has had upon the particular child's heart, gearing his presentation to the child's intellectual ability to grasp the information. In any discussion with the child he is honest, avoids unjustified reassurance but emphasizes the optimistic, positive aspects of the situation, placing the emphasis on what the child *can* do rather than on what he cannot do.

As an additional important protection against unwarranted anxiety, the doctor also talks to the parents, attempting to correct any misinformation they may have, and again giving them as optimistic a picture of the future as is honestly warranted. In preparation for the child's return home, he relates the child's ultimate level of recovery to the long-range planning of the family or clinic physician by whom the child will subsequently be treated. The more adequately the institutional management of the case can be correlated with the management during the acute phase of the postconvalescent period, the more confidence the parents will have in the physician to whom they return and the care the child will have during his convalescence.

The institution program itself tends to allay some of the child's anxiety. Herrick House has studied the effect of a more flexible and often more rapid rehabilitation of the child during the convalescent period than was practiced in the past. This study and a follow-up of the children who were allowed an accelerated schedule have been reported elsewhere. After the child's present cardiac condition as well as cardiac potential is evaluated as accurately as possible, the doctor interprets his findings and recommendations to the staff. Gradually the child is allowed to resume activities. He is closely watched for signs that he is pressing beyond his capacity. He is allowed to return to activities compatible with his basic heart condition as rapidly as it proves medically advisable as determined by the physician. The child's activities are supervised in as nonanxiety-producing manner as possible. His activities are programmed at the level of his physical capacity. An attempt is made to keep the child occupied and happy at whatever level of activity he is physically capable of handling at that time. While it is difficult to describe this in any detail, the underlying philosophy is to put the stress on "You *can* do this" rather than "You *cannot* do that." This reassures the child in several ways. He finds himself having a good time at the activity level that is commensurate with his condition. Because he is enjoying himself, the frustration of not being able to do more is held relatively, in most cases, at a minimum. (It has to be recognized that there are always children who can really get pleasure only out of extreme physical activity.) Secondly, he sees other children able to be more active than he is and knows that they represent a stage of return to health ahead of his status. In a month he will be able to do more.

The anxiety in many children is also allayed by the benign type of supervision they experience. Some children find real relief from the anxiety when they do not have to carry the burden for determining how much they do. In some cases for instance, the doctor's word alone has not been sufficient because the doctor is not always present. Once it is pointed out to the child that his counselors are well aware of the doctor's recommendation, are familiar with children who are recovering from rheumatic fever, and are therefore quite capable of judging when an activity is permissible, the child feels freer to participate without fear in the program that is allowed him. He knows that he is not in danger because the adults will protect him from injuring himself. One of the goals of convalescent care is to develop in the child an ability to evaluate and control his own activity. This is too great a burden often, early in convalescence, particularly for an anxious child. It is gradually acquired during the child's stay.

As indicated earlier, the child, in addition to his concern

about the illness, may be anxious because of his separation from the home. In many instances this has been handled partially by the child before he comes to the convalescent home, having come to accept it during his period in the hospital. However, it cannot be assumed that the fear is completely mastered. The counselors play a very important part in either the continuance of the child's adaptation to separation or in making it more tolerable for him. One of the chief roles the counselor serves is to meet those needs of the child that ordinarily would be met by a parent. This has to be geared to the actual need of each child and involves the whole question of dealing with the emotionally upset child in an institutional environment, a subject for a separate paper.

It has been observed that a very important contributing factor in allaying the child's anxiety irrespective of its origin lies in the child's capacity to relate to an adult on the staff. In general it has appeared important not only that a child relate to some one individual, but also that he have a sense of a relationship with the total institution. Every staff member, irrespective of his particular assignment, is available to every child as that child needs him. Because the child's anxiety may be focused on his physical well-being, the nurses play an extremely important part in this adaptation to the institution. Any child who has a physical complaint is free at all times to turn to the nurse for evaluation of his condition. This not only reassures him but gives proof of her interest and her nonanxious but sincere consideration of his symptomatology.

Having carried out this type of program over the past eight years, we have drawn certain tentative conclusions. Most children, no matter how frightened they are when they come to Herrick House, soon cease to show anxiety about their heart condition. It has been very interesting to observe what appears to be the child's basic faith in his own health. No matter how much he has been told by others that his condition is serious and extremely crippling, if this evaluation is not considered correct and the contrary point of view is presented by the attending physician, the child tends to discount the previous opinion. An interesting example of this was a child who had been seriously frightened during his acute illness. He commented to his counselor after being seen by the institution physician, "You know, it's remarkable Dr. X is supposed to be such a good doctor and he was so completely wrong in my case. The doctor here seems to be the only one that really understands rheumatic fever." This, in spite of the fact that the original doctor was a very famous physician while the institution physician was at that time relatively unknown to the family. This same acceptance of a more favorable prognosis is observed also in the parents. This in turn reflects back upon the child and decreases the child's anxiety. Because of this human characteristic to accept reassurance it is so important that the physician at the institution not only know cardiology, but also have integrity so that he is truthful with both the child and the parents, as well as fair to the original doctor.

Anxiety will persist in many cases where the damage to the heart is severe and the prognosis extremely guarded. In spite of a program compatible with the child's strength and one that the child enjoys, he persists in giving the impression of being either anxious or depressed. In some instances of such nature where, for example, the child's heart is chronically at the border of decompensation, it has been speculated that the psychological anxiety may be the direct result of the physical condition, not the result of a knowledge of the condition. It is as if the child experienced the emotion of anxiety because his breathing is rapid and shallow and his heart beat rapid—the physiologic counterpart of anxiety. If the normal physiological manifestation of anxiety is experienced even though the cause may be organic, the psychological response occurs. The cart appears to be actually before the horse. These cases need to be studied more thoroughly before any valid conclusion can be drawn as to the meaning of the anxiety observed. Experienced staff often recognize the poor prognosis for a child before the physician reveals it to them because of the personality picture observed,

It has been the impression of the staff that if any anxiety manifested during the early period in the institution (other than that evidenced in the child whose condition is very poor) does not disappear within two or three weeks after the child comes to the institution, exploration of the possibility of other roots for it is indicated. The apparent legitimate cardiac anxiety is in many of these cases actually a displacement. The anxiety has its roots in something other than the actual cardiac condition. Persistent unwarranted cardiac anxiety may be related to other conditions that are realistically frightening, or may be a manifestation of neurotic anxiety caused by unrecognized internal conflicts.

Those cases based upon a reality situation are perhaps never completely free of unconscious conflictual significance. However, there are some cases of persistent anxiety in which the manifest content relates to reality situations. Alleviation of those situations, or an opportunity to discuss them and find some help in shaping a point of view toward them, relieves the concern. For example, if the child is concerned about what is going on at home because the father or mother is ill, or if there is seriously destructive quarreling in the home, he may be frightened by what he fantasies is going on and imagines he could prevent it if he were at home. He may express this anxiety only as fear about his own physical condition. In those cases a discussion of the reality situation, with an attempt to clarify any of the uncertainties the child may have and assistance in accepting that there is no way for him to really help the situation during the convalescent period, decreases his anxiety. Any residual anxiety then is expressed about the real situation rather than in terms of his heart. Obviously, however, in some of these cases, there is no way to alleviate the anxiety completely until the condition is cleared up. For instance, if the mother is ill and has to have surgery, little can be done except to be frank with the child as to the developments in it, provide people for him to talk to when he is worried, and keep him as contented as possible.

Neurotic anxiety displaced upon the heart has been particularly interesting to study in those cases in which it has been possible to unveil what appears to be at least part of the underlying conflict. The following cases are examples of this. They are given in brief form with just a summary of what the underlying problem appears to be.

Alice M. was 14. Among multiple personality difficulties indicative of emotional conflict was a verbal pessimism in regard to her ultimate fate as a cardiac. She had moderate heart damage in spite of two previous attacks of rheumatic fever. There was every reason to suppose that after a reasonable convalescent period she would return to full activity. She was to remain at the institution for the entire winter, primarily because there was no healthy home environment to which she could go. She had had both recurrences during the winter. She accepted the fact that it would be wise for her to stay at the convalescent home for the entire winter in order to have one winter free of a recurrence. In spite of the assurance that there was every likelihood that she would not have a recurrence during the winter at Herrick House, she insisted that even though the physical setup were conducive to health, she would continue to have recurrences, with progressive heart damage, until the disease proved fatal. No amount of assurance on the part of the doctor alleviated the anxiety behind this conviction.

A few interviews with her brought out indications of underlying problems. She saw two possibilities in life. She could be a prostitute like her mother and marry an alcoholic and a brutal person like her father. The alternative was to lead a life similar to that of a maiden aunt and have as her ideal a bachelor acquaintance of hers of whom she was very fond, but who extolled the virtue of an asexual life. Her normal biological maturation resulted in sexual urges that she wished to express in heterosexual relationships. This could only be expressed, however, through prostitution. That had been her mother's answer. Her ideal for herself more closely paralleled the behavior of her aunt, who had always told her the virgin woman was the purest woman. She feared she could not live up to her ego ideal because of her libidinal drives. Her fear was of what she would become; she translated this into anxiety about her heart. This anxiety, however, was unconsciously not so much a fear of a recurrence but a fear that she would not have one. A recurrence and a fatal termination of her disease would result in a final solution of her internal conflict.

She worked this through on a conscious level and became convinced that one could be something other than a prostitute or a virgin. Her cardiac anxiety disappeared. She is now sure that her heart will in no way interfere with her future. This conviction has lasted for two years while she is living a normal life in a coeducational boarding school with satisfactory social contacts with both sexes.

John R. presented a superficial picture of alternation between a deep depression and withdrawal, and violent temper outbreaks. Brief contact with him revealed an underlying anxiety. In view of repeated illnesses it seemed that this might be due to concern about his own physical well-being, particularly as he expressed anxiety about his future. Superficial exploration, however, again brought out a different picture. When John was four years old he discovered his mother murdered, with the father unconscious, the latter having attempted to commit suicide after destroying his wife. The father recovered to be a paraplegic and to serve a prison sentence. He had never revealed the reason for murdering his wife. John had great admiration for his father. His father represented to him an adequate aggressive man. There was some positive recall also of his mother, but he was convinced that his father had a good reason to murder her, an attitude that was shared by relatives and people in the community. He suspected, and again this was confirmed by rumors in the community, that his mother had been unfaithful.

John's anxiety centered around his concept of his future but not because of the effect of his heart disease. To be an aggressive male as he wished to be, in other words to be like his father, a goal which in many ways was desirable, meant that he would murder. To seek a relationship with a woman meant to expose oneself to unfaithfulness. This would arouse his anger and would result in destructive impulses. John was frightened by his own aggressiveness as well as by his desire to form a relationship with a woman. As he was able to talk this out and as he was exposed to contact with men who did not murder and women who were not unfaithful, he gradually became more comfortable with his normal aggressiveness and more accepting of the opposite sex. His excessive cardiac anxiety disappeared. He now takes adequate care of himself, and assumes that his life span will not be particularly shortened, an attitude that would seem justified in view of the degree of heart damage.

Mary L. has already been presented in another context. Mary was a child of alcoholic, promiscuous parents. Her father was brutal to her mother. Mary decided as a small child that she'd be a cowboy because men had a safer life than women. When she discovered that she wasn't a boy, she decided that she'd be a cowgirl, wear boys' clothes, act like a boy and therefore hide her femininity from everyone. She became ill with rheumatic fever. She was told then that she could not act like a boy. Because of her degree of heart damage, she would always be somewhat limited in her activities. At this point anxiety developed, manifesting itself chiefly in severe nightmares every night. The nightmares were always of bugs. In the course of a few interviews with her it became clear that the bugs represented to her the cause of rheumatic fever. Rheumatic fever deprived her of her pseudo masculinity and left her helpless in a terrifying world. While she had considerable concern about her physical condition, the concern was not really about the heart per se. Her heart damage exposed her to a dangerous world, against which she could not defend herself because of her physical limitations. Her cardiac anxiety disappeared as she found evidence that it was safe to be a woman.

Harry O., an eight-year-old, indicated through a story he liked to tell himself the underlying frame of his anxiety. He had spent four of his last five years at complete bed rest. He had no heart damage. At first at Herrick House he refused to participate in activities because he would drop dead if he did. He held his anxiety in check by rigid control not only of his activities but, according to the Rorschach, of his feelings also. The Rorschach indicated no outlet through fantasy living. He told, however, of one fantasy that he recounted to himself over and over again as he lay in bed. He watched the tree outside his window. The leaves were children. The tree trunk and branches were the mother. The leaves wanted to be free of the mother and run and play in the stream and fields. The mother wouldn't let them go. Then the leaves got older and brown and they fell off the tree. They played in the stream and in the field but then when they wanted to return to their mother they couldn't. It is not surprising that the Rorschach indicated that this child was struggling with the wish to be more independent but feared the loss of his dependency gratification from the mother if he did assert this independence. His anxiety was rooted in this conflict.

Summary

Anxiety concerning the heart may be present in children convalescing from rheumatic fever as a result of the reality experiences the child has had during the acute illness. Anxiety from this source responds quickly to the assurance the child gains from his own recognition of his increasing tolerance for activity and from wise interpretation of and management of the convalescent period. Anxiety will often persist in those cases where the cardiac damage is severe and the immediate prognosis poor. If the anxiety manifested is unwarranted by the actual heart condition and if it is not relieved by wise child care during the early period of convalescence the apparent cardiac anxiety is probably a displacement to the heart of anxiety related to another source. The primary source may be another reality situation. It may have its roots in neurotic conflict. Anxiety probably always places additional strain on an already damaged heart. It would appear that when anxiety persists, convalescence will be facilitated if the cause of the anxiety can be eradicated. In such cases a psychiatric study is always indicated.

Discussion

JULIUS B. RICHMOND, M.D. (Professor of Pediatrics, State University of New York College of Medicine at Syracuse): This very sensitive presentation of the problems of management of the child with rheumatic heart disease by Dr. Josselyn and her collaborators is most appropriate at a time when more specific information is becoming available concerning the pathogenesis and the management of the organic consequences of the disease. Without adequate awareness of undesirable physiological consequences of anxiety, the physician may not find it possible to understand why the patient does not progress as he anticipates. Thus, as has been pointed out so well in the presentation, the medical armamentarium is not sufficient for the management of these patients.

This brings me to a significant point raised in the paper and which I should like to extend: that of the special role of the physician or convalescent institution particularly skilled in the case of children ill with rheumatic fever. These children realistically have experienced organic insult of central significance in their total adaptation. As a consequence, unusual professional skill resulting in deeper understanding with its resultant increased confidence is required to provide for the child the support necessary to carry on a maximum activity program as described. Such confidence does not develop without an extended experience in working with such children; physicians or institutions without this background are usually themselves anxious and this anxiety becomes communicated to the patient. I have tended to think symbolically of these children as having, as a consequence of the organic lesion, an ego defect into which the role of the physician or institution staff can fit as a prosthesis. The effectiveness with which the child deals with this defect depends to a considerable extent on how well the prosthesis fits. This visualization of the child's problem respects its uniqueness since we generally regard prostheses as being fitted individually.

In the light of the significance of this relationship with which I am in agreement as I have already indicated, I wonder if Dr. Josselyn could indicate to us how the problems of separation from the institution are dealt with constructively. She has already commented upon the management of separation problems upon the child's entry into the institution; if the institution serves the needs of the child the problem of mastering the separating experience from it can be a considerable one. Or is it more feasible to propose a program embodying a continuing relationship of the patient with the institution after discharge? I present this not as a rhetorical question, to which I have an answer, but rather as one which all who care for these children are concerned with.

A fascinating problem raised in this presentation relates to the effect of physical status—particularly early heart failure which may be clinically undetected—upon psychological status. At the outset I might say that I would strongly reinforce the validity of this formulation from clinical experience and from neurophysiologic information available to us. The sequence of events may be formulated somewhat as follows: early heart failure is associated with visceral change. Minimal cardiac enlargement and minimal pulmonary engorgement and distention occur. The visceral innervation undoubtedly records these changes centrally and since we now know that these autonomic impulses become cortically projected it is not difficult to speculate that personality change may perhaps be a more sensitive index of physiologic status than physical diagnostic signs. These important clinical observations therefore should serve as a stimulus for us to refine our physiologic methods to detect heart failure in even earlier phases than we now can.

I cannot think of this question which has been raised without commenting on some other investigative interests of our group which may seem somewhat far afield, but actually are not. In our studies of autonomic responses in young infants we observe wide individual variation in functions such as heart rate and skin temperature. The logical question is, of course, whether or not those infants with more extreme responses are predisposed to anxiety from less intense emotional stimuli as contrasted to other infants. From the observations of Dr. Josselyn and her collaborators one might be inclined to say yes. Obviously such studies are difficult to conduct and a more final answer must await considerably more data.

Finally, I should like to congratulate Dr. Josselyn and her group on the tenacity with which they have pursued their studies. In an area of study in which data collection is difficult and long-term observations are of central importance, their studies have been adding to our knowledge steadily. Perhaps most significantly we are indebted to them for not engaging in oversimplification of a very complex problem.

TREATMENT OF HYPERKINETIC EMOTIONALLY DISTURBED CHILDREN WITH PROLONGED ADMINISTRATION OF CHLORPROMAZINE

Herbert Freed, M.D., and Charles A. Peifer, B.S.

The observation that overactivity in all types of mental disorders in adults was reduced by the administration of chlorpromazine* suggested its use in the treatment of hyperkinetic, emotionally disturbed children. At present a review of the literature suggests certain areas of agreement that are pertinent to this paper. Following exhibition of the drug: (1) There is a reduction of overactivity in all types of mental states. (2) The adventitious movements in neurological cases are also reduced if not removed. (3) There is production of a state of psychic indifference in which while the individual says he "couldn't care less," he is still capable of sustained attention, reflection, and concentration. (4) "Deconditioning" takes place in rats treated with chlorpromazine.

At this point the question may justly be asked, "Why use such a potent drug on these children instead of psychotherapy?" Fundamentally, the chief reason was the need to improve a situation, such as individual misbehavior in a school room where the authorities could use only limited controls in dealing

---

* 10-(3-dimethylaminopropyl)-2-chlorphenothiazine hydrochloride was supplied as Thorazine through the courtesy of Mr. C. W. French, Smith, Kline & French Laboratories, Philadelphia, Pa. It was originally developed in France by Rhone-Poulenc Special Laboratories, who market it abroad and in Canada as Largactil. We also wish to express our gratitude to the many teachers and counselors of the Philadelphia Public School System who cooperated in this study.

with the student. Twenty of these children (80%) were either illegitimate or came from broken homes. Psychotherapy with the remaining parent was therefore, for economic or other reasons, impossible.

Procedure

Twenty-five children, 20 male and 5 female, ranging in age from 7 to 15 years were treated from 4 to 16 months. They had been referred usually by the school authorities. While all were overactive and apparently emotionally disturbed, almost half were combative with their classmates or teachers. Five had not been allowed to return to school. From a diagnostic classification, 18 exhibited primary behavior disorders, 2 were classified as psychoneurotic, 2 as ambulatory schizophrenics, and 3 as reactive behavior disorders associated with organic brain disease.

Initially a battery of psychological tests was given. It comprised the Wechsler Intelligence Scale For Children, Wide Range Achievement Test, Rorschach Test, Children's Apperception Tests or Symonds Picture Test, House-Tree-Person Test, Bender-Gestalt Test and, in some cases, the Vineland Social Maturity Test. This battery was repeated at the termination of the reported period of observation.

Electroencephalographic studies were carried out whenever the patients would cooperate. Because of one report suggesting hematologic changes in adults, sequential complete blood counts were done.

The patients were then usually started on doses of chlorpromazine of 25 mg. orally, t.i.d. The suitable dose was then determined empirically by the behavioral responses, maintaining the child in a calm state without undue drowsiness. The desirable doses were found to range from 10 to 250 mg. daily. The large majority (92%) of these children were not give any formal psychotherapy, *e.g.*, play therapy, in addition to the medication. However, superficial therapy was necessarily instituted in the relationship therapy that developed from regular contacts both with the children and parent or surrogate, who reported on changes in behavior, etc.

Behavioral observations were made not only by the authors and parents but also by the teachers and school counselors who cooperated fully in the study. An effort was made to evaluate properly the effect of the drug by the utilization of placebo therapy during some interval of treatment extending from 4 to 6 weeks. Full realization of the occasional effect of placebo therapy alone was kept in mind.

Observations

Improvement was evaluated on the basis of: (1) changes in antisocial behavior in school; (2) behavior in home environment; (3) school achievement; (4) the psychological test battery. Improvement was observed in 21 patients (84%). The behavioral improvement was marked in 18 cases (72%). The outstanding manifestation was the lessening of overactivity, ranging from restlessness to combativeness. The children spontaneously commented that they did not fight anymore. This was confirmed by the teachers who added that these children were now more cooperative.

The faculty for learning was reported as improved in the majority of cases and markedly improved in 5 (20%). Two children who had been excluded from school were returned and have continued to make a satisfactory adjustment. Another outstandingly hard to manage child, J. L., has accepted a visiting teacher to his home and his improvement has been so marked that his case is given below in greater detail.

J. L., white male, aged 11, had been ill for 4 years with symptoms characteristic of schizophrenia. There was restlessness and unpredictable combativeness in school associated with bizarre mannerisms and masochistic behavior at home. He was suspended indefinitely after trying both the parochial and the public schools. Five months of psychotherapy at St. Christopher's Hospital was terminated by his combativeness toward the therapist. The patient's mother was also considered an ambulatory schizophrenic, paranoid type. He was then referred by the juvenile division of the municipal court to our clinic after tentative arrangements had been made for placement in a state hospital. He was placed on chlorpromazine medication, 100 mg. daily and seen on an average of once per 10 days for the next 8 months.

His behavior in the clinic and at home improved significantly. He was able to make a much better play adjustment with neighborhood children. A comparison of the battery of psychological tests before and after this course of treatment is instructive. That given before treatment required 3 days to complete; that administered after, 3 hours. The I.Q.'s were the same—87. The memory spans, however, changed, showing marked improvement. Before it was 4 digits forward and none in reverse. After, it was 7 forward and 3 in reverse. Both Rorschach's showed him to be psychotic with the potential for uncontrolled and explosive behavior. P. responses increased from 1 to 4 and there was an absence of bizarre and contaminated responses present initially. Fk responses appearing in the second test would suggest development of awareness of his problem. The FM responses showed diminished hyperkinetic activity in this content. Finally, the Wide Range Achievement Test showed reading to be 1.4, spelling 1.5, and arithmetic 3.1; the previous readings all being at the baseline of 1.0.

The comprehensive picture obtained from the study of the retest results outlined certain conclusions and suggested other trends in personality functioning: (1) The basic character picture remained the same, the same types of defenses were utilized, and the core conflicts persisted. (2) Although the intelligence quotients were significantly unchanged, there was usually evidence of improved intellectual functioning (increase in F responses, M. replaces FM responses). This had to be evaluated with an appreciation of the changes that can be expected in the normal intellectual growth of the child in contrast with the findings in the disturbed child. The norms reported by Ames *et. al.* and Ford were used. (3) Facilitation of the learning process is suggested by improvement in the Wide Range Achievement Test and in the memory spans. (4) There is a trend toward greater self-acceptance and an associated urging toward closer interpersonal relationships. (5) Trends were also noted in the strengthening of emotional controls both quantitatively and qualitatively, *e.g.* Rorschach responses scored as evidences of hostility were replaced by those indicating only aggression, *e.g.* fighting cats were replaced by crawling cats.

Drowsiness was the chief side effect noted. Seven children (27%) complained of it at some time during therapy. As might have been expected, both the parents and teachers were so much relieved by the comparative underactivity in contrast with the previous disturbing overactivity that sleeping in class was rarely a complaint by the teacher. Significantly, drowsiness never interfered with play. One boy of 12 with a diagnosis of primary behavior disorder, who did complain of occasional nightmares, was finally standardized on a single dose of 10 mg. at night. This very small dose resulted not only in the establishment of a more wholesome sleep pattern free of nightmares, but also in a more relaxed and productive routine in school. This small dosage was unique. The average dose which did not produce drowsiness was 25 mg. t.i.d. We came to the conclusion early that children required larger doses in proportion to the body weight than had been suggested initially, and that undesirable side effects were minimal when compared with the findings in adults. The only other possible by-effect was a localized itching macular eruption which appeared in 2 colored children. The drug was discontinued temporarily and the eruptions subsided. One was subsequently attributed to sensitivity to a local atopen and drug treatment was renewed. The sequential complete blood count studies did not reveal any significant abnormal responses.

In 5 patients enuresis had been one of the complaints. Improvement in this symptom ranging from diminution to complete cessation was reported in each of the patients. No explanation is offered at this time. It is our impression that the improved mother-child relationship was a more potent mitigating factor than possible alterations in the autonomic innervations to the genito-urinary tract.

The responses to placebo medication were interesting in that 5 patients continued to maintain their improved status while on placebo. This raises the important question, "To what extent can the positive response be attributed to the development of a therapeutic interpersonal relation resulting from kindly attention from a therapist, school counselor and, possibly, others in the child's environment?" The observation was frequently made that while the child would insist that there was no change in his behavior and adjustment during the placebo phase, a return of the restlessness of the hyperkinetic aspect was observable to the therapist.

An outstanding case was a 15-year-old boy with a diagnosis of ambulatory schizophrenia. The significant clinical manifestations were multiple tics of the upper half of the body associated with ideas of reference and occasional hallucinations of a mildly threatening nature. The ideas of reference and hallucinations were relieved initially. The tics, essentially magical defense gestures, then were largely controlled. On placebo medication the tics first reappeared and then the patient began again to complain of the same type of ideas of reference.

Discussion

It has been suggested that the development of chlorpromazine has ushered in a new era in psychiatric treatment. We would seem to have a therapeutic adjuvant which will relax the apprehensive subject, immobilize the hostile one, and simultaneously make them receptive to verbalization, or at least not produce a clouding of the sensorium. A number of reporters believe that the drug does permit "sustained psychotherapeutic rapport."

There is now evidence from the reports of Hiebel *et al.* and Terzian that this type of response can possibly be explained by the effect of chlorpromazine on the reticular, activating system of Magoun which controls the reaction of arousal. This reaction can be considered a continuum of behavior which extends from the sham rage reaction of Bard through hypervigilance and ordinary alertness to stupor and deep coma. Magoun describes this system as having an over-all effect on the consciousness because when activated it also exerts pronounced facilitory influences on lower motor outflows so that it functions normally both to promote central alertness and to facilitate motor behavior. Animal experimentation offers evidence that chlorpromazine produces a "medicamentous hypophysectomy," *i.e.*, chlorpromazine "blocked the hypophyseal reaction to aggression."

We suggest the possibility that activation of this system is the neurophysiological mechanism which gives rise to the primitive behavior we have labeled the fight-flight response. The drug seems to moderate the intense fight or flight responses to new situations. If such is the case, we have at last been able to exhibit a drug that alters such primitive behavior and also makes the patient available for psychotherapy.

The responses to placebo medication alone and the positive changes noted in both behavioral and psychological test responses suggest to us that the interpersonal relationships and their modifications are at the core of therapy. Further observations on the diminution of anxiety and tension in these patients, in both clinical and psychological aspects, are being pursued. Certainly the quieter child makes less demand on the environment. Parental giving is more freely offered when placidity abounds. Learning is facilitated when teachers are not frustrated.

The degree to which tension is lessened, perception and memory improved, etc., by the basic neurophysiologic changes, must be determined. Realizing that the reserpine fraction of Rauwolfia serpentina has also been found effective in a wide range of disturbed patients although the neurophysiologic responses differ somewhat from those of chlorpromazine, it was decided to treat a comparative series of children with reserpine. This study will be reported later.

We emphasize that therapy was a "combined procedure" in which the drug effects were facilitory to the interpersonal relationship which was established. It is thus complementary to psychotherapy when emotional growth ensues. There are indications that the drugs like chlorpromazine, reserpine, and LSD 25, may have helped initiate a new era in psychiatry, the era of combined therapy where drug therapy and psychotherapy are complementary to each other.

Summary and Conclusions

Twenty-five hyperkinetic, emotionally disturbed children were treated with chlorpromazine for periods lasting from 4 to 16 months. They also served as their own controls by receiving placebo medication for 4 to 6 weeks during some phase of treatment. Response was determined from the following observations: (1) Clinical changes noted by the clinic staff which included the social worker and psychologist as well as the therapist; (2) data from the home environment; (3) reports from the school counselors; (4) changes in the battery of psychological tests done before and after treatment.

Improvement in varying degrees was noted in 21 cases—84% and was marked in 70%. Diminution in hyperactivity was the outstanding phenomenon. Combativeness was reduced considerably. There was definite improvement in willingness to learn

The psychological testing suggested that the learning process was facilitated. Trends toward increased emotional control were evidenced although the basic personality seemed unchanged.

The procedure was effective because an "improved interpersonal relationship" could be established and exploited for the sake of the learning process.

The side effects were minimal compared with those of adult and did not necessitate the termination of treatment in any case. Sequential blood count studies were negative.

It is suggested that, perhaps for the first time, we have a drug which dampens the primitive fight-flight responses, possibly actuated by the "arousal system" of Magoun. It is further suggested that by controlling this basic mechanism without im pairing consciousness and the learning process, we can now do more effective psychotherapy.

We seem to have entered the era of "combined therapy" where drug therapy and psychotherapy are complementary and can be combined to change the personality most effectively.

Discussion

Thaddeus P. Krush, M.D. (Waltham, Mass.).—Some time ago a professional worker curious about our work with children on an inpatient basis, spoke to one of our residents, and, in tones of mildly horrified disapproval said, "I understand that Doctor Krush uses drugs in the treatment of the children at the Met," to which she received the answer, "Why yes, we do." After a moment's hesitation, she condescendingly excused us with the remark, "Oh, but then I suppose he has to; they have such sick children out there."

It is, of course, true that we do receive children under 16 years of age having the most severe behavioral disturbances in the Commonwealth, and I sometimes grow weary trying to clarify the point that as physicians we have a wide range of therapeutic agents at our command.

It may be redundant to mention it, but it seems to me that we utilize a therapeutic agent, be it psychotherapy, drug, or whatever, to produce an effect modifying the reaction of the patient, or patients, with whom we are working; and, that treatment is planned, not so much on the basis of exclusion until only the most drastic measures remain for the most disturbed, but as an expression of opinion on the part of the physician as to what is needed to promote a state of health or to meliorate the ravages of a continuing state of disease. Varying forms of psychotherapy and medications are not mutually exclusive of one another, but frequently lead to more rapid progress with the patient and his human constellation than might be expected if anyone were used singly.

I therefore read this paper with considerable interest and

pleasure. Inasmuch as Doctor Brian Hunt and I have been conducting a similar study during the past 4 months with 58 hospitalized children, I should like to draw from our brief experience with chlorpromazine (Thorazine) comment relevant to the paper under discussion:

We especially confirm the clinical impressions of: (1) A greater self-acceptance on the part of the patient toward his problems; with a trend toward improved interpersonal relations; (2) a strengthening of emotional controls; (3) the best results, in the nonpsychotic group, were obtained with those children having hyperactivity as a more important clinical manifestation; (4) the transient nature of the drowsiness.

At the start of our trial run the pills were presented to each child as "a means of helping you to get along better." During the first day the children, as they were able to compare observations, got the idea that these were actually vitamins to pep them up and a large number became much more active whether on placebo or drug. On the second and third day word got around that they were getting a sleeping medicine and a large number of the children spent much of these 2 days asleep or dozing, again unrelated to whether placebo or drug.

While the basic problems of the patient remain the same unless psychotherapeutically manipulated, a more florid expression of the illness (marked regression in latent schizophrenia, marked depression in strongly hostile and aggressive character disorders) is occasionally encountered.

Continuing blood studies have revealed no remarkable changes, but in addition to the drowsiness and one urticarial reaction, we have encountered 3 cases of mild edema (two face, one ankles) and in 2 other instances reactivation of seizures, both having an increase in number of seizures. Our range of medication spanned from 50 mg. to 600 mg. per day.

We should be interested in further observations regarding the "facilitation of learning" effect; and whether any further side reactions are encountered.

Response to the Foregoing

In answer to the questions of Dr. Krush, we did not observe any further side reaction than we have reported above.

In our opinion the facilitation of learning was shown by:

(1) The increase in the Wide Range Achievement Test in all 13 patients who were studied for longer than 6 months to a degree that was greater than might be expected in the normal course of events; (2) by the improvement in the memory span in many cases, an effect which should improve the "climate for learning"; (3) the reports of the teachers and councilors of the improvement in grades of the students.

ON TREATMENT BY HYDROXYZINE OF NERVOUS CONDITIONS DURING CHILDHOOD

J. Bayart, M.D.

I. Introduction

The physician, and above all the pediatrician, is often consulted because of young patients for whom he should obtain tranquillity. When not prescribing specifically sedative medications, until now he has had to call upon substances that, besides chiefly having a general soporific effect, pacify the patient because he finds himself in a condition close to sleep. But what the physician really sought, and had seldom or never found, was to obtain peace of mind, and emotional stability.

The possibilities of chemical synthesis have permitted placing at the disposal of physicians what they have long sought, the discovery of hydroxyzine* has finally solved this problem. In short, hydroxyzine can remove all excessiveness of reactivity; it quiets excessive emotion, it avoids outbursts of temper in the overnervous and those suffering from mental overstrain; it calms the distressed and brings confidence to the embittered and anxious. The person treated with hydroxyzine retains full consciousness of the stimuli, affective or otherwise, that released his disturbance. He reports their nature and their intensity but his reactions have become those of a completely balanced individual.

---

* Chemical Name: 1-(p-Chlorobenzhydryl-)-4-(2-(hydroxyethoxy)ethyl) diethyl enediamine. Trade Name: Atarax—Union Chimique Belge, Brussels; J. B. Roeri and Company, Divn. Chas. Pfizer & Co., Inc.

II. Pharmacology

Examination of the structural formula shows that it belongs to the group of antihistamine products, for it comprises a tertiary ethylamine coupled to a radical having two symmetrical rings, which form the essential constituent of those products. By effecting important modifications of the aminic group, one has been able to give hydroxyzine the special properties that distinguish it from other preparations.

The most general use for antihistamines is for treatment of allergies, by action against the histamines. However, their employment in this indication and in others, brings about secondary reactions of varying intensity according to the product and the patient.

The most disagreeable secondary reactions from these medicaments are sedation, which is the most common, and is followed in order of frequency, by lassitude and muscular weakness. As in certain industrial processes, the by-products, heretofore considered as being useless, come to be regarded more highly than the original product; thus, with hydroxyzine, sedation and lassitude are no longer injurious results, but very much those by which one profits and which serve as a base for all its therapeutic indications.

III. Pharmacological Study of Animals

The method generally used for sedatives consists in observation of the movements of the laboratory animals to which the substance has been administered. The classic techniques are confined to recording by a special method the spontaneous movements of the animals under test, compared with a control group; for example, the footprints left by the animals on blackened paper or even the kymographic recording of the movements communicated to a cage by the animal that finds itself imprisoned, etc.

For the study of hydroxyzine, the method was different; it

was based on observation of the attitude of the animal, a method that was shown to be very responsive. After having received the nerve sedative, the experimental mice became motionless and completely relaxed. It is important to note that the animals retained their vitality intact and their escape reflexes during violent excitement remained unchanged.

The method of procedure for the class of products to which hydroxyzine belongs is certainly different from that used for the barbiturates, for example; for even by greatly increasing the dosage, one never obtained the stage of sleep. Therefore, it is not a question of hypnotics.

Experiments upon animals have shown that it is not at all a question of an effect comparable to that of curare. The control has been employed in different tests; excitation of the sciatic nerve causing contraction of the rabbit's foot; head drop of the rabbit; a separate preparation of the phrenic diaphragm nerve of the rat; rectus abdominis of the frog; curarization of the whole frog.

IV. Basic Clinical Action

The sedative action noted during experiments on animals is comparable to that in humans, and therefore differs from that of the neuro-sedatives most employed in practice, such as barbiturates, bromides, and chloral hydrate, of which the sedative action results from their hypnotic power. These medicaments can induce neurolepsy, and real narcosis by increasing the dosage, and affect to a greater or lesser degree the conscious state. On the other hand, hydroxyzine never affects the conscious state and never causes the somniferous effects caused by the former. It actually is related to a new pharmacological effect recently recognized with the discovery of chlorpromazine and which, in turn, has been found in reserpine and, recently, in hydroxyzine.

In order to convey this new idea for chlorpromazine, one invented the word "neuroplegia" but Delay in his study on reserpine, proposed the term "neurolepsia" for the medicaments that diminish nervous and psychic tension and which induce quiet and mental peace, and not paralysis of the nerves, as the word "neuroplegia" suggests.

In accordance with Delay's proposal, endorsed by Farah, we prefer the designation "neuroleptic agents" for the three mentioned products.

V. Clinical Action on Nervous Conditions in Childhood

Among the numerous investigations we have made on treatment with hydroxyzine, in nervous conditions in childhood, we have chosen the conditions where any well defined nervous illness was the cause of the outbreaks we wished to ameliorate.

All our tests have also been made on children who were ambulatory cases, in order that the previous conditions of life and surroundings should be identical with those during and after the test of the treatment.

The number of cases studied totaled 187, and comprised the most diverse nervous conditions (nocturnal nightmares, incontinence of urine, crying spasms, tics, unbalanced children, etc.) that one meets in children between 1 and 12 years of age.

Two very definite indications, especially—nervous tics on the one hand; nervous children, unbalanced, consequently poor scholars, on the other hand—have especially attracted our attention, because under these conditions our results have been most spectacular and the most regular.

The first series comprised 70 children whose age varied between 5 and 12 years, with a majority from 8 to 10 years; it was composed of 47 boys and 23 girls and relates to $2/3$ facial tics and $1/3$ other localizations.

On 90% of our little patients the tics disappeared after 10 to 12 days' treatment; the remaining 10% did not show any improvement.

The dosage administered was 30 mg. daily, in three doses. In all the little invalids, the hydroxyzine treatment was maintained at the same dosage and uninterruptedly for three months, then it was continued by intermittent treatment for 10 to 15 days, with, after each treatment a progressively increased rest period.

In 78% of the cases, the recovery was complete and the tics did not reappear. In 22% of the cases, the tics reappeared during the three months of the treatment and most often for an emotional reason. To benefit these relapses, it was necessary to double the dosage originally administered, for instance, 60 mg daily, for 15 days. Sixty per cent of the relapsed cases responded to the treatment, and the tics definitely disappeared; the others were in no way changed.

The second series comprised 56 cases, 36 boys and 20 girls whose age varied between 7 and 12 years. All were unbalanced children, nervous, consequently poor scholars.

The treatment set up was analogous to that of the first series.

Thanks to the help of the parents and above all of the teaching personnel, who gave us their valuable cooperation, we have been able to follow very closely the improvement in these children, which usually commenced 10 to 15 days after starting the treatment. The calming effect of hydroxyzine was remarkable and allowed several of our little patients to attain distinctly more regular and more favorable scholastic results.

In the opinion of the teaching staff the calming action of the product showed itself by more regular and neater handwriting as well as by a distinctly livelier and more sustained attention and a very much improved application to studies.

We have also been able to estimate the happy effect of hydroxyzine in another form of childhood nervousness. It is known that the first days of hospitalization or of admission to a day nursery are always distressing and filled with many difficulties. The loneliness of these children after their parents leave, the sight of strange people and of the nurses in white uniforms disturb the children to the point where they neither sleep nor eat. When administering hydroxyzine, during the first four or five days of hospitalization or admission to a day nursery, one notes that, instead of the tears and complaints generally noticed, the children are definitely calmer, sleep quietly, and eat almost normally.

The action of the product is definitely superior to the classic sedatives barbiturates, bromides, chloral.

VI. Conclusions

In the course of our tests with hydroxyzine on the various nervous conditions of children, we have especially been able to note its remarkable effects in two well-defined indications: nervous tics, on the one hand; unbalanced, nervous children, therefore poor scholars, on the other hand.

In the first cases, the tics disappeared after 10 to 12 days of treatment, in 90% of our patients, not reappearing (in 78% of our cases). The dosage administered was 30 mg. daily, divided into three doses.

In the second series, at the end of 10 to 15 days of treatment, we were able to appreciate, at the examinations, together with the parents and the teaching staff, the remarkable calming effect of the product, which allowed several small patients to attain definitely more regular and favorable scholastic results.

To summarize the results obtained, the hydroxyzine treatment is maintained at the same dosage without interruption during three months, then it was continued by intermittent treatments of 10 to 15 days, with, after each treatment a progressively increased rest period.

The digestive and general tolerance was perfect. The appetite and digestion remained normal and, whatever the dosage administered, we have never noted either somnolence or slowing down of the mental faculties.

For the most closely observed cases, we have never noticed a bad influence either on the blood pressure, except for a slight temporary rise in the first 3-4 days of the treatment, or on the blood counts; the number of red and white corpuscles and the hemoglobin count remained practically unchanged.

IMPAIRMENT OF THE SENSE OF REALITY AS MANIFESTED IN PSYCHONEUROSIS AND EVERYDAY LIFE

George Frumkes, M.D.

According to the psychoanalytic theory, the reality principle is an outgrowth of the pleasure principle. It has the same ultimate aim of avoiding pain and achieving instinctual gratification. Human behaviour is determined by the pleasure principle, but control is necessary, and reality must be considered so as to facilitate behaviour which will actually yield pleasure rather than pain.

The modification of the pleasure principle in the interest of a realistic adaptation is not an easy process. The development of a sense of reality requires time and effort; the postponement, alteration, and even the sacrifice of enjoyment is often necessary. The maturation of a sense of reality does not depend upon the individual alone. Education takes place in a human milieu. We are dependent upon other people not only for support during the learning process, but also for training and for facts about the surroundings. The development is never complete because of man's limitations in the face of the wide world, and because the environment is in a constant state of flux. The organism's biological needs recur; the universe poses infinite changing problems; therefore we must regard the sense of reality as being relative. It is a process of shifting equilibrium.

"Eternal vigilance is the price of liberty." It is also the price of a good sense of reality. Only in sleep may vigilance be relaxed, because in sleep motility is temporarily arrested. The unconscious manifests itself in the distortions produced by the formation of the manifest dream from the latent dream, and achieves an illusory wish-fulfilment. Reality testing is impaired in neurosis and psychosis, the symptoms of which have been compared to the dream; they are distortions of behaviour produced by inroads of the unconscious into the ego.

Reality testing is an essential part of the conscious and belongs to the core of the ego, which, utilizing perception, memory, and control of motility, performs an integrative function. Even in Freud's early formulation of metapsychology, which opposed the conscious to the unconscious, there were two distinct mental processes; the primary process with its unmodified pleasure principle and mode of unconscious thought, and the secondary process which included reason, judgment and the censor. Later, this fundamental dichotomy was retained despite its modification by making part of the ego unconscious (i.e. the repressing forces) and the introduction of the concept of the superego.

In 1911 Freud demonstrated the importance of the subject of reality in understanding neuroses and psychoses. Normally, the pleasure ego develops into and is safeguarded by the reality ego, which learns to defer pleasure for future reward and recognizes that it is impossible to persist in unrealistic behaviour. The hallucinatory wish-fulfilments of the pleasure ego are abandoned as awareness of the world is forced upon us by the sense organs and the fact that effort must be exerted to obtain real satisfaction becomes inescapable. This process requires the development of attention, memory, thought, and the ability to make impartial judgments. This means that motor discharge must be postponed, restrained, and otherwise converted into action directed towards changing reality rather than merely discharging tension.

The sex instincts are less subject to the reality principle than are the ego instincts, since they are most easily gratified by autoerotism and more readily displaced on to substitute objects. Besides, sex phantasies may be repressed without immediate danger to life, whereas ego drives may not. But repression represents a defect in the psychic structure which leads to the denial of truths merely because they are painful, and this tendency can interfere with the operation of the reality principle in all types of thought.

The sex drives cannot be sharply separated from the ego drives with which they co-operate during infancy; the pleasure principle continually interferes with the reality principle. A measure of unrealism may be tolerated even for the ego instincts if the organism has sufficient reserve of strength, and if it is not threatened by any imminent or overwhelming danger. The prolonged human infancy may be used to foster unrealistic thinking in regard to both types of instincts. A long childhood is required for optimum mental development. The situation is paradoxical and the risk unavoidable.

Freud exemplified the tenacity with which we hold on to sources of pleasure by pointing out that wishful thinking persists in phantasy-making and day-dreaming. Religion teaches us to postpone all pleasure for reward in heaven, and is therefore useful for learning renunciation at the price of too much unrealistic thinking. Science offers intellectual pleasure and practical gains. Art reconciles the two principles, since the artist expresses his phantasy in a way that will bring him real rewards as well as the wish-fulfilment and the participation of the audience in his gratification. Education promotes the reality principle by using love as a reward, and will fail if the child is loved regardless of its behavior. In relation to this last, it must be added that human development requires a margin of security. The child must feel free to play and experiment, safe in the knowledge that it will be loved even when it is naughty. It is true that development of the reality principle will be retarded if there is too much indulgence, but, on the other hand, mental growth will be stunted if the child must anxiously accede to all commands and teaching.

Freud described realistic thinking as opposed to wishful thinking. He illustrated certain types of neurotic disregard for reality, such as omnipotence of thought and the assumption that the wish is the same as the deed. He did not, however, indicate the essential process involved in the sense of reality, nor did he describe the steps in its development. The missing elements were supplied by Ferenczi, who based his considerations partly on the paper which I have just discussed, and partly on an earlier paper by Freud. He postulated that a sense of reality consists in a clear recognition of the difference between the ego and the outside world, between the organism and its environment. In 1914 Freud elaborated this concept further in another paper which has since become of cardinal importance in psychoanalytic theory.

The infant does not clearly distinguish between itself and its surroundings. Since its desires are satisfied without the need of making them known and without any effort on its part, it assumes that the wish is sufficient. Ferenczi called this the period of unconditional omnipotence. Trying to "feel himself" into the soul of the infant and using an idea of Freud's, he hypothesized that the child's first wish is to return to the womb and that the nurse's attempts to create womblike conditions by supplying warmth, darkness, and quiet cause the child to feel himself possessed of magical power to realize wishes by merely imagining. This is called the period of magical-hallucinatory omnipotence, and Ferenczi suggests that a parallel exists in the delusions of the psychotic.

Next, according to his theory, comes the period of omnipotence by the help of magic gestures, when the infant thrashes about and cries to obtain satisfaction, though it still has no idea of cause and effect. Both these stages are correlated with the introjection phase in mental development, during which the child takes the world into himself. This is followed by the projection phase, in which his own characteristics are ascribed to the outside world. Ferenczi called this the animistic period. In it the child projects his own ego on to external objects. He becomes increasingly aware of a hostile, unfriendly world which will not yield to his wishes. This frustration is the original incentive for the development of a sense of reality, but not all magic is given up. The child can still obtain satisfaction from the mother by merely informing her of its desires, and it enters what Ferenczi named the period of magic thoughts and magic words. The omnipotence of thought of the obsessional neurotic is a regression to this stage, as is the use of religious prayers and magical formulas.

In the development of the sense of reality, Ferenczi, like Freud, differentiated between the ego instincts and the sex instincts. The illusion of omnipotence, he said, persists in sexuality long after the ego has become familiar with natural forces, and may even be lifelong, since narcissism is a constantly accessible way of regression after every love disappointment. On the subject of neuroses, Ferenczi made a valuable contribution by emphasizing the role of faulty reality testing in the formation of symptoms.

A good reality sense may be expressed in various terms, such as a strong ego, instincts which are not too powerful, no loss of ego boundaries, or good object relations. There are criteria by which its development in an individual may be determined, and I enumerate ten of them. These standards are not independent of each other, and may, in fact, merely denote different manifestations of the same process. They are:

(1) The ability to defer action. This implies not only control but the ability to think and substitute thought for action until action is feasible.
(2) The ability to employ action in accordance with natural laws in order to bring about a desired change. This is different from action which merely discharges tension.
(3) A clear realization of the difference between the self and the not-self. When a person has such a realization he does not attempt the magic of willing an external motion in the same way as he wills his extremities to move.
(4) Awareness that the need for a satisfaction does not guarantee the satisfaction, as in unconditional omnipotence.
(5) Realization that wishes in themselves do not bring about satisfactions.
(6) Realization that symbolic actions do not bring about satisfaction, and that external objects in spite of certain re-

semblances to portions of one's body are not influenced in the same way.
(7) Awareness that the symbol and the object are different.
   A. Identity or mutual influence are not established because objects were once in contact, as in contiguous magic.
   B. That two objects have something in common, such as name, appearance, origin, does not mean that they are the same, as in homeopathic magic.
(8) Awareness of the temptation to deny reality because its recognition would bring pain. A person with a good sense of reality is able to tolerate a fair amount of tension.
(9) Continuous alertness to the dangers involved in ascribing omnipotence to anything. When an object is regarded as omnipotent one may seek to regain one's own omnipotence by identification with it, thus reviving the illusion of the identity of the self with the outer world.
(10) Other evidence that the ego is effectively performing its integrative function—that it performs this function not only for the conflicting impulses of the id, but that it recognizes the demands of its other masters, the superego and reality. The subject can only be mentioned, since details would finally include criteria for successful termination of analysis. These include a minimizing of symptoms, capacity for full sexual enjoyment, work, and play. I would like to add one other characteristic which may be particularly pertinent in this discussion, i.e. the courage to form phantasies, to play or joke, which denotes sufficient confidence in one's soundness of mind for one to feel that one can safely abandon reality temporarily in the sure expectation of finding one's way back. There is a flexibility of affect.

Keeping these criteria in mind, I should like to give briefly some illustrations of more or less disguised magical thinking taken from psychosis, primitive religion, and psychoneurosis. All these examples may be considered in terms of the degree of awareness of difference between the self and its surroundings, and of the means employed to bring about satisfaction when the operation of the laws of nature is disregarded.

The psychoses furnish the most flagrant examples of the denial of reality. In postpartum psychosis the new mother may insist that she never bore a child or that the child which is shown her is a changeling. A widow may not permit the removal of her dead husband. Bleuler relates that a schizophrenic patient would regularly perform this ceremony at the time a train was scheduled to leave: he would study his watch intently, and at the correct moment raise his arm in a signal to the driver. The train would puff away, the patient would replace his watch in his pocket and return to the hospital convinced that it was he who had dispatched the train.

Frazer has given many examples of a similar magical reasoning in the ceremonies which had for their purpose to make the sun rise. It was believed that if the Egyptian king or the Brahmin priest omitted the rites, the world would be left in darkness. The clouds were considered to be evil spirits, intent on arresting the sun. The priests thwarted these fiends of darkness by burning their effigies. Other primitive magical practices include rainmaking by pouring water through a sieve. To ensure bountiful crops from Mother Earth, certain primitive peoples would set her a good example by copulating in the fields.

Freud showed many analogies between the practices of obsessional patients and primitive magic in the use of symbols, rituals, and magic formulas. In spite of their intelligence these patients are superstitious. They believe in the omnipotence of thought, particularly in regard to hostile impulses. They feel as guilty about a wish as if it had been a deed. Ferenczi remarked that the feeling of omnipotence of thought in a compulsive neurotic arises from his own sense of powerlessness against his drives. In other words, the illusion comes from identifying oneself with the instinctual drive. The world is assumed to be as powerless as the patient.

The obsessional neurotic may project his guilt on to a symbol and persuade himself that in working with the symbol he is working with the object of his guilt. An official of whom Freud wrote always presented cleanly washed and pressed paper currency to compensate for his 'dirty' sexual habits. The obsessional doubt may also serve a magic function. The doubt leads to inaction, which may have the same effect as a hostile deed. The obsessional may try to deceive himself, by his denial of overt hostility, but unconsciously he is aware of his motives and he feels guilt which is often displaced on to another idea.

In the phobias, fears may be displaced from one object to another. There is magical thinking involved in the idea that by avoiding the secondary object one will avoid the anxieties raised by the primary object. Little Hans had a phobia of horses rather than fear of his father. Because of certain resemblances in the way of strength and passion, the horse was a symbol for the father. The magical trick is based upon the equation of symbol and object. A patient avoids the street in an attempt to escape from her repressed sexual wishes. Because of the similarity in a word, fear of the street and fear of street-walking are equated and the avoidance of the street is adopted in the hope of controlling prostitution phantasies.

There is another bit of magic, the displacement of internal fears to external fears, probably based on the fact that we know the external world only by perceptions which are in our minds. Since the internal fears are also in our mind, we may say that both have similar origins, both outside or both inside, interchangeable whichever way suits the moment. A patient of mine who had hysterical vomiting unconsciously and magically thought that he could solve his conflict about being dependent upon his wife for support by expelling the food she served to him. The bridge was, "I can't take it," then by rejecting the food he also rejected the support.

Impairment of the reality sense is also found in the psychoanalytic resistances. Every psychoanalytic case history is concerned with the more or less disguised methods used in seeking instinctual gratification, and the ways in which the patient attempts to deceive himself as to the nature of his drives. We analyze action or thought in terms of its libidinal or instinctual component, as well as in terms of the defences, the ego and the superego.

Freud classified the resistance to psychoanalysis into five groups, of which three derive from the ego, one from the superego, and one from the id. The one most familiar to us is repression resistance. The pressure of a repressed impulse to become conscious is felt as dangerous since its attempted gratification would cause a conflict with reality or with the superego. The ego prefers to keep the idea unconscious and maintains control over the psychic apparatus by its threat to produce the anxiety signal. To avoid the pain of anxiety and in conformity with the pleasure principle, the repression is maintained and the idea remains unconscious.

Repression resistance is distinguished from transference resistance, which has the same general character, but is evident in more definite ways, since in analysis transference revives a repressed idea instead of merely recalling it. Transference resistance, like repression resistance, serves the pleasure principle in its attempt to avoid the anxiety signal. It misinterprets the actual situation, and in a surreptitious way seeks for instinctual discharge by disregarding reality. On the other hand a patient may construe any unwelcome interpretation as a rejection similar to one sustained in childhood. By assuming the analyst to be hostile, the patient automatically invalidates the interpretation of current behaviour.

Now if we take the justified step of admitting that transferences have a part in all interpersonal relationships and are not confined to the analytic situation in which they are most intensively studied, then we can grasp the extent to which the reality principle may be inhibited in all domestic and social behaviour.

The third ego-resistance may be traced to secondary gain, and to the inclusion of the symptoms in the ego. The break with reality, in this case, consists in the belief that the illness or character deviation is assumed from free choice, when in fact it consists of a compromise with, if not a reversal of, instinctual drives. Reality is distorted to justify the alteration in aim or object, and there is falsification of both inner and external reality. As an example, a girl might deny her hate for her mother and not only behave in a loving way but even seem sincere in her praises of the mother's generosity, beauty, and tolerance, when, in fact, the mother has none of these traits. The obsessional neurotic denies internal reality twice over in regressing to anal erotism, then reacting against it, then believing that there was free choice of behaviour and misinterpreting the environment so that his character may seem suitable. A man who is excessively orderly and punctilious in all that he does may choose book-keeping as his vocation, and then claim that it is his work which has trained him to be painstaking and exact.

A fourth source of resistance from which several classes of unreality may arise derives from the superego. A person who can fulfill the role of parent surrogate, or can be identified with the ego-ideal, is not perceived realistically. In this sense, the type of unreality resembles those which occur in transference, but there are special characteristics arising from the special position of this form of ego alteration. The superego has a large unconscious component and utilizes aggressive instincts. Freud thought it derived from the sense of guilt and the need for punishment, and we know that a sense of guilt is capable of producing extraordinary distortions in the appreciation of reality. Witness the large number of self-confessed murderers who offer to give themselves up after every publicized crime.

The fifth resistance, that of the id, contributes to the difficulties of reality testing because it represents the drive of the pleasure principle for expression without regard for reality. It represents the pleasure principle in its least adulterated form. A quality of the id resistance, the repetition compulsion, is also 'beyond the pleasure principle'.

Having reviewed ways in which the sense of reality is strained in the struggle with instinctual drives, we should then consider the effects of the outside world. Thinking is an ego function, and the ego is formed through the influence of reality on the id. External agencies include the physical environment and the customs, practices, and beliefs of people, especially the parents, with whom an individual comes in contact. An attempt should be made to evaluate ideologies and customs in terms of the criteria for an efficient sense of reality, and to ask why harmful myths are perpetuated.

In this paper, instead of extending the range of the investigation, I will expand upon some of the clinical material to which I have alluded.

A government official, one of Freud's earliest cases of obsessional neurosis, whose symptoms included extreme scrupulosity, invariably paid Freud with apparently new paper currency. Freud remarked that one could tell a government official by the brand new notes that he drew from the State Treasury. The man corrected Freud and said that on the contrary this money had been ironed out at home. He did this from consideration for the people with whom he would have dealings. Money was often dirty, and he did not want to be responsible for transmitting disease.

Since Freud had already formulated his ideas concerning the sexual etiology of neuroses, he thereupon questioned the man as to his sexual life. The official replied that his sexual needs were taken care of, in spite of the fact that he was a bachelor. He knew several families where there were young daughters, and he played the part of a dear old uncle to these girls. He would arrange to take one of these girls on an outing in the country, and at weekends, when they missed the train, they would be forced to stay at an inn. He prided himself on the fact that he always engaged separate rooms for himself and the girl, and that he was not cheapened in this regard. During the course of the evening he would enter the girl's bedroom and caress her, and manipulate her genitals. Freud then asked if he did not think this action was dirty. The patient indignantly denied this, and was angry at Freud's attempt to connect the feeling of dirtiness in his sexual life with the feeling of dirtiness in the money that he passed on. As a matter of fact, the patient insisted, he had not harmed the girls, who had later succeeded in making good marriages.

PSYCHONEUROSIS AND EVERYDAY LIFE

Now in this case there was no gross misrepresentation of reality. The patient did not say that money dirt and moral dirt were the same, but his behaviour showed that he seemed to believe the two were equivalent. The unreality is not openly admitted, as might be the case with a psychotic. It is concealed, and it is only on interpretation that we may see that the patient mistakes a symbol for an object or a symbol for a phenomenon, or that he considers the two phenomena the same because they have something in common. In this case the idea or the word "dirty" affords a semantic confusion which is used by the neurosis.

The following example of the confusion of two phenomena, just because they have one item in common, is taken from the treatment of a case of anxiety hysteria. A young married woman had a severe agoraphobia. She was afraid to go out in public conveyances; she thought that people knew that she was nervous. She feared that she would be sexually attacked or seduced. She was afraid to walk down alleys because men might dart out of the houses and snatch her away. The sexual nature of her fears was explained to her. The patient improved during treatment. She later became pregnant and delivered a fine boy. She was happy in her married life, her sexual pleasure increased, and she had orgasms.

One day she came to the hour in great distress; it was with great difficulty that she had refrained from calling me during the night. She was very nervous and tremulous. She could not sleep or solve trivial problems. She felt that all her previous improvement had been wiped out. During the course of the hour she gave illustrations of her inefficiency and inability to decide the simplest questions. Among the problems she mentioned was her indecision about an eighteen-dollar cheque she had received from the insurance company. She herself spoke a good deal about this cheque and the problems it raised. She had burned a cigarette hole in an inexpensive dress, and was advised by the members of her family to exaggerate the cost of the dress when she put her claim in for insurance payment, if she wished to get back what she had paid for it. The patient then valued the dress at $20, about twice its cost. After the insurance adjuster appeared and asked how much wear she had had out of the dress, she replied about $2 worth, and to her surprise she received a cheque for $18. She thereupon became very anxious; she felt that she had been dishonest. This was a feeling rather than a conviction. She excused her peccadillo by all sorts of rationalizations; for example, how much it would cost to replace the dress in the present market, the fact that she had suffered previous little damages that she had not reported to the insurance company and was therefore justified in receiving a larger cheque for the present accident. She acted as though she felt very guilty. She did not know what to do with the money. She did something that for her was very strange; she offered to give the cheque to her husband and to let him use part of it to apply to some sort of payment, whereas until then she had tried to get as much money as she could from her husband. She acted as if it were "hot money."

Now this patient had had a great many prostitution phantasies; she had played with the idea of being unfaithful to her husband, that is, cheating him. In this case the switch word is cheat. The patient had cheated the insurance company, but the guilt that she felt was as if she had cheated her husband. Because she did not actually admit the circumstances of her money dishonesty, she could not understand the situation clearly, and her doubts as to her money dishonesty were transmitted so as to become doubts as to her sexual virtue. The patient could be helped only when she could be made to realize clearly what she had done in securing the overpayment in the money matters. When she knew her guilt in one respect she could be convinced of her actual innocence, so far as actual deeds were concerned, in the other. The incident is useful also to illustrate another characteristic of the operation of the unconscious, which has no regard for quantitative considerations and no sense of proportion. A sin is a sin, whether it be murder or the theft of a piece of fruit.

The patient was one of the younger children in a family of ten. Her father had died when she was very young and the mother had had a difficult time raising the family. The sons had to work; the patient was very docile, the mother was able to maintain discipline in the family by arousing the children's fears; she threatened them with various punishments and encouraged all sorts of superstitious beliefs as to the omnipotence of the punisher and the omniscience of the detector of any infringements of her rules. Since there was not always enough food, the children would raid the market basket when it ar-

PSYCHONEUROSIS AND EVERYDAY LIFE

rived, each trying to take an extra piece of fruit and hiding it. When the patient was six years old, she was enticed into the cellar by a neighbour, a boy of twelve or fourteen. He exposed his penis and told her that if she sucked it, she would find that it was an ice cream cone with two scoops of ice cream. After she complied, she felt duped at not receiving the ice cream; although she says that she was innocent of the significance of what she had done, she must have had some guilt, since she never mentioned the incident to her mother or sisters. In the cheque incident, the switch word was cheat, as I said, and the patient reacts to the cheating of a few dollars in the same way as though she had been an adultress.

Now in religious practice, the same equation of various sins is made. St. Augustine said that the new-born infant was sinful and he described the sinful practices of the baby in loudly demanding and crying for milk; it was only the infant's powerlessness which made it innocent; as far as its intentions were concerned it was no more innocent than the adult, and unless a child was baptized the sin would be sufficient to condemn it to eternal hell-fire. So the new-born baby is sinful and a murderer is sinful; the same word is used for both. Politicians and demagogues make use of this semantic confusion to exact severe punishments for petty offenses and, on the other hand, to appeal for mercy when they wish to condone crimes.

A young married man was referred to me by a roentgenologist. He had been vomiting after meals; a diagnosis of peptic ulcer had been tentatively made, but not confirmed by the X-ray examination. The patient had no suspicions of any psychic cause. He came only because the doctor had sent him. During the course of the treatment, he told about himself. He was an orphan, brought up in a Jewish Orphan Asylum; he had been a good boy. At the age of sixteen he had been discharged. He had been able to support himself by securing a clerical position. Periodically he would return to the Orphan Asylum to show his former teachers how well he was doing as an independent citizen. After he married, his wife continued working as a secretary and they had a small apartment. They lived happily together and he would help with the dishes after she cooked the meals. Unfortunately in an economic recession he lost his job. He assiduously sought work. At first he was confident that he would find a new position, but as time went on he became more discouraged.

The first eight or nine hours of the treatment were taken up with a discussion of the patient's early life, his aspirations, his plans for the future, his love for his wife and his wish to support her, his sexual life, and the details concerning his vomiting. The vomiting began after he had become discouraged about the prospects of finding a new position. He vomited only in the morning or evening, but he himself had no idea of the possibility of any connection between the two except that being without a job was distressing. One day as he was relating the day's activities, he mentioned that he vomited after the meal, and used this phrase: "I can't take it" when he referred to his shame at eating food his wife had earned. Asked what he meant, he said that he could not accept the fact that he had to take support from his wife and that it was her food which she had earned, which he was eating. I remarked to him: "Just consider the phrase which you used. Do you see what you have done?" He chuckled and then berated himself and called himself an ungrateful wretch. He now realized that he had done in pantomime what he wanted to express in words. Literally, he rejected the food his wife gave him by vomiting, hoping by ejecting the food to do away with his dependence. Since he was an orphan, he was especially sensitized to the idea of being dependent, and he found the situation specially intolerable.

The unreality consists in using the same phrase "I can't take it" for the mental attitude and for the physical food, and in thinking, because they have this phrase in common, that the action which would be applicable to the one phenomenon would be applicable to the other. A faulty perception of unreality arises through the confusion of objects because of their symbolic connection through a common phrase. But there is another mechanism at work. The patient tries to deal with an internal problem by externalizing it and then reacting to this externalized substitute.

Likewise in Freud's case of little Hans, the boy tried to deal with his fear of his father by equating his father with a horse and then avoiding horses. In the case of the agoraphobic, she tries to avoid her sexual impulses by avoiding the streets where she might be tempted.

This mechanism has its basis in the fact that external objects are perceived by the mind just as are internal impulses. Therefore the possibilities are presented of equating the two in position, since both are represented in the mind. The external problem may be considered an internal one and the internal one is made external. Then the patient may try to deal with the internal problem as he does with the external problems, by avoiding them. The patient may either avoid the internal problem directly by repression, using the analogy from his dealing with external problems, or he may change the internal problem into an external problem and then avoid the external substitute. This incident of the hysterical vomiter who tried to eject his dependency problem is especially interesting, because he literally tried to externalize something. Little Hans or the agoraphobic externalized their problems only figuratively. As this patient vomited only in the morning and in the evening, a clue was provided to the fact that he was vomiting only the meals that his wife had prepared. The patient's vomiting ceased when he recognized the pantomime meaning of his action.

Another example of the impaired reality-sense in the obsessionally neurotic is shown in the following observation. The patient, a gifted college graduate, spent many many hours in giving material which could be interpreted as revolving around the one theme: that he was very intelligent and the world was unjust in giving greater rewards in the way of money, position, or love of women to other less gifted individuals. He behaved as if he thought that intelligence *ipso facto* entitled him to rewards. He did not act as if he realized that intelligence or the intelligence quotient was only a potential. If it was highly prized in childhood, it was only because it promised that he could eventually accomplish intellectual work when he was an adult, and that this intellectual work would in some way serve other individuals and they would be willing to pay for satisfactory work. He confused the promise of one aspect of the phenomenon of intellectual performance with the performance itself. As a child, he could have only the potentiality, and there may have been some justification for the indulgences which were accorded to him because of his cleverness. This view was entirely erroneous for an adult. This patient's confusion or error was only a more obvious expression of the confusion which is probably quite widespread, and is probably encouraged and developed by the distinctions between manual and mental workers.

I will illustrate the same thing by the behaviour of his mother. She aspired to become a concert pianist and she considered herself very cultured. When she rented an apartment she would stress her culture to the landlord and use it as a bargaining point, implying that she was an asset as a tenant, clean, quiet, and pleasant. Instead she was very noisy, quarrelsome, dirty, vulgar, and destructive. The landlords were always glad to be rid of her. But she could never believe the validity of the criticism of her behaviour, because such behaviour was uncultured, and she was cultured because she played the piano very well and her sister was a member of the Browning Society. Other professional people may make the same error in not realizing that their rewards are for services which they are expected to render rather than for their degrees.

Sometimes even doctors feel they are entitled to certain rewards just because they are doctors and not because of the work they do. An amusing if trifling example of this can be seen in the following anecdote. One of my patients has several doctors in her family, and she used to receive her drugs from the pharmacy at a discount. One day she asked that her purchase be delivered. The pharmacist said that if he was to give her the discount, he could not afford to deliver the drugs, and made the point that he does not give discounts to doctors just because they are doctors; he gives them in the hope of getting business, and since my patient's relatives did not refer him any accounts, there was no justification for their expecting preferential treatment.

PSYCHONEUROSIS AND EVERYDAY LIFE

These are illustrations of the impaired sense of reality as revealed in transference:

A. The "Rat-man" mistook a female in Freud's house for Freud's daughter, and interpreted the meeting as evidence that Freud wanted him for a son-in-law. Because of his wishes he did not see reality correctly. In addition, he used the mistake to gratify repressed wishes and to distort what had happened in the past. He used the transference mistake to gratify the wish that his father were still alive and looking after him; he also used it to deny his guilt in not having married the woman he himself had preferred. He escapes guilt about his own ambivalence. Transference is used to deny not only present but also past reality.

B. A female patient of mine had had very harsh treatment from her supervisors in the Orphan Home where she had lived during most of her childhood. When interpretations were made which she did not like she reacted to me as if I were the old enemy. But she used this device to rob my critical remarks of all validity. If I tried to show her that she had actually been very demanding and even obnoxiously competitive in her present dealings with her fellow workers, she merely interpreted the criticism as hostility and assumed a tearful or martyred demeanour. She would react in the same way if her requests were not granted, or if she were kept waiting even for two minutes. My behaviour was interpreted by her as dislike, and she was accustomed to being persecuted. So transference could be used as a means of denying the present reality and the actual unpleasantness of her own behaviour. She always hoped to find a saint-like father, and when I was pleasant, this meant that her wish had come true.

The transference is a magical situation wherein not only old thwarted aspirations are gratified, but also retrospective falsification denies that there ever was a painful situation.

Concluding Notes

Freud said, "The development of the ego consists in a departure from the primary narcissism and results in a vigorous attempt to recover it."

Psychoanalytic authors recognize the necessity for relaxation and the indulgence of phantasy and play. Ferenczi mentions the vicarious joy experienced by parents in reading fairy stories to children. Jekels and Bergler comment upon the deep psychic regressions which accompany love, including the return to the womb and the restoration of the dual-unity of mother and child. Zilboorg demonstrates the fallacy of a crassly materialistic interpretation of human behaviour. He indicates that in psychological "culturalism" there is concealed a return to animism in the projection of omnipotence on to "society." Helpless against the cosmos, man seeks refuge in one or another form of animism. Laforgue goes so far as to deny that religion is an illusion. He considers that there were three types of reality; magic, religion, and science, and that religion can no more justly be called an illusion than the science of yesterday. As a stage in development it had its validity as a theory of causality.

Lewin observes that some of his male patients with great castration anxiety equated reality with the female genital. "Reality" meant the absence of the penis, and "illusion" meant the illusory penis. He quotes a passage from the work of one philosopher which is surprisingly reminiscent of his own patient's association.

We cannot escape from some form of magical thinking; from the old desire for omnipotence, for renewal of something like the ideal situation when one need not work but merely wish to have one's desires gratified. I saw an example of this in an advertisement for a retirement plan. The reward for a life of thrift is pictured above the caption, "What is *so right* about this picture?" An elderly man sleeps peacefully and smilingly, his knees drawn up as in the foetal position. A sign, "Do not disturb," is above his bed. The alarm clock is silenced and swathed in ribbons, and the sixtyish wife looks on benignly from the door of the bedroom. It reminds one of Ferenczi's description of the baby's first sleep and his wish to return to the womb-like environment where effort is not necessary and the wish is sufficient.

Summary. This paper attempts to:

Review the development of the sense of reality, the clear recognition of the difference between the ego and the environment.

Give criteria for evaluating impairment in its development.

Describe the manner in which magical thinking persists in psychopathology, particularly in neurotic symptoms and psychoanalytic resistances.

Demonstrate that the sense of reality is a relative process and that some relaxation of reality testing is inevitable.

THE NEUROSES OF EVERYDAY LIVING

David C. Wilson, M.D.

Ecology is the name given to that branch of biology which deals with the relation of the organism to its environment. Medicine in the past has had the tendency to look on man as an animal and to carry over into the study of man those things learned from the study of other animals. Human physiology has been the most important subject studied in our medical schools and this science has been based to a large degree on the animal reactions of man. Man is undoubtedly an animal, but also an animal that has built up an artificial environment with which he has interacted for ages. Man's personality is to a large extent the product of this interaction. Therefore, the writer predicts that human ecology will soon have as important a place in medical teaching as physiology does today. The study presented here could be considered as an exercise in human ecology: the relation of man to his environment.

The dichotomy of mind and body has disturbed thinkers over the centuries. The concept of the personality as a whole was created to combat this dichotomy and to emphasize the unity of all human behavior. This idea of oneness has been carried along by the terms psychosomatic, which, in a paradoxical way, again emphasizes the dichotomy of mind and body because the word is so constructed that it intimates that psyche and soma are separate entities. Recently, investigators in the fields of psychology, sociology, and psychiatry have returned to the concept of the person as a whole as an object for study. They emphasize the unity of his behavior and emphasize that the dichotomies rest in the eye of the beholder. It is the difference points of view that make the difference between psyche and soma. The difference depends on the field of reference, not on any innate character of the human being himself.

If you wish to approach the subject from the point of view of physics you follow the laws of physics. If you wish to apply biochemical tests, you use biochemical formulas. When the study is made of the behavior of the person as a whole, you apply the laws of psychology. When you are considering this total behavior in the terms of the individual person, your study is psychological; but you use the laws of sociology when you study the actions of groups of individuals. At all times, it is important to remain in one's field of reference, so that confusion will not arise from applying laws which hold in one area to another where they do not necessarily apply.

The idea of the integration of the whole personality brings this out quite clearly. There is the subatomic level, the atomic, the molecular, the anatomical, then the biological, and finally, the total individual. Yet the individual is again a part, when we realize that he is part of a community and is influenced by pressures from without as well as from within. Each level of integration can be considered discretely, only if considered in a special field of reference, since each, while a whole from one point of view, is always a part of a greater whole. It is important in the study of the stomach to know what kind of a person it is in, just as it is important to know what kind of a community a person lives in to understand that person. In studying the stomach, we apply the laws of physiology; when we study the kind of person the stomach is in, we apply laws of psychology. If we study the influence of the community, we apply sociology when we approach from the community standpoint, but psychology, if from the standpoint of the individual. The person as a whole, therefore, while an individual unit, is under the influence of his parts and is at all times acting as a part in a larger whole.

The study reported here is of the behavior of the individual as a whole when he acts as a part of a group, or at least when he responds to the pressures of his culture. The field of reference is at all times that of the total individual. The effects of culture-pressure on the delinquent and on those definitely mentally ill have been reported frequently; but this study differs in that it attempts to show how exaggerations, which are considered normal, may cause distortions which have injurious effects on the normal individual. There seems to be a tendency of humans to exaggerate. If some of anything is good, then more is better, and so on, until the exaggeration becomes painful. These injurious exaggerations trap individuals to their hurt so that they act in a manner which is, for them, unreasonable. The writer has called this resulting irrational behavior the neurosis of everyday living.

The term, neurosis, is applied to behavior which is irrational to a sufficient degree to disturb the individual in his relations to other individuals and to behavior which the individual may recognize as irrational but of which he does not know the cause. A neurosis is distinguished from a psychosis by the fact that neurosis is irrational under a definite set of circumstances while a psychosis is behavior which is irrational under all circumstances.

The influence of the general culture on the individual is well known. The impact, on the individuals concerned, of specific pressures within the culture has usually been considered for its intrapsychic implications and not from the points of view of the general characteristics of the behavior of the person under the specific pressures. When a juvenile delinquent is studied, the effects of the impact of culture are presented in great detail as far as the structure of that delinquent's behavior is concerned. Also the effects of war, the crime movies and the comics on the same delinquents are frequently investigated, but there is very little consideration given to what cultural pressures, drives, obsessions are doing to normal everyday people who make up our world. The behavior of these people is more important than that of those who are definitely sick

THE NEUROSES OF EVERYDAY LIVING

We shall now consider the interaction of these everyday people to a few of the trends in American culture.

This year (1956) is especially outstanding because of the presidential election. One group of voters will be vying against another to win. Most of the voters of the country will consider themselves Democrats or Republicans. They will do as the party of their choice instructs them and they will feel the way they consider Republicans or Democrats should feel. They will become members of groups which control their lives and determine their destinies. The analysis of why a person joins one party and not another would lead far afield. Indeed, it would be necessary to study the details of each individual's life to determine the reasons for joining and being carried along in any particular mass movement.

There are many group activities similar to political party behavior which influence the lives of everyday Americans. Sometimes the group influence works out for the good of the individual involved and sometimes both the individual and the community are injured. Disturbances of health and happiness, which may lead to gross behavior disorders in both the individual and the group, often follow.

Sociologists and social psychologists have been studying the characteristics of groups and group activity. They have reached several conclusions regarding the nature of group behavior. According to Kreck and Crutchfield in *The Theory and Problems of Social Psychology,* a group does not mean a collection of individuals characterized by some similar property. Thus, for example, a collection of Republicans or farmers or Negroes, is not a group but a class of people. The term, group, refers to two or more people who bear an explicit psychological relationship to one another. A collection of Republicans working together to win an election becomes a group. A farmers' co-operative is a group. The various members exist for each other in some significant way. The criterion for recognizing a group is whether the behavior of other members in the supposed group has any direct influence on the behavior of the given individual and whether his behavior has direct effect on the other members. Such influence may be slight and vague. It is psychological, not material, but is definite enough to be recognizable.

A person, a community, a state or national organization, can act in a manner so distorted and so full of danger that the action must be considered diseased, even though no one seems aware of the diseased state. Football as a sport, for instance, has many values both for those who play and for those who watch; yet, of late, the game with all that goes with it has become a monster which menaces the integrity of our youth and distorts to an alarming degree the behavior of our colleges and universities. The behavior of some religious sects amounts to masochistic orgies when self-sacrifice and suffering are exaggerated to an extreme degree. Labor unions have done much for the working man, yet they, in turn, may evidence abnormal behavior which is a menace to the nation. It may be concluded, the writer believes, that, just as individuals behave at one time in a normal fashion and at another in an abnormal manner, so groups may evidence well-balanced behavior at one time, yet at another show most unusual and bizarre conduct.

To the individual caught up in such a mass movement, nothing seems to be wrong. This individual attitude of innocence makes it worth while to study the situation of the individual caught up in a group which has ceased to act in a normal manner. Mass behavior of any sort is composed of individual behavior of a similar nature, which is as badly diseased as the group action is diseased. If we observe this individual, however, he shows no signs of suffering. He is not thought to be abnormal by his fellows, or by those who are not caught up in the mass movement. He is not suspected of either neurosis or psychosis.

Individual neuroses and psychoses are forms of behavior which arise from within the person and are developed on an individual basis. While a person sick with a neurotic reaction may be a member of a group, and while his neurosis may lead him to aid in the group distortion, yet, at heart, he is antisocial since he wishes to control others by his own methods for his own ends. His reaction is one that cannot be shared with anyone else. He is a person who attempts to solve life's problems in his own individual way by his own techniques. These techniques are often exaggerated to such a degree that they irritate the group. The group shuns, excludes, ostracizes, and often attacks, this individual who dares too much individuality.

The actions of these individuals—of the person suffering from an individual neurosis and of the person taking part in a group distortion—have many similarities. First, in each, there is an exaggeration of a form of behavior beyond the limits of what, to the clear-thinking individual, seems warranted by the circumstances. In the individual neurotic, the pain or the paralysis cannot be explained by anatomical structure or by reasonable disease. In the group distortion, the best interests of the individual are obviously sacrificed beyond the demands of rational needs. Second, both forms of behavior injure interpersonal relations. In the long run, each tends to make more difficult the ability of people to live together. This trend may lead to infringement on the laws of the land, to the impoverishment of people, or to actual conflicts—within individuals, between individuals, or between groups of individuals. The first type of behavior, when the law is broken, is called criminal. The second, where people are impoverished materially or spiritually, is often disguised as public welfare or deficit spending. The third form of neurotic behavior, arising from conflict, may be made manifest in symptoms, such as headaches, on the individual level; as race or religious prejudice on the community level; and as war on the international level.

The similarity of individual neurotic behavior and neurotic behavior produced by group pressure is that the cause of the excess is not known to the performer of the action. The neurotic headache is said to come from a bad tooth, but the real cause is hatred of a mother-in-law. The prejudice against the Jew is said to be because the Jew has all the money in the world, while the real reason is the group's own insecurity—

and perhaps a need to escape from feelings of self-hate. The cause for war is often said to be for the sake of democracy, while the actual cause is the lack of self-confidence which produces fear, and the hate fear engenders.

Finally, causes for this exaggeration common to individuals and to groups of individuals may be understood by both the individual and the mass; yet neither the individual nor the group is able to modify the irritating behavior sufficiently to end the irritation. This fact represents a resistance to change resulting from the long period of training which produces the abnormal behavior, and from the many secondary gains which accumulate, as the creation of the reaction is effected. War offers a very good illustration of this situation. The causes of war are well understood: Everyone agrees that war as a technique for solving man's hostility to man is outmoded, yet we live under a constant threat of this form of group psychosis.

The neurosis of the individual caught up in a group exaggeration, and the neurosis which is entirely a result of the individual's own efforts to get along in life, have many differences as well as similarities. One of the outstanding differences is that the perpetrator of group action has no idea that he is sick, nor is he considered to be odd by anyone in his social setting. In fact, he may be looked upon as an example of correct behavior. He may win medals and be promoted by members of the group to places of leadership. The adoration of the group often calls for the senseless selection of such a hero for a position for which he is in no way qualified. Also, persons not entangled in the group distortion consider the behavior of individuals involved to be acceptable. What is more unreasonable than a mass of rabid individuals of late middle age rushing pell mell over the highways, where death lurks at every turn, just to be in on the "kick-off"? Few would consider these persons neurotic even when they sit out on concrete seats in a blizzard, while other men whom they hardly know and can scarcely see, run up and down a frozen field assaulting one another. The causes for this abnormal exaggeration of behavior are also behind the force that makes some college presidents perjure themselves for the sake of winning football teams. No one considers such a president's action proper, although it is condoned, while the actions of middle-aged alumni are not questioned. Indeed, the abnormalities of behavior of individuals carried along by groups are so common to everyday living that it is difficult to designate the point at which the disorder becomes a disease. This depends, the writer believes, not so much on the behavior of the group but on the significance of the behavior to the individual concerned. Therefore, this condition is not a neurosis of the group, but one of individuals, and our field of reference is still the person as a whole who acts as a part.

A definition that would cover the idea embraced in the discussion just given can now be developed. A neurosis of everyday living occurs when socially-accepted behavior is exaggerated to such a degree that it interferes in an injurious manner with interpersonal relations, and the performer is unaware of the actual cause for his behavior, or—if he becomes aware—is unable to modify the exaggeration. In contradistinction to a person with an individual neurosis, the persons showing the reaction do not consider themselves sick. They are not considered sick by the others in the group or by the bystanders who observe their behavior.

The attitude of a large number of individuals toward the game of football represents this form of neurosis. The behavior of many Americans at Christmas offers another example. "Keeping up with the Joneses" represents another exaggeration that disturbs comfortable living. The influence of labor unions and of big business on interpersonal relations is worthy of study. The mass hysteria on New Year's Eve is an example of a variation in the same disease. Deficit spending could be considered a neurosis of everyday living at the national level. This unreasonable behavior probably developed as an exaggeration because of the long training given to citizens of this country in buying on the installment plan. When the citizens of Virginia are referred to as Democrats, that is a classification. When they elect a candidate, that is normal group behavior. But when citizens as Democrats allow a self-perpetuating organization to control their destinies over a generation in spite of the fact that this organizations often acts contrary to their wishes, then they as individuals are suffering from a neurosis of everyday living. War represents the example of an international exaggeration of socially-accepted group hostility which is called nationalism. There are many such distortions which affect the lives of us all. Country club life may destroy some individuals. The idea fostered by many merchants that society demands a yearly crop of debutantes is a racket for some, and a neurosis for others. How can one expect to end the abnormal relations between the colored people and the white as long as many of our churches draw the color line? Understanding the causes and effects of such behavior does not help many individuals who are swept along in the group. They must be able to act on their knowledge. They must divorce themselves from the area of pressure.

Recently a middle-aged man came into the psychiatric clinic of the University of Virginia Hospital. He complained that his right arm was paralyzed. The arm hung in a limp fashion. Apparently he could not move it. Also, when the arm was examined further it was found to be anesthetic to pin prick. Sharp instruments could be driven through the skin while the patient sat smiling. He declared he could not feel any pain. All examinations of the arm failed to show any defect. The blood flow was normal, the nerve supply was normal. Reflex activity was normal. The man was cured rapidly. He left the clinic with a normal arm but he was not quite so happy. In the course of clinic work with him, it had developed that he hated his wife. She had demanded that he cut wood. His paralyzed arm had enabled him to frustrate her demands. He had unconsciously separated his arm from the rest of his personality so that no will power of his could make it move or feel. In the case of the individual this is known as a hysterical reaction. The arm is said to be blocked off, or excluded, from the rest of the person. The cause in this case was the hatred and fear of the wife and the determination to frustrate her wishes. There was perhaps, also, a dislike of wood chopping!

In 1865, a constitutional amendment made the colored man a citizen of the United States. The southern states were forced to ratify this amendment. There were many feelings of hatred and hostility toward their recent deadly enemies who now demanded that their former slaves be recognized as their political and social equals. The acceptance of the role demanded was too much, and a hysterical sort of blocking off, known as segregation, came into existence. By means of this reaction, the white citizen was able to exclude the colored man from his life. The colored man didn't exist. He was put in special places that could be ignored. He could not come out of these areas unless he assumed a role of servility or appeasement which might be called the "Uncle Tom" reaction.

Segregation became a fixed pattern of behavior, probably initiated because of the hostilities engendered by the War Between the States and by the stupidity of those in charge of the reconstruction period. The colored man of that day was illiterate and dependent. He was totally unprepared for citizenship or for a position of social equality. Segregation was a method of defense created by the white man to thwart a hated order and to help solve an intolerable situation. Segregation was accepted by the colored man as an escape from many situations that were embarrassing to him. The similarity of the hysterical blocking off of an arm and the excluding of colored people must be apparent to everyone. Segregation could be called a form of neurosis of everyday living. People of the south are caught up in this reaction and carried along regardless of their own reasons for acting the part assigned to them. Certainly they could not be called sick because they act out their roles. Yet by doing so, they are perpetuating a form of behavior which is contrary to the fundamental principles of our democracy.

Segregation is like individual neuroses in many ways. The debacle of 1861-1870 may have precipitated the disease, but its roots lie in the distant past. The reason for its present existence is found in outmoded ideas of one sort or another and to secondary gains that accrue to certain individuals, thus making it worth while to sustain the reaction. As in all other forms of group neurosis, each individual has his own reasons for joining the movement. In one case it is ignorance; in another, fear; in another, insecurity; and in another, a shrewd awareness that segregation reduces competition, thus making more jobs available to less efficient people. To others, segregation gives, or preserves, a false pride based on feelings of unwarranted superiority.

A certain amount of race prejudice can be considered normal; but when it develops to such a degree as is manifested toward the colored people in the United States, it interferes with interpersonal relations and so becomes a neurosis of everyday living. The treatment of this disorder can be attempted by individuals, but group therapy would be much more effective.

The best attack would be on the causes which are grounded in race prejudice. The emphasis should be on democracy and the assault on the false concept that the American is always a Protestant Anglo-Saxon. Although there are many kinds of people, there is only one type of citizen and that is a first-class citizen. In the army, race prejudice was often forgotten, because men worked together for a serious cause. Groups devoted to a cause would have no place for prejudice. The ability of persons to get along with each other depends to a large extent on their ability to identify. Their ability to relate depends on their ability to accept the qualities of one another. Their relatedness, therefore, depends on the possibility of their knowing each other as individuals, so that they can find acceptable qualities which will permit identification. It is impossible to identify with a stranger; but if that stranger has value in promoting a common cause, the strangeness disappears, and identification is possible. The church with its group activities, and the mental hygiene socities—since they must deal with minority groups—

are excellent organizations to undertake the therapy of this disorder.

There is another form of segregation existing in our midst. The reaction of the individual is similar to that just described. It is a blocking off similar to that seen in hysteria. The reaction the writer wishes to discuss is that of the person who considers himself normal toward all those who are labelled as having mental disease. We might call this "the great segregation."

As soon as the patient begins to show symptoms that are out of line, he begins to be excluded. This is true in the family when the existence of the mental distortion becomes a family disgrace to be hidden—a skeleton in the closet. In the community, this same reaction occurs, but it is most marked in a general hospital, especially if there is a psychiatric ward attached to it. As soon as any patient becomes disturbed on a general ward, he must be transferred to psychiatry forthwith. There is an attempt to exclude the psychiatric ward from the rest of the hospital and to consider the psychiatric staff as separate from the rest of the medical school. It has been only recently that medical schools have begun to consider mental illness as a type of human disease. The medical profession at large still does not consider the mentally sick as its responsibility. A patient came to the University of Virginia Hospital psychiatric service the other day because of back pain of 20 years' duration. She had had four operations on her back and three on her abdomen. The note on the chart by the referring doctor stated that he thought they should operate again, but that, if that didn't work, he was "afraid" they would have to call in a psychiatrist. This patient had presented a definite psychoneurotic reaction since childhood. The medical refusal to consider an evident neurosis is a variant of this blocking off reaction ("the great segregation"), where the disease is blocked off but not the patient. If the doctor accepted the disease as a neurosis, he would have to block off the patient lest he become contaminated because he treated such disorders. He would be afraid that he would "lose face" in the community.

The schizophrenic feels the community hostility, so weaves it into his fantasy. He takes advantage of the desire to isolate what is queer to get what he wants—isolation. Thus the ostracism of the mentally ill aids and abets the development of many psychotic reactions.

The reaction toward the mentally disordered has all the characteristics of a neurosis of everyday living. It is an attitude that upsets interpersonal relations in a tremendous fashion. It prevents the proper care of those thought to be sick and heightens the fear and prejudice of those who think themselves well. The person taking part in the segregation is often not aware that he suffers from an exaggeration; and, if he is aware, cannot modify his attitude. Finally, he is not considered abnormal by any of his group.

Not only do the persons caught up in this exaggeration exclude the mentally ill in "the great segregation," but their reaction is so great that they also exclude the hospitals for the mentally ill, their staffs and, frequently, the very existence of mental illness. We know now that people who are mentally ill can never be well until they have learned to get along in the community without the use of their illnesses. Therefore, a return to the community is as important to all of the mentally ill as it is to those maladjusted individuals called alcoholics. It is essential that we as psychiatrists, for the good of our patients, recognize and attack this neurosis of everyday living, the hysteroid exclusion of the problems connected with mental illness. We can apply to this larger field what has been learned in the handling of those whose common symptom is the inability to handle alcohol—the value of group therapy. The way to break down the individual attitude is to organize groups which understand and no longer fear the mentally ill. The community must go to the hospital, but groups in the community must also accept the mentally ill sufficiently to identify to such an extent that they cease to have prejudice, fear and a need to ostracize.

If we understand these reactions of everyday life, not as mass movements, but as examples of individual behavior in response to culture pressures, then the psychiatrist can remain in his field of reference which is that of treating the personality as a whole. Such an understanding will facilitate clear thinking and permit application to these "caught-up" individuals of those techniques used successfully in the treatment of other forms of distorted human behavior.

OCCUPATIONAL NEUROSES

A Study in Dependency Reaction

John W. Bick, Jr., M.D.

The incidence of demand for compensation for industrial accidents has grown as insurance coverage has been extended. With increasing awareness of psychiatry as a specialty, legal representatives of the injured often turn to us for assistance. Our help is especially sought in those cases where a disability is claimed but where no physical evidence of trauma exists. Being asked to retire from our traditional tasks as therapists and to assume a judicial role, is to many of us, a new and untried experience. Our task is sometimes made more difficult by the patient's attitude. He does not wish treatment. In fact, the sole purpose of the claimant usually is to sustain his illness. He frequently feels that submitting to therapy would be tantamount to admitting to malingering. As a result, he persists in his symptoms until the award or denial of a cash settlement.

Too often, when examining a patient seeking compensation for a neurosis allegedly precipitated by an industrial accident, the psychiatrist adheres to an exceptionally narrow view in the interpretation of the patient's presenting symptoms. For example, we still hear of the term "railroad spine" to describe back symptoms in a railroad worker. This often implies an occupational etiology and ignores his many domestic and emotional loads which are usually of far greater significance than his job. During the war we glibly spoke of combat fatigue even though maternal dependence or unresolved hostility were usually of greater importance than contact with the enemy. We carelessly affirm that patients suffer from a "lightening neurosis," an "irritable heart," "endocrine unbalance," all implying a simple etiology while ignoring the many complex factors that enter into the formulation of a personality disturbance.

Probably our desire for simplicity causes us to glibly use such terms as traumatic neuroses of industry, occupational personality disturbances or compensation neuroses. The use of such nomenclature carrying with it the implication of a single definite etiology is often puzzling and bewildering to judges, jurors and personnel directors who seek our guidance. Further, the persistent use of such diagnostic entities often focuses our attention upon a trivial injury, at the expense of the patient as a whole, his loves, his hates, his fears, his resentments and above all, his dependency needs.

This report is a brief summary of a group of sixteen patients who sustained minor industrial injuries. They were all examined months or years after injury, just prior to their appearance in court in an effort to secure financial compensation. Litigation was already in progress and the desire for a cash settlement was paramount. It is not our wish to go into various semantic and psychological discussions of such terms as traumatic neuroses and compensation neuroses but rather, we wish to briefly mention some of the conclusions drawn from this group of patients, their backgrounds, their motivations and their personality structures.

A review of the patients' developmental history, their school record, occupational adjustment, their social and marital status all reveal the presence of marked pre-traumatic psychopathology. We cannot agree with those writers who frequently stress that preexisting neurotic behavior is uncommon in these patients. In practically every instance each patient, as he entered the consultation room, showed considerable anxiety, marked hostility, aggressiveness, narcissism and above all a desire and need for dependency. I believe that narcissistic behavior in the post-accident neurotic patient is familiar to all of us. To quote from a recent article by Dr. Herbert Monheimer, "It gradually becomes apparent to us that he acts as though he is in love with his body, especially with the traumatized area and its adjacent parts. He looks at it lovingly, strokes it, squeezes it, fondles and caresses it even at times touches it to his lips with a kiss-like gesture, treating his own body in the same way as otherwise the body of a sexual object is treated." It is easy to see how important such an attitude can become in the formation of the presenting set of symptoms.

All our patients revealed some degree of anxiety. We take exception to those psychiatrists who after a brief examination attribute an accumulation of anxiety directly to the accident. It seems obvious that excessive narcissistic behavior, marked aggression, unusual dependency, all occur in individuals whose emotional functioning was already under great stress prior to the accident and occurred in individuals already well prepared to seize upon a minor trauma to bolster their weakening ego defenses.

Hostility, marked aggression toward the employer, the various physicians involved, the company representatives were encountered. In most instances the patient seemed to adopt an attitude of "you caused all this." It impresses the examiner as though a life-long accumulation of unspent hostility is directed toward the one he holds responsible for the accident. Suddenly there appears a channel for the relief of old aggressive impulses and dependency needs. In an unconscious fashion the patient finds in his injury and its sequelae the equivalent of mother love and father care. It is as though all of his mixed up feelings of love and hate suddenly come to the fore. At times he seems to be trying to verbalize "you have been a bad parent, but you will take care of me. That will make things right." One of our patients is now serving a life penitentiary term. When the court rendered an unfavorable verdict in his compensation suit he became panic-stricken. Unable to find any one individual in that vague entity which he called "the company" on whom to vent his wrath, he turned to the one toward whom all of his hostility could be expressed. He blamed his wife for all of his misfortune and following a minor argument shot her fatally through the chest.

Most interesting perhaps of all the features shown by these patients is the way in which they handled their dependency prior and subsequent to the accident. One middle-aged patient had functioned well in a Northern industrial center until his wife, who had been adopted in infancy, suddenly discovered her real parents. She grew dissatisfied and wanted to be near them. Our patient left his job, his chief source of security and satisfaction, his aged parents and migrated South. Numerous adjustment difficulties followed the discovery of his new in-laws which disturbed a prior adequate relationship with his wife and children. Being a passive husband with a controlling, hostile wife, afraid of expressing his dissatisfaction with his new environment, a minor back injury provided the stimulus necessary to bring his difficulties to the fore and to focus all his hate and hostility upon the construction company which employed him.

New job responsibilities often pose a threat to a long established dependency reaction pattern. One pile driver operator was apparently well adjusted in his work, performing so efficiently that he was brought into the office and given an assignment as an estimator. Back pains, nervousness and apprehension greeted his promotion. He was out of place with executive personnel, did not understand their conversations, their small talk, their hobbies and their interests. During the examination his conversation frequently turned to his pleasant moments on the driving rig and his happy days with the old gang. His symptoms cleared a few weeks later when he was returned to his former assignment.

The psychiatric expert is, at times, called upon to testify regarding the compensation angle in these cases. Frequently we are tempted to turn our attention toward the accident and its immediate results. Perhaps we too seldom realize that by so doing we are fixing a pattern of adaptation in neurotic directions which will become increasingly difficult for rehabilitation.

Possibly unaccustomed to the judicial role we forget that our principal task should always be the alleviation of suffering, not rewarding discomfort or regressive dependency tendencies with financial gain. More important, however, an early decision that a patient's symptoms are primarily the result of a trivial industrial mishap, a stumble, a bruise or a sprain, is usually an indication that traumatic events in the past history or that a long standing period of adjustment difficulties have all been lightly passed over in our examination. We are not aiding the patient, or our social structure, if we continue to reward neurotic behavior with ready financial gain. This fact should be brought home to all of us when we hear of the reluctance of some of our colleagues to administer electro-convulsive therapy to depressed patients for fear that a later neurotic disturbance may be attributed to a complication of this form of therapy.

What can we say of the pre-traumatic personalities of this group of patients? If we consult the writings which so well describe the pre-traumatic behavior of accident prone individuals we find similar features in the group seeking compensation. LeShan aptly describes their outstanding features. He emphasizes lack of warmth in their relationships with others, tension over their own health and over the state of their physiques and more important, a persistent attempt towards a higher social status which has failed in the past or is being undertaken with little hope of success. They also show aggression toward authority and finally, poor and erratic planning for the future. It is our contention that such factors are of far greater importance than any so called precipitating cause, namely the minor industrial accident.

It is unfortunate that we use the term precipitating cause so glibly in psychiatric reports. To the legal mind and to the juror it carries a connotation of greater significance than is intended. A case will illustrate.

A 42 year old white male had been orphaned at six, left school at nine, spent long periods of unhappiness in orphan homes and was discharged from the Army for inadaptability.

He held numerous jobs, leaving each because he always became nervous when he met people. One marriage ended in failure. Pursued by debts, by demands for alimony, his situation was momentarily solved one day when he stumbled, but did not fall, while working as a paper hanger's assistant. There was no injury but he claimed that his subsequent unsteadiness caused such anxiety that he was unable to resume his former occupation; hence he claimed that he was entitled to compensation for total and permanent disability. It seems obvious that in the evaluation of such a case, the lifelong picture of adjustment difficulty is of more significance than the alleged precipitating cause.

The following case, while not in the group of patients who sustained industrial injuries, illustrates several points of interest.

A 40 year old physician on military service in World War II provides an example of how a trivial injury with a resultant disability award can, by satisfying dependency needs, sabotage needed psychotherapy and make impossible a more healthy adjustment to a series of difficult circumstances. This officer had been having difficulty with his wife, a demanding, aggressive and dominating individual. He entered upon an extramarital relationship with a female army associate, became guilt-ridden and depressed. While on maneuvers he slipped and sprained his right wrist. There was no evidence of physical injury but long periods of hospitalization, consultations and observations, the entertaining of such diagnoses as causalgios, reflex dystrophies and the like, eventually ended in the diagnosis of hysteria with resultant retirement. For ten years this physician, previously accustomed to an income of $25,000 per year, has been content to subsist on one-tenth that amount because it allows him to be taken care of, and to deal with a hostile wife on the only basis that he has found, namely by assuming the attitude of a sick, hurt child and by being cared for as such.

The educational records of these patients, excluding the physician just mentioned, are interesting. Four completed the third grade, one the fourth, two the sixth, four the seventh, two the eighth and three completed the tenth. None completed high school. Five of the sixteen could be classified as mental defectives but it is felt that other factors interrupted the education of the remaining eleven, chiefly aggression and hostility which caused difficulties at school.

What criteria should we use in deciding whether neurotic symptoms that occur after an accident are deserving of financial compensation? Certainly, many factors must be considered. Often the psychiatric examiner is placed in the position of having to give an exact answer—a yes or no response to the question posed by the court, namely, are these symptoms due to the accident? From our experience it is felt that the psychiatrist should be a broad observer, an advisor of the court, who gives interpretations and suggestions rather than infallible answers. Our first motive should be to get the patient in therapy, to point out the undesirability of the gains which monetary compensation offers as contrasted with the advantages of genuine therapy and rehabilitation.

We feel that compensation for psychiatric disability should be limited to those patients who have suffered from a genuine and severe threat or trauma. We feel, too, that we should avoid being a party to the award of financial compensation to those with trivial symptoms or who have experienced only a minor accident. The complaints noted in this group suggest symptoms of mild anxiety and tension, chiefly insomnia, fears, tension, profuse perspiration and the like, plus various pains and discomforts. With few exceptions these symptoms were not disabling and were little different from those commonly experienced by patients on their first visits to doctors.

We should also avoid encouraging the patient's neurotic hostility toward his employer or his representative, whom he usually feels bears the responsibility for his injury and for his resulting symptoms. I have often found that the patient's attitude towards his symptoms is a valuable criterion for our decisions. I asked all the patients in this series if they would consider psychotherapy to alleviate their symptoms. Every one refused. Their attitude can be summarized in the response of one patient. "The company is responsible for this; they should pay through the nose. And they should pay me, not another insurance doctor."

Too often, this desire for financial gain, a fully conscious wish seems to be the outstanding content of thought presented in the post accident patient engaged in litigation. This has led Dr. Gordon Kamman* to suggest the term "Attitudinal Pathosis," rather than "Post-traumatic Neurosis" for this group. This was first suggested by F. C. Thorne in 1949. According to these writers, such patients often have a nuclear core attitude which can be summed up by, "I have been injured and cannot work." This reasoning can be carried farther with the thought, "My employers carry compensation insurance and I have been injured. Therefore, I am entitled to compensation." Possibly, this concept can be of assistance in evaluating these patients. The conscious desire and need for financial gain does not prove that a patient is suffering from a "compensable neurosis."

Some may object to a concept of attitudinal pathosis which emphasizes the conscious desire for remuneration. Should we wish to adhere to the concept that such patients are suffering from a neurosis, I am sure we all agree that the neurosis has been of long standing and that more personal factors than a trivial injury are usually responsible. Are we not being naive in our knowledge of psychopathology when we say that a sprained ankle caused a neurosis and ignore an orphaned childhood, an inadequate school and vocational adjustment, marital failure, divorce, sexual impotence, to mention a few factors found in one case?

It seems obvious that there is an alarming tendency for individuals to seek financial gain because of an alleged neurosis resulting from industrial accidents. It is questionable whether the trivial accident may be considered as causative in the presence of conscious attitude, frankly demanding secondary gain or in the presence of a life replete with neurotic traits. Perhaps our legal associates need education at our hands. By encouraging such suits, attorneys often harm their clients' adjustments.

* Archives of Neurology and Psychiatry, Vol. 65; pp. 593-603, 1951.

INSTINCT OF SELF-PRESERVATION AND NEUROSIS

Siegfried Fischer, M.D.

The terms love, affection, self-esteem, rejection, self-consciousness and insecurity occur frequently in books and articles on dynamic psychology and abnormal psychology, and often in psychoanalytic literature. It is proposed here to investigate the underlying principle of the dynamics connected with these concepts and their significance in neuroses.

One may choose as an example a relatively simple case of a neurosis.

Case 1

A man now 50 years old, came to this country about 12 years ago. He worked first as a stock clerk. As he wanted to become independent, he took a course in sign painting, a trade which he liked and for which he was qualified by natural aptitude, as well as through some training in art which he had had when he was younger.

As soon as he began to work as an independent sign painter, he suffered from nightmares almost every night. He would wake up in great fear, his heart pounding, and only after an hour or two was able to fall asleep again.

He also complained that he was constantly afraid of delivering signs to his customers, because he feared they would tell him the signs were not satisfactory or, even more important, would say there were better sign painters. Although he wanted to increase his business, he was afraid to ask a prospective customer for work for fear of being rejected. When he finally gathered courage to interview a new prospect, he was immediately discouraged if he was told that the proprietor was too busy to see him, or something similar. His fears became so great that, as he said, he sometimes played with the idea of "jumping off the bridge."

The history of the patient in brief was as follows. He was the second of five children. His oldest sibling was a sister. He had two younger sisters and a younger brother, Harry, who was born when the patient was six years old. In the second interview, the patient mentioned his distinct memory that, "When Harry was born I was pushed aside. Harry was the apple of my mother's eye and was favored by the whole family. Everybody bragged about him, how handsome he was and how intelligent. Nobody paid attention to me. Even my father made me feel that I was not as intelligent nor as good-looking as my brother."

After he finished high school, he went to an art school for about a year. He then entered his father's store. At that time he already suffered from the symptoms described. He was afraid that his father or his customers would blame him for being inefficient, and, therefore, he lived in almost constant fear.

It is obvious that this patient's present suffering was caused by his childhood experiences. Let us first look at the fear from which he suffers today. According to his description, the fear was often unbearable. Sometimes it was so strong that suicide seemed to be the only way out. What was this man afraid of? Anticipation of rejection by his customers, or of being told that another man was better than he, gave him, in his own words, "the feeling of being worthless." And the feeling of being worthless is unbearable; it can be so strong that death appears to be a deliverance. Our patient, therefore, anticipated an impending unbearable danger when he foresaw that he might feel worthless.

Going back to the origin of his neurosis, we know that he was "pushed aside" by his family, and particularly by his mother, from the time he was six years old, when his younger brother was born, through the years of his later childhood and adolescence. His family made him feel that he was no good and, particularly, that he was not so good as his brother. He felt he was not accepted by his parents, as was his brother.

One can see that as a child the patient evaluated his own

worth according to the way he was treated by his parents. The writer has pointed out in other reports, that *the child has no other measure of his own value but recognition*. In other words, independent of the actual value of the child, whether he is handsome or ugly, intelligent or stupid, healthy or crippled, he *feels* about his own value *only* according to the amount of recognition (time, affection and love) given by his parents. To mention only one example: Crippled children who usually get much attention and time from their parents, *feel* valuable despite their *knowledge* of physical inferiority

What is termed *recognition* here is only what the child accepts as such. Recognition is, first of all, the amount of time we spend with the child; second, it is the interest we show the child during this time by doing something with him which he enjoys; third, it is encouragement; fourth, it is the verbal approval the child receives; fifth, but not least, it is the affection we give the child.

In the writer's opinion, knowledge of the fact that the child has no measure of his own value other than recognition is a basic prerequisite for the understanding of children, as well as for the understanding of many neurotic patients. If a child does not receive the time, interest, attention and affection he needs, he does not have the feeling that he is worth while. Worse, he feels worthless. And the feeling of being worthless is unbearable. Therefore, the child has to blind himself to the feeling, otherwise he cannot go on living.

From Case 1, we also learn that the feeling of being worthless, which is created in childhood, is carried over to adulthood When this occurs, a neurosis exists. The adult patient, despite knowing better, is not able to fight the feeling of being worthless, and he must adjust his whole life to this fact. The feeling of being worthless deprives the subjects of any self-confidence or self-assurance, and, as a consequence, of any real security Feeling secure is *the* prerequisite of everything else in life. This is true of both human beings and animals, mature and im

INSTINCT OF SELF-PRESERVATION AND NEUROSIS

mature. If a person or animal feels insecure, all other interests, and even other drives, disappear; if the feeling of helplessness or insecurity is strong enough, even the sex drive may vanish.

It seems necessary to clarify what is meant by the terms: feeling of security and insecurity. The person who is really adult feels insecure or helpless only when he is confronted with an actual danger to his life from which it is impossible to defend himself.* Just the opposite is true of many neurotic persons and of children; their feelings of security or insecurity are *not* based on any actual dangers existing in the external world. A very good example is the statement of a war correspondent who suffered from a neurotic feeling of insecurity. Once during World War II when he was under terrific bombardment, he looked at the tense faces of some officers and said smilingly to himself, "If they only knew what it is to try to cross Market Street in San Francisco." We can understand these feelings better when we think of the emotional reactions of children: A child walks with his mother in a crowded street and suddenly finds himself without her. The child becomes panic-stricken in a situation where no actual danger exists. On the other hand, his mother may take him in her arms and leap from the twentieth floor of a building in order to escape a fire, yet the child feels safe because he is in the arms of his mother. In the first instance, although there is no actual danger, the child is panic-stricken. In the second, the greatest danger exists, but the child is unafraid.

It is obvious that the child derives his feeling of being secure from the outside world through his parents or their substitutes. When the child feels that he is unprotected, whether an actual danger exists or not, he feels insecure. He derives his feeling of security from the same source from which he derives his feeling of being worth while. The same is true of many neurotic individuals. They too derive their feelings of being secure, as well

---

* It should however be remembered that the psyche of the adult contains protective devices which prevent excessively traumatic effects following emotional blows.

as of being worth while, from other people, not from themselves as the mature adult does.

There are different degrees of the feeling of inadequacy, of inferiority or of being worthless. The basic quality, however, is always the same. Every child feels inadequate and consequently insecure when he believes he is not recognized or is not sufficiently recognized. The same is true of the neurotic adult who has carried over to his adulthood the open wound of the feeling of being of no value or of being worthless. *Each of these persons is afraid of being hurt again on the wound that was inflicted on him in childhood and that has never healed.* Therefore, he is careful and is alert for any possible danger, like a man with an open wound who tries to protect his injury from further harm. He watches so that it shall not even be touched again. In all these cases, the individual has the fear of becoming aware of being worthless or of thinking that other people might find him worthless (projection).

Whereas the child is helplessly exposed to such feelings, unless he makes himself blind to them and escapes in daydreams, the adult is not supposed to be dependent on the recognition of other people for a sense of his own value. *The diametric contrast between a child and an adult in this respect lies in the fact that recognition is vital, essential for the very life of the child. For the truly adult person, however, recognition, while pleasant and comfortable, is never essential to his life.* Recognition may be pleasant but it can never change the feeling of the real adult about his own value. This feeling lies within himself. He has the feeling of being valuable when he fulfills his duty to the best of his abilities; and the opinion of others cannot change his feeling, unless he accepts a criticism as justified. Only neurotic people—who have not reached this adult stage because they were hurt in childhood—react like children to rejection (and more often to anticipated rejection) with fear and anxiety, and to recognition, approval and acceptance with relaxation. Recognition and acceptance not only cause a pleasant feeling in neurotics, but result in a feeling of safety and security as if, for the time being, they can go on living.

As a consequence in such cases of neuroses, we deal with a power that is much greater than any other drive, including the sex drive: namely, the drive for self-preservation.

Insecurity and helplessness, of course, may arise from other causes, but this discussion is limited intentionally only to the feeling of insecurity that results from the feeling of being not valuable.

Realizing that we are dealing here with the fear of annihilation, or on the other side of the coin, with the drive for self-preservation, it becomes evident why some people with such a background are shy, why they retreat and become self-conscious. It is also obvious why other persons develop such tremendous reactions as rebellion against everything and everybody, why they have a lust for power or are greedy for money.

The importance of this concept for the understanding and the treatment of some neurotics is exemplified in the short description of the following two cases, a compulsion neurosis in a woman and a case of exhibitionism in a man.

Case 2

An unmarried woman, 24 years old, had the following complaints: She felt compelled to wash her genital organs and anus for hours until she felt clean. Similarly, she was impelled to wash her hands frequently. She was panic-stricken when she was near any bottle that might contain alcohol because she feared she might drink the contents, become drunk and forget what she was doing. She was also in terror of contact with any bottle that contained acid or a caustic fluid for fear she would get it on her face and be hurt and disfigured. In such instances, she had to assure herself over and over again that nothing had happened to her. Her greatest fear was of losing control of her bowels and bladder, because if that happened she would be soiled and could never again feel that she was actually clean.

Both the patient's parents were of Italian descent. Her father showed no interest in her; he never had time for her and never was affectionate. She could not remember that he had ever kissed her. He frequently told his wife not to play with the children because that would spoil them. Her mother was always busy with the household and her many children. She was strict and the patient often heard her saying, "If you ever have anything to do with a man before you are married, you can never come home again."

From the age of 10 to 12 years, the patient frequently indulged in childish sex play with her brother, who was two years younger than she. Because this was, she said, the only pleasure in her very unhappy childhood, she continued the sex play, even though she felt extremely guilty about it. Although she realized that her parents knew nothing about these acts, the patient felt that she was neglected because of her bad behavior with her brother. At the age of 18, she kissed a young man, pressed her body against his and, although fully clothed, experienced a clitoral orgasm. From that day on, she felt extremely worthless because she believed she had gone against her mother's injunction and done the worst thing possible. Yet, at that time and through all the following years, she always had the hope that there might be a slight chance to gain the love and affection she had missed during her whole life. She believed this would be possible if she could be entirely clean and if she could keep her appearance from being spoiled by an irreparable physical injury. In other words, she hoped that if nothing else were added to make her *completely* worthless, she might still have a slight chance.

A few days after the experience just described, the patient began to have compulsive symptoms which developed more and more as time went on. She could not keep from cleansing her sexual organs, anal area and hands. She had to wash herself for hours. When she saw a car going by her window she was panic-stricken for fear it might injure her head and spoil her appearance so that she would no longer be acceptable. She was afraid of the electric light, of hairpins and, as mentioned before, of liquor. It became necessary for her to "check," over and over again to see that there was nothing near which could cause her injury.

The patient was first treated with electric shock by a private psychiatrist. When she showed further deterioration, he sent her to a hospital. She remained in the hospital for about 18 months, but became steadily worse, particularly after the following incident. She liked the doctor who treated her, except

INSTINCT OF SELF-PRESERVATION AND NEUROSIS

that "he never talked." One day she felt that it would help her in her distress if the doctor would show interest, in other words, if he would show that he accepted her. During an interview, she got up from her chair and put her arm around the doctor, wishing to be embraced by him, but the doctor did not move. The patient's immediate reaction was that, obviously, he did not accept her. The apparent rejection increased her feeling of being worthless. About the same time, she received a further blow which resulted in a tremendous handicap in later treatment. She was told that the staff of the clinic considered performing a lobotomy, an operation which, to her, indicated that she would become worthless beyond repair. The idea of being forced to undergo such treatment haunted her for months. When she finally came to the author for treatment, she was in a desperate state and was so worn that she looked 15 years older than her actual age.

The patient was treated according to the following underlying principle. It was realized that she felt almost entirely worthless and lost because of a lack of recognition and acceptance throughout her entire childhood and adolescence. This feeling referred to her whole personality, as well as to her appearance. It had come to a climax after she had committed the act of embracing the young man, which, according to her mother's teaching, was unforgivable. In spite of her guilt, she still believed that she might lose this unbearable feeling, that she might be acceptable and accepted if she did not become more unworthy because of uncleanliness, physical or spiritual, or through an irreparable physical injury or disfiguration. To her, such events would have implied that she had reached complete worthlessness. In this case, she would have been entirely lost, or in her own words, "unable to go on living," without any hope. The patient, therefore, was striving to avoid the feeling of complete worthlessness or complete annihilation; she was fighting for her life.

In time, this patient lost almost all symptoms. She also found a young man who gave her much of the love and attention she needed. After she was practically cured, he married her, and, as far as it is known now, she is happily married. Whether her husband's love will continue to compensate for the lack of previous recognition, particularly for neglect in her childhood, is not known. Even if it does, the neurosis has not been entirely cured, since a husband's love certainly should not be needed to satisfy the childish wish for feeling valuable.

Although sex factors were involved in this case, they were not basic for the understanding of the patient's problems and were not important in her treatment. The dynamics became entirely comprehensible to the patient when she realized that her symptoms resulted from her feeling of worthlessness or, in the last analysis, from the drive for self-preservation. The more the patient realized the effect of the injuries she had experienced in her childhood, and the more she felt that her worth today did not depend on the estimation of her mother, or on external sources, the more her condition improved.

Case 3

This patient, a 29-year-old happily married man, suffered from a tremendous urge to expose his genital organs to women, especially young girls. His pleasure was considerably increased if he masturbated at the same time. He imagined that he was providing a performance no woman had ever seen before. If the woman saw him and perhaps smiled or giggled, the climax of his ecstasy was reached, since he interpreted her laughing as approval and confirmation of the fact that he had shown her something out of the ordinary. As long as possible, he avoided an orgasm. Often, however, he continued exhibiting his genital organs after having had an orgasm. In explanation he stated that, "When I don't have any sex desire, I still have the tendency to exhibit, for instance, after I have had an orgasm. The sex desire only increases my desire to exhibit."

The patient had visited foreign countries while serving in the merchant marine, but had no urge to exhibit himself during this time. He remarked spontaneously that he felt so superior, because he was an American citizen, that the thought of exhibiting never occurred to him.

He daydreamed frequently of masturbating in front of a group of elegant and exquisite women who admired him for giving them a wonderful performance such as they, even though

INSTINCT OF SELF-PRESERVATION AND NEUROSIS

they were rich and had seen everything, had never encountered before.

The patient also suffered from another symptom which dated back much further than his tendency to exhibitionism. As long as he could remember, he had always been oversensitive to any slighting remark, particularly those referring to his physical strength. Whenever such remarks were made, he flew into a rage. Any comment, no matter how far-fetched, which could be interpreted as derogatory or humiliating caused the strongest resentment. He then indulged in daydreams and imagined that he attacked and hit his detractor. When he felt that his employer "looked down" upon him, he imagined setting the store in which he worked on fire. His favorite daydream, which, with some variations, he had imagined since childhood, was that of breaking out of prison after having attacked the judge who sentenced him and the policeman who took him there.

He always tried to impress people by showing off when he swam or ice skated. Several times, he applied for a job as truck driver, a job which was for him, the symbol of strength.

A short time ago a dramatic change occurred in the patient's neurosis. He was promoted at work. Since then, he has not once thought of exhibiting his sexual organs, even when the opportunity was offered; he has not indulged in his usual daydreams of revenge. Also, his outlook on life has changed entirely. The members of his family and the people with whom he works have remarked frequently that he has changed since his promotion and that he has lost his irritability and grouchiness. He himself was surprised at the complete loss of any desire for exhibitionism.

In brief, his history was as follows: His brother, who was four years younger than he, was always his "mother's boy," "the good boy," and the favored child. In contrast, the patient was always blamed by his parents, particularly by his mother. He was even blamed for the mischievous actions of his brother—because he had not watched him. His mother was never affectionate with him. The patient did not have much respect for his father. He grew up resenting his father because he could not protect him, as the father was, in the eyes of the patient, weak himself. At the age of 10, the boy's greatest wish was to grow up so that he could be independent of his parents. He was not interested in his schoolwork, fought against his teachers and did not care whether he was punished or not.

When he was 13 years old, his feeling of inadequacy was increased when another boy, on the occasion of mutual masturbation, said, "When are you going to grow up?" meaning that the patient's penis was not large. Shortly after this incident, he developed the impulse to exhibit his genital organs.

The sexual part of this patient's neurosis was only one branch of the whole neurosis. It is obvious that the *sexual* pleasure he derived from exhibitionism was of secondary importance. The important factor for this man was the need to be recognized, approved of, admired as valuable, primarily physically, but also in other respects. He had two ways of counteracting his feeling of being inferior; to imagine that he was admired, and to daydream of revenge and destruction. The latter was his way of saying, "If you don't accept me as I am, then I will be bad and tough, and outstanding as such."

For almost his entire life, this patient has fought to attain the *feeling* that he is good, as good as others. That is the main goal of his life. Because he had to battle over and over for this feeling, there was little energy left for the fulfillment of his daily duties.

When he was promoted at work, he found, for the first time in his life, recognition in reality. This gave him the feeling of being worth while. All his tendencies to gain recognition in childish and neurotic ways, in his imagination and through self-deception (including exhibitionism), stopped automatically when reality gave him what he had craved his whole life. This certainly is not a cure, but it provides evidence of where the patient's real conflict lies.

In this case again, it is apparent that it was not the conflict with the sex drive that made this man unhappy, but his striving for self-esteem and self-preservation, a striving which was necessary because the feeling of being inadequate was intolerable.

This frustration originated in childhood when his mother did not give him a feeling that he met with approval or was as good as his brother. It was increased when other boys humiliated him for having a small penis. He carried this feeling of not being equal over to his manhood. The feeling of not being good enough, or worthless, was deeply integrated with the feeling of being insecure.

The feeling of insecurity may have other causes than those described here. But whatever the cause may be, its root is always the lack of satisfaction of the most powerful drive, the drive for self-preservation.

We now understand why a child needs recognition, love and affection and what it means to a neurotic individual to feel worthless and insecure. Love and affection are not only pleasant for the child, they are essential for his very life. And neurotics who feel worthless do not strive for pleasure but for something vital, for being able to go on living.

The Oedipus complex now appears in a different light. The desire of a son for his mother is not necessarily primarily sexual; it may not be sexual at all. The son needs his mother, first of all, in order to feel secure and valuable. The same is true of many neurotic patients. Such neurotic men want to have their mothers, so that they may feel safe and valuable through their mothers' protection, love or approval. It is true that in some cases a neurotic person wants to have sex relations with his mother. The deeper analysis, however, shows that it is not primarily the gratification of a sex desire that these neurotics anticipate, but the feeling of being accepted entirely. Sexual intercourse of the son with the mother would be the extreme proof that the mother loved him and that would make him feel secure and valuable. In such cases a fusion of two instinctive drives exists.

Summary

It is the goal of every uncovering method in psychotherapy to make the symptoms of a neurosis comprehensible through uncovering that of which the patient is unaware, which in most cases consists of childhood experiences. In three cases it was demonstrated that the symptoms became completely comprehensible by uncovering the feeling of being worthless and insecure, which was created in childhood by the patients' parents. All three patients felt worthless because they did not get the recognition they needed from their parents.

The child—in diametric contrast to the mature adult—has no measure of his own value, other than recognition. Recognition is *essential for the life* of a child, whereas it is pleasant, but never vital, for the mature person.

On the basis of these observations, the Oedipus complex appears more of a tendency to gain security from one's mother than to satisfy a sexual desire.

It is also shown here that therapeutic effects can be accomplished by applying this theory without emphasizing sexual problems; that is, by making the neurosis comprehensible through comprehension of the power of the instinctive drive for self-preservation. It is true that, in at least two of the three cases described, strong sexual problems were involved. The proportion might even be greater in a greater number of cases. We have to assume, therefore, that in such cases a fusion of two instinctive drives exists. At the present time it is not entirely clear why this fusion exists, and what the relationship is between these two drives in neurotic individuals. For purely practical purposes, however, it seems possible to base the treatment of such patients exclusively on the theory of the instinct of self-preservation and to deal with the sex problem as of secondary importance.

FACTORS INVOLVED IN THE GENESIS AND RESOLUTION OF NEUROTIC DETACHMENT

Montague Ullman, M.D.

Although the term "detachment" is in fairly common use, both descriptively and dynamically, its precise implications still elude a complete understanding. It is the object of this paper to attempt a close scrutiny of this particular defensive reaction in a patient who presents many of the typical problems encountered.

Many terms are used in conjunction with and in close relation to detachment. A detached person is said to rely heavily on the mechanism of withdrawal from reality. Depending on the person and the situation, he may be regarded as distant, aloof, untouched, preoccupied, removed, or remote. When there is a greater affective coloring, his detachment may lurk under the guise of arrogance, cynicism, superiority, or snobbishness. Autism and dissociation are other terms that are related to the problem. As considered here, detachment is a way of reacting to one's environment, based on the illusion that it is both possible and necessary to disregard the real needs of people and to exist in a state of isolated independence. Fundamentally, it is an attitude toward the self, projected onto others, of extraordinary disregard and unconcernedness. This definition can be made more specific by a comparison of detachment with other neurotic devices. Any neurotic trend implies a "detaching process." Through the particular trend, the individual detaches himself, or attempts to detach hmself, from what at the inception of the trend must have been a painful area of experience. In the case of neurotic trends other than detachment, however, there is an attempt to restore the equilibrium and compensate for the experiential handicaps by the use and misuse, manipulation and accentuation of real ways of influencing people. People retain their value, and it is still necessary to do things in relation to them. For the mechanism of detachment to come into being, the area of experiential injury must be so great that people are experienced as valueless, and for it to remain in existence, people must continue to be experienced as valueless. It is at great cost to the potential of the human being that this leap is made from the solid ground of human contact to the rarefied atmosphere of splendid (sometimes) but precarious (always) isolation. Once this leap is achieved, the road back entails all the difficulties of any other neurotic trend, in addition to the specific problems involved in countering the conditioned shrinkage from meaningful contact which these patients automatically experience. Having placed themselves beyond the pale, people are willing to pay any price but one, that of psychosis. Unchecked, the end-result of detachment is psychosis, and it is the fear of "insanity" which, when real and intense enough, creates for the first time for these patients an alternative which heretofore did not exist, namely, that of getting well.

As just stated, any neurotic development includes a "detaching process" in the sense of an alteration in the appropriateness and directness of the reaction elicited by the situation. But in these individuals the detaching process is a means to an end, the end being to reach people. In neuroses where the detachment is a significant feature, the detaching process is not only the means, but—evolving out of its function, which is to delay or ward off appropriate contact—becomes the end in itself. The demands for contact are so great in the genesis of human development that almost all of the creative potential has to be invested in the establishment of a character structure which can carry the burden of endlessly maintaining the fiction of isolation. Detachment is in essence a controlled experiment in mental derangement, and so dangerous that the focus remain only upon the experiment. At some point, either the test tube breaks, or one manages to divert some attention to the experimenter. Unfortunately, by the time these situations are ferreted out, the experimenter has become little more than an automatic vehicle attempting to breathe a semblance of human aspect into the façade he has created.

Detachment, then, involves a profound alteration in the perceptive processes, resulting in the substitution for "reality as it is" of a "reality which can be ignored." It results from facing serious deprivation, and once initiated, occasions serious deprivation. Threats to the maintenance of the detachment become the only serious reality; and since the detachment is so invincible a weapon, immediate realities succumb before it and, in so doing, strengthen the defensive structure.

What happens characterologically to these people when the injury is severe enough to result in detachment is still not clear. Although applicable in a meaningful way, the concepts centering around narcissism and the failure of libidinal cathexis serve more of a descriptive than an explanatory function, and seem too generalized for dealing with a condition which can be understood only when broken down, not only into complicated genetic factors, but also into operational techniques whereby it is maintained and propagated. Horney's evaluation of detachment, while stressing the resultant handicap and the compulsivity involved, does not sufficiently assess the unique qualities of this defensive maneuver, namely, the inexorable way in which the positive aspects of the personality are overshadowed, and the bearing this has on therapy—in short, the all-pervasive effect, the powerful, serious, and uncompromising break in the relatedness of the individual to his surroundings which is quantitatively, and eventually qualitatively, different than in the case of the other neurotic trends. The consideration given to the problem in this paper incorporates more of the serious implications of the Freudian views, namely, the earliness and severity of the causative trauma, with an outlook which is not so pessimistic as implied by Freud, nor so accessible and so manipulable as implied by Horney.

Essential to the understanding of defense by detachment, is the realization that neurotically detached patients have been subjected to environments where their treatment and recognition would have been far more appropriate had they been *objects* rather than *developing human beings*. The child encounters rigidity in the human environment to the point where his relatedness is contingent upon automatic conformity. The parental influence, appropriate for an imaginary "animate object," is totally inappropriate for the needs of the child. When the pressure for conformity is so great that the possibilities for genuine spontaneity are wholly lacking, there is an effort on the part of the child to adjust at the level of being an automaton or, in effect, a human object. Since this is impossible, he can only reach his goal by a process of simulation, based on his ability to disguise, ignore, or restrain all impulses that would be incongruous with this goal. Detachment, then, is the general term encompassing those characterologic changes designed to establish and maintain the profound degree of self-alienation necessary to make this type of adjustment.

Detached patients fall into two main, although not sharply defined, categories, depending upon the severity of the syndrome. In the first group the child is hit tangentially by the neurotic conflicts in the home. Although he may be exposed to them in the most devastating fashion, his own existence is not significant to the operation of the neurotic drives of either or both parents. He is the innocent bystander who gets hurt. He is hurt, but not crushed completely. When the situation in the home approximates the conditions outlined here, the hurt results in detachment, but the injury, since it is partial, does not preclude some area of activity capable of yielding gratification. We see in these patients the severe handicap of detachment side by side with the potentiality for growth and an almost indestructible optimism. The patient to be presented here typifies this group.

In the second group, the child not only experiences the impact of the neurotic conflicts in the home, but actually bears the brunt of the disorder. His existence forms the focal point of a destructive, neurotic fixation on the part of one or both parents. In the face of unrelenting pressure of this type, character development can take place only in defensive patterns. The total creative drive of the personality is spent in the service of maintaining the one mechanism *par excellence* capable of meeting this type of threat, namely, detachment. Any tampering with the detachment results in paranoid hostility and suspicion. Owing to the limited scope of this paper, this latter type of development—seen in psychotics and borderline psychotics—will not be illustrated by case material.

Case Presentation

Analysis in Progress 16 Months

The patient is a 30-year-old man who came to analysis in the midst of the following life situation:

He is an artist of a modern school whose work had achieved considerable recognition during the previous five years. About a year prior to coming to analysis, his first marriage had broken up, and the ensuing months had been characterized by feelings of despair, confusion, and frustration. Anxiety had become intense, and the patient had sought some relief through alcohol. Involved as he was, not only in painting and exhibiting, but also in writing, editing, and lecturing, he was forced, with great reluctance on his part, to participate in a round of social activities and parties which had come in the wake of his recent successes. He was beset with almost unbearable feelings of awkwardness and self-consciousness in these situations, as well as in his ordinary dealings with people. He began to feel more and more harassed and was finally incapacitated by a prolonged bout of chest infections. At the time of his first visit to the analyst, he had begun to recuperate a bit from a morass of physical and mental debility, though he still had considerable anxiety. He was concerned about his drinking and frightened lest the old feelings of confusion and panic return.

The patient's father had been an eminently successful business man. The patient recalls his childhood as characterized by a profound sense of isolation and the feeling that he simply did not belong. Both parents were concerned with possessions to the point where their protective attitudes seemed to operate more spontaneously in relation to possessions than in relation to the needs of their child. Orderliness, neatness, cleanliness, and conformity seemed to comprise exclusively all that was virtuous. The father's drive for power and prestige in the business world was matched by the mother's efforts to mold the home life in accordance with the pressures and demands of her husband's activities. She was a highly imaginative woman who in her ordinary dealings with people was flighty and ineffectual. The patient has often characterized her emotionally as primitive. The patient was an only child.

The patient was much alone during his formative years, with no close friends and very little group activity. At college he proved to be a brilliant student whose chief interest was English literature. Following his graduation he studied both in this country and abroad, and finally accepted a teaching position in a leading eastern university. He held this position for a short time, and it was during this period that his interest turned to painting. In his middle twenties he left the university post and came to New York. He became acquainted with artists and soon began to paint on his own. He had had no previous experience in painting. When he did begin to paint, it was with an intensity and fervor he had never before experienced. Within a few years his work drew serious attention and at the time he came to analysis he was considered one of the leading *"avant garde"* artists in the country. He was continually in economic jeopardy receiving only occasional sporadic financial returns from his paintings and writings.

The early analytic situation was as follows: The patient had a very pleasant, agreeable approach. He was over-polite, how ever, almost to the point of obeisance. He would say "thank you" at the end of each analytic session. Anxiety about the therapy manifested itself by concern with the duration of treatment, efforts to manipulate the hours, and the repeatedly expressed hope that the treatment could be terminated in three to six months so that he could embark on a projected European trip. Analysis of these early features brought out his fear of involvement, his immediate reaction to a new situation as limiting and restricting, and his need to control, manipulate, and delimit any situation that was not of his own creation. He then began to focus more clearly on what heretofore had been but dimly sensed, namely, the feeling that there was something basically wrong with himself (something about himself which he characterized as inhuman) which filled him with a feeling of futility and at times desperation. He was referring to his detachment and the resultant inability to enjoy direct, relaxed contact with other people. This seemed in marked contrast to the optimism and inspiration he consistently felt in relation to his work. Despite his growing respect for the analytic process, his deferential, formal manner persisted, and there was little affective coloring to his productions except for the feeling of being trapped and helpless.

Several months after the start of the analysis, he began to broach the question of divorce. He struggled with considerable inertia evolving out of his reluctance to sever even for a brief time the round of activities in which he was engaged in New York, to hazard a trip to Reno by himself. In addition to this, he was hampered by inflated notions of his responsibilities to his wife. He had little money of his own, and her support would devolve upon his mother. Despite these difficulties, it was felt that the move was not only right, but necessary at this time to clear the path for his own future development. He was actively encouraged, and finally did make the trip. He returned to New York two months later, having successfully carried through the arrangements with regard to the divorce. He had withstood the onslaught of his family, and he had in the interim become interested in another young woman.

During the next few weeks he spoke a great deal about this girl. Several things became apparent. He found himself drawn to her for qualities which he had either never noticed or which were not there in the other women he had known. He was greatly taken by her warmth, her directness, and the undemanding nature of her attachment to him. There were moments when he would experience a positive sense of responsibility and commitment in relation to her, but these were, at least in the beginning, lost sight of in his fear of treading outside the sphere of art and art personalities. He feared the reaction of his friends to someone who had no special interest in art. For a time the relationship was stalemated and almost completely lost sight of.

The pressure to establish himself on more secure economic grounds—a theme which had recurred from time to time since the start of the analysis—was again considered, but this time was followed by definite action on his part. He had in the past received offers of academic posts, one of them as a professor of art, but he had rejected all of them, as he considered himself ill-suited for the quiet, and what he regarded as the restricting conventionality, of academic life. He did aspire, however, to have his own school of painting, although he had, up to this point, shied away from the idea. He greatly feared his own awkwardness and impracticality in effecting even the simplest and most ordinary business affairs. In addition to this, all the advice he received indicated that setting up his own school was the sort of venture in which only an older and more established painter could hope to succeed. On the other hand, he did enjoy teaching and was successful at it, and he felt that he had original and significant ideas to present.

Again it was felt that the movement here was in the right direction, despite the fact that the outcome could not be certain. Analysis of the factors in his way, and encouragement and reassurance resulted in his taking the first steps. Within a few months, the school was a going concern and working out more smoothly than had been anticipated. Once this was accomplished, he seemed eager to resume and come to grips with the relationship with his girl. The two things about himself which disturbed him most—his compulsiveness about his work and his general aloofness and lack of concern for people and activities unrelated to the art world—now began to disturb him more than ever because of their specific destructive potential in relation to this girl. It was at this point that the fetishistic nature of his attachment to his own talent specifically, and to the world of art in general, was developed as a central analytic theme. His compulsive and all-engrossing concern with the art world was seen as a substitute means, although a necessary one, of relating himself to other people, a means born out of revulsion to, and intolerance of, the world as he had experienced it.

Although his talent was recognizable and real, he seemed to relate to it as if he himself were helpless, insignificant, and virtually nonexistent. He actually seemed to be trapped by the pleasure he experienced in the *act* of painting, a pleasure which seemed so all-consuming and powerful that it excluded any concern with the painting itself, that is, with the finished product. Whenever he discussed his work it was in terms of the *act* of painting; and only an occasional reference was made to a finished picture. He was impervious to the impact of his paintings on others (aloof and indifferent to his critics and his followers alike) and showed no genuine concern with an effort to harness some of the fruits of his creative energy in stabilizing his own life from the financial point of view (his economic situation having been precarious until he opened his own school). In short, he was relating in an inhuman and slavish way to his own creativity.

Once these matters were established, he began to struggle less against the recognition of his own need for the qualities which the girl had to offer. They were married within a year after his return from Reno. The marriage took place during the summer and he was seen two months later. Despite the fact that he was still profoundly disturbed over his conflicts, the early period of his marriage had resulted in greater closeness with his wife, more real respect for her, and a greater eagerness to achieve some mastery over his own problems.

In the fall, he was again faced with the mounting pressures of preparing for exhibits, meeting editorial deadlines, arranging his school program, and participating in numerous other ventures in which he had become involved. In addition to this, there was the problem of setting up a home and studio. He became more and more aloof and distant toward his wife, lost interest in their sexual activity, which up to that point had been highly gratifying, and even at times felt reluctant to return home at the end of the day. His need to reject, withdraw, and remain uninvolved gave rise intermittently to almost paralyzing feelings of hostility. He felt discouraged and futile in the analysis. The stage was thus set for a renewed effort on his part—although at a different level, by virtue both of his marriage and the self-confidence attendant upon his venture into teaching—to achieve his neurotic goal, namely, the pursuit of gratification in art at the expense of self-effacement and through the relinquishment of all responsibility in relation to other human beings. This attempt was again subtle and, like the initial attempt, became manifest by his efforts to control and delimit the analysis. He became preoccupied with the idea of moving to the West to free himself from the tensions and pressures which he experienced in New York, and thus be in a position to devote himself to painting in a total and more sustained way.

This material was analyzed as follows: It was pointed out to what extent his drive both toward marriage and toward analysis had incorporated within it the effort to become more human by osmosis, so to speak. Still laboring under the oppressive influence of his detachment, he had not relinquished the hope that his attachment to another human being in a passive, helpless, self-effacing sort of way could substitute for the task he faced, and conceived of as impossible—that of overthrowing his detachment and becoming a human being. Interpretations along these lines took the edge off the escapist impulses and brought out into the open his hope that what he had failed to do by himself, namely, to work out a way of life that would leave him unhampered and unfettered, he could now accomplish with his wife by severing all their ties here and attempting a more simplified existence away from the pressures of civilization.

The fantasy of "one against the world" had evolved into "two against the world." It became apparent to what extent he was buffeted about by the importance to him of the act of painting, and to what extent this forced him to maneuver and overpower those to whom he felt closest. This understanding eased the situation in the analysis; but it was not until a short time later, that a very intuitive observation on his wife's part eased the tension at home. It occurred in the course of a conversation which took place at a time when their relationship had deteriorated to a critical level. She succeeded in pointing out to him that she did not take exception to his interest in and enjoyment of painting, but that she was puzzled by two things, first the fact that this interest seemed to be exclusively centered in the preparations and arrangements that went into the making of a picture, and not in the picture itself, and second, that it seemed to crowd out the possibilities of any other interests. It was the first time for the patient that what was most important to him was shared, accepted, and critically evaluated by a significant person. It also fanned the first genuine sparks of hope in his struggle to change himself.

The attitudes with which this patient will ultimately have to come to grips have to do with his concept of people either as dehumanized automatons, ruthlessly pursuing their predatory impulses and relating to others as if they were capable of being owned and manipulated (his perception of his father), or as basically parasitic and venting their emotionality in an aimless and uncontrollable way (his perception of his mother). His real impotence as a child in relation to this state of affairs gave rise to a negativism which, coupled with his sensitivity, resulted in a critical rejection of his own human environment and the values it represented. His existence seemed to hinge upon his ability to subjugate, not other people, as in the case of the powerful adults who surrounded him, but himself. The waste, the cruelty, and the alienation wrought upon himself and others by this attitude make a virtue of unawareness, blind him to the vulnerability of his detachmnt, and make an inexorable necessity of it. His talent and creativity, in forcing their way through these barriers, are cast out with little direction or goal, in hateful defiance of the oppression and melancholy that pervades his life. In rejecting the values about him, he devotes himself to a search for absolute values. His sensitivity to line and color is a real attribute developed in his struggle to abstract beauty from the world of objects.

In summarizing the analytic process thus far, one sees that despite the fact that there has been very little analytic activity in the ordinary sense of the term, and despite the fact that the detachment is still operating, although not so effectively as it did in the beginning, the analysis has witnessed and supported some measure of real growth.

1. In the step toward marriage, the patient risked the first definite break with the kind of relatedness he had with the art world.

2. In the establishment of his school, he made the first wholehearted attempt to alter for the better the financially precarious, socially irresponsible, and generally unstabilized character of his earlier mode of existence.

3. The fact that both the analysis and his marriage have withstood his subtle but powerful efforts to manipulate and abort them has made him somewhat less fearful of his own destructive potential. It is this fear which must be mastered before he can experience his own neurosis as a reality rather than an abstraction, and can come to grips with his own terrible distorted attitudes toward people, attitudes which his detachment serves.

Although the detachment has not been fully resolved in this patient, it is no longer a bulwark against analytic progress, and some inferences may be drawn as to the factors involved in its resolution.

It is important to note that in the case of the more benign syndromes, the analysis itself actively challenges the defensive structure. In the case of the detached patient, the elements of struggle can be successfully hidden, at least in the beginning. In fact, the analysis is set up as a citadel against struggle. The analyst is not a significant figure to the patient. The latter is capable of experiencing people as significant only when they directly relate to his own area of creative function, and here their significance as people is overshadowed by their significance as manipulable and maneuverable objects. In the light of this, the steps in the process of resolution may be outlined as follows:

1. In a situation where no genuine human relationships have previously occurred, the analyst can only ally himself with a reality tool rather than a real ego. In the patient presented, this would refer to his talent and sensitivity.

2. Relatedness to people must be initiated by someone significant to the patient in relation to this reality tool. In the case of the patient presented, the neurotic component of his marriage (and by far the strongest component) was the hope of solving his human needs by blind, passive attachment to his wife. His wife thus became a significant figure to him. It is the pressure of this relationship, interpreted and handled within the therapeutic situation, which undermines his detachment and necessitates an active struggle against it. Not until the patient can actively identify himself with this struggle does the therapist become a truly significant figure for him.

Summary

1. Genetically, detachment develops as a defense against the enforced transformation of human potential into automatic, mechanical responsiveness.

2. Resolution depends on the full understanding of the fragmentary means of contact established by these patients and the ruthlessness with which it is protected.

3. A case is presented illustrating the analytic problems encountered in the therapy of a severely detached personality.

THE MEANING OF ANXIETY

Edward Podolsky, M.D.

Primitive man related everything to present circumstances; he had no notion of future events. He practiced hunting for the impelling present needs, but not agriculture nor any form of saving to provide for future needs. Only immediate dangers were avoided by him. He experienced fear when frightening stimuli were present but he was not anxious about future happenings. Anxiety came into man's awareness when he acquired a conception of time as the carrier of future events.

The existence of man is essentially finite. Limited by death, his existence is a "being for death." Although our existence is characterized by the fact that there are things possible for us, the moment will come when there will be no more possibilities, when there will be no more ahead of us. This, of course, is the moment of death. It is this fact of our being in a finite and limited time which accounts for the tragic character of anxiety.

We go beyond ourselves toward the future. Each of us is always in front of himself. We are always planning, and we project ourselves into the plan. Man is a being who has to exist. The time of existence begins with the future. Comprehension is always stretched toward the future. It is thus that we are always filled with anxiety and care. We are always concerned with something which is yet to come; and Being, in so far as we seize it in existence, is care and temporality.

Anxiety thus exists essentially as a time element. It is the reaction to a threat to the existence of one's self as a human being, or to the values that one identifies with that existence.

It is well known that every individual tends to reach a level of integration maximal for himself; he seeks to defend the particular level he has attained against any threat or danger, because any lowering of this level constitutes a vital injury to his ego. Accordingly, anxiety may be expected to arise whenever the individual feels threatened not only by actual danger, but by a situation which threatens his personality as a whole.

Anxiety appears when gratification is frustrated. It is because of the frustration that a reality factor, the ego, is born. Hence the ego is born and develops out of the pain of frustration. The antithesis between instinct and anxiety becomes the antithesis between id and ego.

As the organism becomes more complex the reactions of the primitive ego to external reality became more complicated by its having to turn its attention to states of instinct tension which would threaten its freedom from within. It may be torn between adopting reality to suit its instinct demands, and suppressing instinct demands when these would endanger its relationship to reality. The problem is also complicated by the existence of the superego, which must also be placated in the course of ego adjustment.

Anxiety is the tension or continuing discomfort experienced when reality frustrates the gratification of an urge or desire (the neutralization of a chemico-physical condition). The anxiety leads to an abandonment of the pleasure principle, which is inoperative on account of the frustration, and causes an automatic mobilization of all the resources of the organism to deal with the cause of the frustration. This usually means a concentration of attention upon reality. From this concentration on reality the ego comes into being, and at the instigation of further reality frustrations, it develops. As instinct gratification is accompanied by pleasure, this process of instinct frustration and ego development is accompanied by anxiety. The degree of anxiety will naturally vary from imperceptible faintness, when the ego is in the process of successfully coping with reality and removing frustrating obstacles of instinct gratification, to heightened tension when the ego is failing and frustration is persisting.

Both anxiety and freedom arise from the same capacities of man. The planning function of the nervous system, in the course of evolution, has culminated in the appearance of ideas, values and pleasures. These are the unique manifestations of man's social living. Man alone can plan for the distant future and think ahead. For this reason man alone can be anxious. Anxiety accompanies intellectual activity as its shadow.

The very nature of human living evokes anxiety. Man is always looking ahead of himself. He has to find himself constantly. His future is limited by the fact that at the end there is always death. Thus he moves ceaselessly from his future to his past, from his anticipations and plans to memories, regrets and remorses and this is usually accompanied by anxiety.

Anxiety is purely a human manifestation. Man alone has to make decisions and each decision is a risk. Man is always surrounded by and filled with uncertainty and uncertainty and risk give rise to anxiety.

The human being exists as a mortal; he is the only being who knows, who can know—that he is mortal. It is this inexorable limit, mortality, finitude and death which determines and characterizes man. It is this awareness of his mortality and uncertainty of the future, the constant threats to his career as a human being that is the source of all anxieties.

CHRONIC ANXIETY SYMPTOMATOLOGY, EXPERIMENTAL STRESS, AND HCL SECRETION

George F. Mahl, Ph.D. and Eugene B. Brody, M.D.

Previous experiments demonstrated significant increases in HCl secretion during experimentally produced chronic fear in dogs and monkeys and during sustained "examination-period anxiety" in undergraduate students. Indices of the HCl secretion of a chronically anxious patient were higher during five very anxious psychoanalytic hours than during five relatively nonanxious hours. Other investigators, largely in studies of single subjects, have reported similar results. Evaluation of those studies reporting a negative or a variable relationship between HCl secretion and anxiety is hindered by a lack of either adequate experimental controls or sufficient data. The primary interest of this report is the implication of these results for the unqualified use of Cannon's emergency theory of emotions as a basic concept in psychosomatic theory.

The apparently consistent finding of increased HCl secretion during sustained anxiety in controlled experiments is just the opposite of what one would expect if the extension of Cannon's theory from acute-emergency to chronic emotions were valid in psychosomatic theory. According to this position, in both acute and chronic anxiety there is sympathetic-epinephrine excitation and parasympathetic inhibition. Thus, vagus-excited increased HCl secretion should not be a component of either acute or chronic anxiety. Several proposals have been made to resolve the contradiction between this conclusion and the experimental findings cited above.

Alexander and Szasz have assumed that the dogs in the study referred to above were not primarily frightened but were primarily regressed. They believe that the concept of "vegetative retreat" adequately accounts for the findings. It has been shown, however, that the animals anticipated painful shock stimulation with avoidance behavior, developed phobic avoidance of their cages where the experimental stimulation occurred, trembled and startled to extraneous stimuli—in short, behaved in a manner usually considered to be motivated by fear. Increased HCl secretion accompanying this behavior was also associated with increased heart rate. In the subsequent study with monkeys, independent judges agreed that their behavior was "fearful" at the times HCl secretion increased. Blood sugar measurements in these animals showed no hypoglycemic changes interdependently related to the increased HCl secretion or the behavioral changes.

Not only is the skeletal behavior of the dogs and monkeys contrary to the "withdrawal from action" of the vegetative-retreat principle, but the multiple autonomic changes do not support the picture of a generalized shift from predominantly sympathetic-epinephrine to vagus-insulin excitation hypothesized in this principle.

One of us (G.F.M.) once proposed that HCl secretion during fear may have been erroneously subsumed under the emergency theory. This suggestion was made because the total amount of data on HCl secretion considered by Cannon was limited and only one observation (Le Conte's) seemed clearly to be of secretion during fear. Although not yet ruled out in human HCl secretion by experimental evidence, this suggestion now seems less likely than the following.

Exploratory observations in the study with dogs suggested that increased HCl secretion was associated with chronic, but not with acute, fear. The experiment with monkeys systematically investigated the nature of HCl secretion during acute-episodic and sustained fear. It was found that HCl secretion did not increase during brief fear episodes but that it did during relatively continuous, sustained fear. Both animal studies showed that mere repetition of discrete pain-fear stimulation and response was not sufficient for the appearance of increased gastric acidity. HCl secretion increased only when continuous, sustained fear developed or when sudden conditioned fear was evoked after sustained fear had been learned in response to a stimulus pattrn and not extinguished.

The results of the two animal studies support the hypothesis that increased HCl secretion is associated with sustained or chronic anxiety but not with acute anxiety. This hypothesis directly implies that the extension of Cannon's emergency theory to chronic anxiety is not valid and thus resolves the contradiction stated at the onset of this discussion.

In a reinterpretation of the results of studies of human HCl secretion it was found that the majority of them agree with the above hypothesis. An attempt to study this hypothesis directly in humans seems desirable, however, because none of these studies had systematically controlled the acute-chronic anxiety variable.

Aside from this theoretical goal, it also seems important simply to obtain more empirical data on HCl secretion and emotions in humans. Varying etiological importance has been attributed to dependency conflict, hostility, anxiety, and HCl secretion in peptic ulcer development. Yet there has been only one study in humans of anxiety and HCl secretion that included in itself more than one subject, control measurement, and a quantitative analysis of the reliability of the findings. There has been no published study of dependency conflict or hostility and HCl secretion meeting these minimal criteria.

The reader will soon discover that this experiment failed in its attempt to test the acute-chronic hypothesis in humans. The write-up follows the original prospectus of the experiment, however, to clarify the description of the study and certain methodological problems encountered.

Present Experiment

1. *The Problem.*—The theoretical problem is to test in humans the validity of the hypothesis that HCl secretion does not increase during acute, but does during sustained, anxiety.

The ideal condition for testing this hypothesis is one in which the experimenter can control the variation from acute to sustained anxiety by manipulating the anxiety-evoking stimuli and the conditions of learning that determine this change. This is possible to a large degree in experiments with lower animals but is not feasible in the majority of conceivable human studies.

An alternative procedure of "controlling" the acute-chronic anxiety variable determined the design of this experiment. The intent was experimentally to induce anxiety responses for a brief period of time in a group of already "chronically anxious" people (experimental group) and in a group of subjects not reacting with sustained anxiety (control group) up to the moment of the experimentally induced anxiety episode.

If these conditions are met and the acute-chronic hypothesis is valid, one would predict the following:

(*a*) Independent of the experimental anxiety condition, the gastric acidity of the experimental group will be significantly greater than that of the control group. This would demonstrate further that chronic anxiety and HCl secretion in humans are positively related.

(*b*) The gastric acidity of the control group will not increase during the acute experimental anxiety condition, and this secretory response will be significantly different than that of the experimental group. This would demonstrate that in humans acute anxiety is not accompanied by increased HCl secretion.

The procedure of the experiment cannot guarantee, however, that the intended differential pretest conditions of sustained anxiety would actually obtain between the two groups, but practically guarantees at least a difference in degree of pretest anxiety. In such a case, the effect of variation from acute to sustained anxiety cannot be tested, for there is no basal condition of no, or very slight, anxiety to change into a sudden, acute anxiety episode in the control group. Prediction (*a*) would still be made on the assumption that the positive HCl secretion-chronic anxiety relation is an increasing function and not simply an all-or-none relation. Some slight evidence from the monkey study already cited supports this assumption.

It is not possible to predict precisely the HCl secretory responses of the experimental subjects or of the control subjects if the latter anticipate the experimental stress with anxiety. If the interaction of the prestress and the stress-induced anxiety is cumulative, one would predict increases in HCl secretion during the experimental anxiety episode. But a cumulative interaction is not necessary, or the only possible, consequence here, and there is no adequate way available at present to measure such changes in the anxiety variable under these particular experimental conditions. The nature of these HCl secretory responses is left as an empirical subquestion of the study.

The experimental problem is to test the appropriate predictions and investigate the empirical subquestion cited above.

II. *Procedure.*—(*a*) Subjects: Before anyone was accepted as a subject and tested under the experimental conditions, he was evaluated clinically to see whether he met a priori criteria for assignment to the experimental or the control group. The criterion for assignment to the experimental group was a presenting history of chronic anxiety symptomatology which included repeated subjective anxiety experiences and at least one of the group of physiological symptoms generally regarded as an indication of "free-floating" anxiety. The criteria for assignment to the control group were that the person was not undergoing psychiatric treatment at the time of the study and the absence of a history of chronic anxiety symptomatology.

The experimental group consisted of six psychoneurotic patients, five of whom were being treated as inpatients and one as an outpatient, and one person who was not a patient but who expressed some need for psychiatric treatment and whose life history was one of chronic anxiety reaction. The control group consisted of seven subjects who met the criteria. One of these had been under psychotherapy for a brief time but had interrupted it voluntarily two years before the experiment.

The clinical evaluation of the patients was based on the intake interview and additional material obtained during the course of therapy. The evaluation of the nonpatients was based upon one anamnestic interview and the subject's responses on a check-list questionnaire.

An attempt was made to match the control group with the experimental group with respect to sex and age. Each group contained five women and two men, but the mean age of the experimental group (36 years) is slightly greater than that for the control group (31 years). The influence of this factor will be assessed in presenting the results.

All subjects were first contacted about five days before the experimental sessions. At this time they were told that the study involved their "swallowing a stomach tube" and an investigation of their stomach secretions. The controls were also told that it would be necessary for them to be interviewed by one of the authors (E.B.), whom they knew to be a psychiatrist, and that the experimental sessions included a mild "stress" situation.

It was realized that the controls' foreknowledge of intubation, of the psychiatric interview, and of the use of a "stress situation" could produce anticipatory anxiety in them, maintain it up to the time of the experimental sessions, and so prevent the study of HCl secretions during only an acute-emergency anxiety episode. Yet experience with exploratory subjects convinced us that it was necessary to tell them these things to insure even the available source of controls, their cooperation as subjects, and freedom from contamination of the testing periods with strong affect evoked by the "surprise" of intubation. In order to reduce their anticipatory anxiety, the controls were reassured extensively about the procedures and were asked to consider the request for their services for two or three days before committing themselves.

During the interviews and the preparatory period on the first two experimental days, references by the controls to the pending experiment were noted. These observations form the basis for assessing whether or not the controls anticipated the experiment with anxiety, and thus which predictions could be tested.

(b) Measurement of HCl Secretion: Fasting gastric samples were obtained by aspiration through a Levin tube, which was introduced nasally in the majority of cases. The subjects had not eaten for a minimum of nine hours, or taken water for two hours, preceding any of the experimental sessions. The gastric samples were titrated against 0.1 N NaOH, using Töpfer's reagent and phenolphthalein as end-point indicators for free HCl and total acidity in the usual way.

(c) The Testing Conditions: With two exceptions, the subjects were tested under three different conditions on three successive mornings. In one exceptional case, one week separated the control from the remaining two conditions. In the other, an experimental subject left the hospital on the third morning and was tested only on the first two days.

1. Control condition, Day I: After the Levin tube was introduced, the subject lay quietly for five minutes. Then the stomach was "cleared" of residual contents.

The examiner then told the subjects that a buzzer would sound occasionally during the next period of time but that nothing else would occur. During the next 20 minutes a buzzer of 15 seconds' duration was administered in accordance with the schedule shown in Table 1.

At the end of this period all of the gastric contents that could be obtained was aspirated. Then a second, and final, 20-minute period ensued in which the buzzer was administered at the times shown in Table 1. At the end of this period a second gastric sample was obtained and the tube withdrawn. The mean of

TABLE 1

SCHEDULE OF EXPERIMENTAL STIMULATION* DURING THE TWO TWENTY-MINUTE TEST PERIODS

First 20-Minute Period	Second 20-Minute Period
3' Buzz-pain	4' Buzz
7' Buzz-pain	8' Buzz-pain
10' Buzz-pain	12' Buzz-pain
13' Buzz	13' Buzz
14' Buzz-pain	14' Buzz-pain
18' Buzz	18' Buzz-pain

* On Day I and Day III only the buzzers were administered; on Day II the buzzers and the pain stimulation were both given.

these two fasting samples was taken as the control condition gastric acidity measure for each subject.

2. Pain-pain anticipation condition, Day II: A 2 by 2 in. (5 by 5 cm.) area of the distal portion of the arch of the right foot was painted with India ink, and the foot was then so placed that it rested comfortably against the tip of a Hardy-Wolff-Goodell pain stimulator. Immediately after intubation, a "pain-adjustment series" of buzzer and heat stimuli took place to establish the intensity of painful heat stimulation that would be used during the testing periods on this day. It was arbitrarily decided to use for each subject that intensity of heat stimulation producing rapid foot withdrawal on three successive stimulations.

A timing device was used whereby the buzzer was sounded for 15 seconds, and the shutter of the heat stimulator opened automatically four seconds before the end of the buzzer. A shutter opening of four seconds' duration was used throughout. At the end of this pain adjustment series, the stomach was cleared of its residual fasting contents.

Two 20-minute test periods then followed, as on the first day. But on this second day some of the buzzers were paired with the pain stimulus of the intensity established in the adjustment series. The actual sequence of buzzer and buzzer-pain stimulation is shown in Table 1. The subjects, of course, did not know which buzzers were to be paired with the pain stimuli. Gastric samples were obtained at the end of each 20-minute period, and the mean acidity of the two samples was taken for the acidity measure for each subject for this condition. The difference between the acidity of the first and that of the second day was taken as the HCl secretory response associated with the pain-pain anticipation condition.

3. Pain anticipation condition, Day III: The subject's foot was again painted with black ink and adjusted to the heat stimulator tip just as on the preceding day, but not as it was on the first day. The subject was again intubated and the stomach "cleared" five minutes later. During two subsequent 20-minute periods the buzzer was administered in accordance with the schedule of Table 1. No painful stimulation was given, but the subjects had no prior knowledge of this fact. Gastric samples were again obtained at the end of each 20-minute period. The mean of these two samples is taken for the gastric acidity measure for this condition for each subject, and the

difference in the acidity of the first day and that of this day is taken as the HCl secretory response of the pain anticipation condition.

When questioned at the end of this condition, all subjects stated either that they did not know whether the "hot foot" would come on this day or that they had expected it to come. This shows that they did in fact anticipate the pain stimulation on this day, as intended by the experimental design.

The testing conditions of all three days also included the application of a blood pressure cuff to the right arm, a pneumograph to the trunk, and electrodes over the heart for the periodic measurement of blood pressure and the continuous recording of respiration and heart rates. (These multiple autonomic measurements are not reported here for the sake of clarity.)

III. *Results.*— (a) Anticipatory Anxiety of Control Subjects: Three of the seven controls indicated directly or indirectly in the psychiatric interview that they were concerned over having to "swallow a stomach tube." Five of the controls were judged to be apprehensive in the control condition, and six were judged to be apprehensive at the beginning of the pain-pain anticipation condition.

The increasing proportion of controls showing observable signs of anxiety as the time prior to the experimental sessions decreases is indicative of anticipatory anxiety that increases in strength as they approach the "goal" of the experimental sessions. The reality and strength of this anticipatory anxiety and its gradient nature are illustrated by the following observations: A control manifested little anxiety over intubation when first contacted but reported a "nightmare"—an event described by the subject as very unusual—the night before the first experimental session. Another subject indicated diffuse anticipatory anxiety in the preparatory period of the first day by asking whether he was to be shocked through the cardiac electrodes—after he had been told they were for picking up his heart beat—although this person was highly motivated to serve as a subject and was not observably upset when first contacted.

The judgments about the anticipatory anxiety of the controls were made prior to the stress situation, and thus independently of knowledge about the nature of the HCl secretory response during stress.

In view of these observations, one must conclude that the anxiety stimulation of the second and third experimental days was not of an acute-emergency nature for the controls but interacted with their anticipatory anxiety reactions. Therefore, only prediction *a* and the empirical interest in the secretory responses of Days II and III are applicable. The latter is considered first.

(*b*) HCl Secretory Response to Anxiety Situations: The mean gastric acidity of both the control and the experimental group increased on Day II and Day III over the level of Day I.

TABLE 2

MEAN GASTRIC ACIDITY, IN CLINICAL UNITS, ON CONTROL AND EXPERIMENTAL DAYS

Day	I. Control Day		II. Pain-Pain Anticipation Day	III. Pain Anticipation Day
Test samples	Total acid	19	29	34
	Free HCl	12	30	23
Clearing samples	Total acid	23	23	25
	Free HCl	12	12	14

N = 13. One subject (experimental group) who did not return for Day III has been omitted from this summary for clarity of presentation. Inclusion of her data for Day I and II increases the Day II-I difference and the reliability of this difference.

Reliabilities of Test-Sample Differences		Reliabilities of Clearing-Sample Differences
Total Acid	*Free HCl*	
I vs. II $P < 0.02$	$P < 0.02$	All differences insignificant by inspection
I vs. III $P < 0.01$	$P < 0.03$	
II vs. III $P > 0.30$	$P > 0.40$	

Reliabilities of Net Differences Between Test-Sample and Clearing-Sample Differences

	Total Acid	*Free HCl*
I vs. II	$P < 0.02$	$P < 0.02$
I vs. III	$P < 0.01$	$P < 0.09$
II vs. III	$P > 0.30$	$P > 0.40$

There were no significant differences between the two groups in their secretory responses of Day II or Day III. Consequently, the data of all the subjects are pooled for the most sensitive assessment of the HCl secretory response. These are presented in Table 2 and Chart 1. The mean gastric acidity of test samples

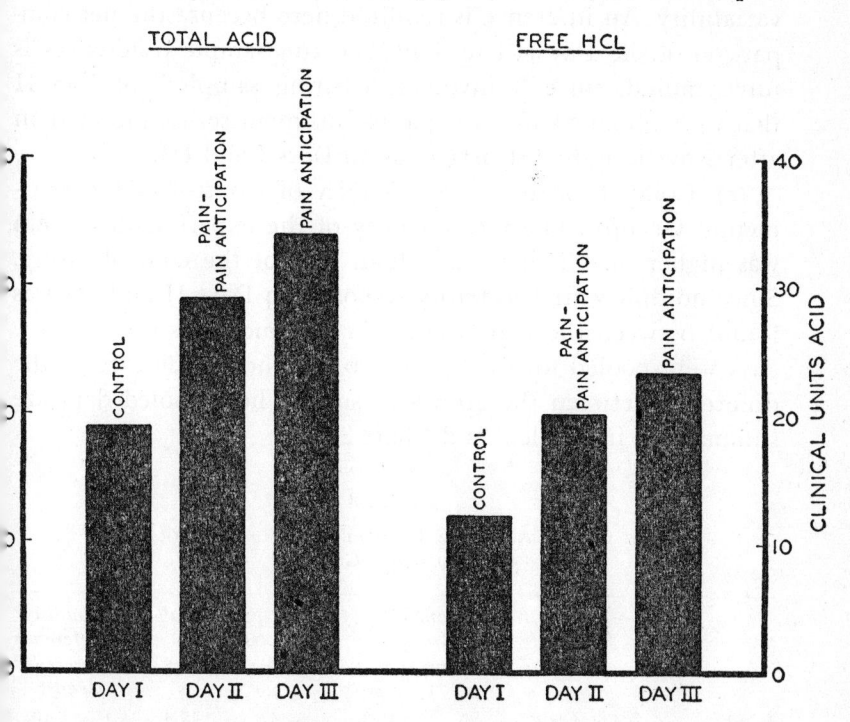

Chart 1.—Mean gastric acidity of 13 subjects during control, pain-pain anticipation, and pain anticipation conditions.

during the pain-pain anticipation condition of Day II and the pain anticipation condition of Day III is significantly higher than that during the control condition of Day I. The difference between Days II and III is not significant.

The mean gastric acidities of the "clearing" samples for these days are also presented in Table 2. There is no significant change in these. Furthermore, the net comparisons of the Day III-I test-sample differences with the Day III-I clearing-sample differences show that the increased gastric acidity of Day III was not due to day-to-day variability but was associated with the experimental stimulation of Day III. Since this net comparison of Day III-I differences brackets Day II, it is inferred that the Day II-I test sample changes are likewise not due to day-to-day variability. An inference is required here because the net comparison of the Day II-I test- and clearing-sample differences is unwarranted, since it involves "clearing samples" of Day II that were obtained after the pain-adjustment series, rather than after a five-minute rest period, as on Days I and III.

(*c*) Comparison of Gastric Acidity of Control and Experimental Groups: The mean acidity of the experimental group was higher on all three days than that of the control group. Since no differential secretory response on Days II and III was found between the two groups, the test measures on all three days were pooled for each group to test the significance of the difference between the groups as such. These pooled data are summarized in Table 3 and Chart 2.

TABLE 3

MEAN GASTRIC ACIDITY IN CLINICAL UNITS OF CONTROL AND EXPERIMENTAL GROUPS

		Control Group $\bar{x}$	Control Group s	Experimental Group $\bar{x}$	Experimental Group s	Reliability of Difference Between Means†
Total sample*	Total acid	25	12.3	37	17.4	$P = 0.10$
	Free HCl	16	11.5	27	19	$P = 0.13$
Restricted sample*	Total acid	21	8.8	39	18.2	$P = 0.04$
	Free HCl	12	7.4	29	19.9	$P = 0.06$

* "Total sample" includes all subjects assigned to the control and experimental groups prior to their participation as subjects. "Restricted sample" excludes from the control group the subject who sought but interrupted psychiatric treatment prior to this study and excludes from the experimental group the subject who felt the need for treatment but was not at the present time in treatment.

† Differences in variability were tested by the F test. None of the variability comparisons were significant at the 5% level.

Significance of differences between means was tested by the t test. P values are for the predicted difference between the control and the experimental groups.

Two summaries are contained in Table 3. The first compares all of the subjects as originally assigned to the control or the experimental group. The Table shows that the mean total acidity and free HCl of the experimental subjects are greater than those of the control subjects. The reliabilities of these differences are only fair.

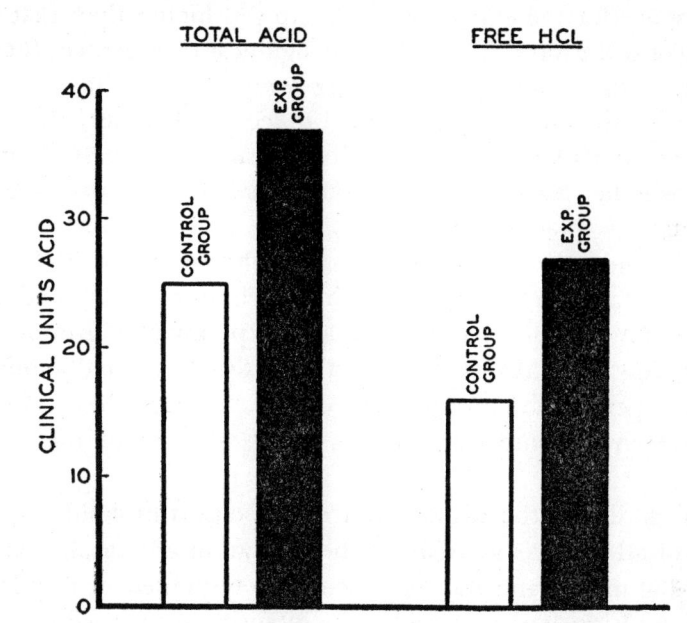

Chart 2.—Mean gastric acidity of control and experimental groups.

The second summary of Table 3 compares the two groups when the subject who was not undergoing psychiatric treatment is omitted from the experimental group and the subject who had started but not continued with psychiatric treatment two years previously is omitted from the control group. The reliability of the differences in gastric acidity between these "restricted" groups is greater than that of the differences of the original control and experimental groups. A possible interpretation of these increases in reliability is presented in the discussion.

The groups were combined and then split at the median age into a "young" and an "old" group to determine the effect of age in the results. If the difference in gastric acidity between the control and the experimental groups is due to the age difference between them, then the "old" group should show a significantly higher acidity than the "young" group because the mean age for the experimental group was higher than that for the control group. There was no significant difference (t-test) in the gastric acidity of the two age groups ($P > 0.50$).

The results were also examined to see whether gastric acidity was related to the pain intensity measured in physical units and whether this relationship contaminated the control-experimental group acidity differences.

The mean response thresholds for the control and the experimental groups were determined. These were 307 and 284 mcal. for the original control and experimental groups, respectively, and 313 and 290 mcal. for the "restricted" control and experimental groups, respectively. Neither difference in the mean response thresholds is statistically significant ($P > 0.20$).

In addition, the distribution of response threshold intensities of all subjects was split at the median of 295 mcal. (range, 250-380 mcal.) and the mean secretory responses on Day II of the resulting low- and high-pain intensity groups were determined. The mean total and free-acid responses of $+$ 10.9 and $+$ 8.9 clinical units for the low-intensity group are practically the same as the mean total and free-acid responses of $+$ 9.1 and $+$ 8.7 clinical units for the high-intensity group. Thus, there was no relationship, over the range of intensities used here, between HCl secretion and the physical intensity of heat.

COMMENT

This study failed to contribute to the primary problem of determining whether there is a change from inhibited to increased HCl secretion in humans associated with the change from acute to sustained anxiety. Both groups presented sustained anxiety at the onset of the pain-pain-anticipation stimulation. This consisted of anticipatory anxiety evoked by foreknowledge of the experiment, which anxiety was not successfully reduced by reassurance and explanation, and chronic psychopathological anxiety in the experimental group. The result was a failure to achieve (in the control group) a condition of no, or very slight, pretest anxiety to change experimentally into acute-emergency anxiety. Verification of the acute-chronic anxiety hypothesis in humans remains an experimental problem. It will require fairly complete control of the pretest anxiety.

The difference in gastric acidity between the original "chronic anxiety" group and the control groups was of only suggestive reliability (total acid, $P = 0.10$). Two factors might be regarded as yielding an attenuated group difference in gastric acidity. First, the anxiety evoked by the prospect and actual occurrence of intubation seemed greater in the controls than in the experimental subjects. It may be that the latter more readily accept an uncomfortable medical procedure perceived as related to their medical study and treatment than the controls, who could only regard intubation as an experimental procedure.

A second attenuating factor may have been a function of variability in anxiety intensities among the individuals within each of the groups. It will be recalled that the experimental group included six psychiatric patients, five of whom were inpatients, and one person who was not a patient but who expressed the need for treatment and who was judged as presenting chronic anxiety symptoms. The possibility raised is not whether or not this person suffered from chronic anxiety, but that including her in this group increased considerably the range of the anxiety intensities represented by the members of the group. A comparable situation seems possible regarding the member assigned to the control group, who had sought, started, and then interrupted psychiatric treatment two years prior to this study. If one assumes that including these two subjects in the groups did have this effect, then eliminating them would increase the difference between the groups in the severity of chronic anxiety. If HCl secretion varies with chronic anxiety, the difference in gastric acidity between these more restricted groups should be greater and the reliability of this difference would be expected to increase. These two expectations were confirmed.

The HCl secretion of the subjects taken as a single group increased significantly upon both pain-pain anticipation and only pain anticipation stimulation. For the reasons stated earlier, the increased HCl secretion on Days II and III could not be predicted. It can be explained by alternative proposals. One is that the interaction between the pretest and the experimental anxiety was cumulative and that the rise in HCl secretion was associated with this increase in anxiety. Another proposal is that such a functional change in the autonomic innervation pattern results from sustained anxiety reactions that any subsequent discrete anxiety stimulus evokes increased HCl secretion. This latter proposal does not concern itself with the interaction between the pretest and the experimental anxiety reactions. The main value of this result is the empirical finding of increased HCl secretion in humans related to a specifiable stimulus that interacts with sustained anxiety.

The condition of pain anticipation (Day III) was just as effective in evoking increased HCl secretion as the condition of pain and pain anticipation (Day II). A similar finding was obtained with dogs and monkeys. These observations demonstrate that increased HCl secretion is part of acquired anxiety reaction (preceded by or evoked during sustained anxiety) that are produced by experimental procedures in dogs, monkeys, and humans. The difference in the gastric acidity of the two groups in this study—the increased gastric acidity in students reacting with "examination anxiety" and the increase in HCl during anxiety-laden psychoanalytic hours in a chronically anxious patient—demonstrates that increased HCl secretion is part of sustained acquired anxiety reactions produced by "real-life" procedures. Studies by others cited in the introduction yielded compatible results.

The consistent finding of increased HCl secretion during acquired anxiety reinforces the belief that the role of chronic anxiety in peptic ulcer etiology requires detailed investigation.

Summary

The evidence that increased HCl secretion occurs during sustained anxiety is contradictory to the unqualified extension of the emergency theory of emotions to chronic emotions. Results of studies with dogs and monkeys indicate that this increased HCl secretion is a function of the change from acute-emergency to sustained anxiety. The problem of the present experiment was to test this conclusion in humans and to obtain further empirical data of HCl secretion and anxiety in humans.

The procedure consisted of (*a*) comparing the fasting gastric acidity levels of seven subjects presenting chronic anxiety symptoms and of a group of seven subjects not presenting such symptoms; and (*b*) comparing the fasting HCl secretory response of these two groups when subjected to one experimental anxiety-evoking situation based upon pain and pain anticipation stimulation and another consisting only of pain anticipation stimulation.

Because of methodological limitations, the desired differential pretest anxiety in the two groups was not obtained. Therefore the nature of HCl secretion during acute-emergency anxiety could not be studied.

The gastric acidity of the original "chronic anxiety" group was greater than that of the control group, but this difference was of only suggestive reliability. When one subject was eliminated from each of these groups on specified grounds in order to make the groups more homogeneous in anxiety, the gastric acidity of the "chronic anxiety" group was significantly greater than that of the control group. When pain and pain-anticipation stimulation and response interacts with the sustained pretest anxiety, there is a significant increase in HCl secretion.

Both these findings are consistent with previous studies of sustained anxiety and HCl secretion. The accumulated evidence (*a*) reveals the invalidity of the unqualified extension of the emergency theory of the chronic emotions involved in psychosomatic disorders and (*b*) reinforces the belief that the role of chronic anxiety in peptic ulcer etiology merits detailed investigation.

ALLERGY AND PSYCHONEUROSES

Frank C. Metzger, M.D.

As one surveys both past and present literature, one is impressed with the infrequency of references to allergic manifestations observed in conjunction with emotional factors. Almost invariably, the conclusions have been that the emotion caused the manifestation, usually asthma. Dr. Warren T. Vaughn even raised the question as to whether or not maladjustments and their consequences and a state of altered reactivity, i.e., allergy, might not be parallel conditions.

Since my conclusion differs somewhat from the generally accepted causative action of the neurosis, I should like to report some of these cases, analyze them and show why and how my opinion was formed.

Many patients consult me for their difficulty in breathing. They describe a tightening of the muscles of the throat and the respiratory chest muscles, with the feeling of tension, tightness and weight confined to the upper part of the chest. These attacks appear usually in public speakers under very easily demonstrable emotional circumstances. Using the word "asthma" to refer in a broad sense to difficulty in the proper flow of air into and out of the bronchial tree, one could call this manifestation "asthma," but I wish to confine my remarks to true atopy, or a protein sensitivity, and in this sense the above is not a manifestation of allergy. The fact that the term "asthma" is frequently confused in the minds of medical men, as well as laymen, is proved by the numerous cases of this sort who are referred to the allergist for treatment. This type of reaction belongs in the realm of the psychiatrist, not the allergist.

When I first started to confine my work exclusively to allergy practically all my efforts were directed toward finding and removing the substances to which the patient was sensitive, i.e., the allergens, but I could not fail to observe the numerous patients who did not improve until a surgeon removed an infected gallbladder, a nose and throat specialist removed badly infected tonsils, or some other infection was eliminated, and therefore I was forced to conclude that this chest, this nose, or this skin I was endeavoring to clear up was only one part of an entire human body and that any infection severe enough to lower the general body resistance also lowered the allergic tolerance. I still believe the weight of evidence points to infections as complications, not causes, of allergy.

As time went on my attention was drawn to another large group of allergic individuals who had manifestations or attacks under circumstances where by no stretch of the imagination could one visualize or prove either an increase in their allergenic exposure or an infection affecting the patient with such suddenness and regularity. I wish to emphasize that in these cases all other efforts to prove the infectious complication in these attacks, including examinations by competent gastro-enterologists, surgeons, laryngologists and laboratory tests resulted in failure.

There are numerous unanswered questions. Why did a mixture of ephedrine, KI and phenobarbital dissolved in a vehicle of simple syrup stop the asthmatic attacks in, say, 100 individuals and when the *vehicle* was switched to lactate pepsin, which is red, it immediately failed to produce the same results in 32% of these 100 cases? Why did a hypodermic of 0.05 cc. of a 1:50 dust solution produce such a widespread variety of bizarre results? Why should a repeat hypodermic of 2 drops of distilled water do the same thing in the same patients? I have produced many asthmatic or hay fever attacks with hypodermics of distilled water. Conversely, I have produced cessation of attacks with distilled water. I am not speaking now of the sudden violent attacks of asthma and hay fever which come quite soon after the inadvertent introduction of a treatment dose into a vein. That bugbear of the allergist is well known and easily recognizable.

The above and numerous other phenomena forced me to another conclusion, i.e., an allergic individual has a mind and if it does not function in the proper channels it can affect the part of the body one is treating (Horne). The case which broke down my resistance and forced this attitude was that of a young woman who had giant urticaria. I found her sensitive to aspirin, eliminated it, and she improved, *but* she had an attack of hives which developed every time I came into the office *with a white coat on,* also every time she saw a man with his collar on backward, i.e., a preacher or priest, in spite of her no drug regime. These hives were usually accompanied by a crying spell. She did *not* get the hives if I left off the white coat.

The first psychiatrist under whom I studied made a definite statement that all allergic manifestations were basically due to psychoneurosis and the consequent nerve exhaustion, yet a survey of 2,000 case reports and patients in his clinic revealed to me only 1.5% had allergic manifestations. Later I read of a similar survey of 7,000 cases in mental institutions in which only 1% showed allergic manifestations. A rather generally accepted figure for unselected cases is that between 6 and 7% have more or less severe allergic spells. My records of allergic patients show that at least 50% of asthma and hay fever victims have definite psychoneurotic symptoms, and 92% of giant urticaria patients are so afflicted. The emotional factor in the hive cases seems to be predominantly a situation neurosis (Horne).

If one is to make deductions from these figures as to cause and effect, the only logical assumption must be the opposite to what the psychiatrist stated, i.e., the allergy causes the psychoneurosis and not vice versa.

I do not believe that the weight of evidence justifies us in assuming that either one *causes* the other. That they are complicating factors however, is quite evident. Let us consider two examples:

Case 1.—Female, age about 56. C. C. Asthma and Hay Fever. History: First attacks at the age of 18 years. Remission at the age of 24 to 40 years. Returned mildly in winter only until age 52, then became severe. Examination: The patient was overweight, otherwise negative except for sibilant and sonorous râles, inspiratory and expiratory bilaterally throughout the chest. No marked evidence of bronchiectasis, emphysema or secondary infection. An allergic survey showed sensitivity to foods and inhalants. An elimination diet was given her, based upon the intradermal tests, and hyposensitization to inhalants also was employed.

She improved quite a bit but continued to have attacks which could not be explained on the basis of an increased exposure to the substances to which she was allergic.

She then told me she "got asthma almost every time she raised her arms and brought her hands together." This was difficult to believe. She brought her arms upward and forward and her fingers almost together and had an asthma attack within two minutes. I gave her adrenalin and stopped the attack. Six separate times, under different weather conditions, I had her repeat the maneuver. Five times asthma followed.

I then obtained the following history: When she was 14 years old her father died. Her mother was an invalid, and she kept the girl in with her, except for her school time, playing cards. The patient's voice conveyed extreme emotion and hatred when she hissed, "playing cards." The mother died when the patient was 24. She married very happily. Asthma became recessive without treatment. The husband died when the patient was 40 years old. At the age of 52 she married a man of 70. He was an invalid and card-playing started "morning, noon and night." A year after her second marriage severe asthma started. The movements of her hands and arms which were followed by asthmatic seizures were exactly those one uses when dealing cards.

Interpretation: A basic atopic asthma, complicated by an emotional disturbance. Raising the patient's tolerance to her allergens freed her of symptoms. The addition of the psychoneurotic consequences to the allergy caused the spells when her hands assumed the position of which she spoke.

Case 2.—Female, age 35: Asthma and hay fever severe during late August and through September and gradually subsiding in October. The rest of the year she had asthmatic and hay fever seizures only on the fifteenth and first days of any month unless these dates came on holidays. Allergic investigation revealed mild sensitivities to foods and house dust and a four positive intradermal test to ragweed. Treatment for ragweed resulted in a cessation of symptoms in August, September and early October, except for spells on the fifteenth and first days of the month.

Her history revealed that her husband occasionally got drunk and came home without his pay check several times. She stated that on pay day she was uneasy, restless and slightly dizzy and nauseated. I then called her husband's employer and had him mail the check to her. On the night of the following 15th she had her usual spell, next pay day a light spell. After four pay days had passed she ceased to have an asthmatic spell on those nights.

My conclusion here is the same as in the first case: A situation neurosis complicating an allergic condition. The resultant double feature took the route to the lungs to which, from previous spells, her attention was directed and asthma resulted.

Sixty-five patients ranging in age from 6 to 19 years, all suffering from asthma, hay fever or hives, some from one and some from more than one of these manifestations, gave the following history:

Shortly after the school term begins, manifestations and seizures either start or become more severe and frequent. Soon after school lets out in the spring their troubles either disappear or become mild. In a search for the causative factors to explain these facts I have failed utterly to demonstrate an increase in exposure to their sensitizing agents in September and have failed to find that their allergens cease to exist or decrease in June.

Having failed to establish an explanation for the attacks in the group of patients referred to above along the allergic lines I was compelled to investigate the nonspecific causes.

The thermal change could be ruled out as in my territory cool weather rarely occurs before the middle of October and warm weather is present for four to five weeks before schools have their summer recess, i.e., late May or early June.

The presence of infection was next considered. Some were found to have bad tonsils, bad teeth and a few other minor troubles, but elimination of these factors did not alter the time or severity of the allergic attacks starting in September nor the remissions in June. In the search for such complications one would have to find a disease or focus of infection which developed only in the month of September and became recessive in June; this is highly improbable.

The exposure to chemical gases in the schools was investigated and found negative. It should be kept in mind that weather changes necessitating artificial heat with the possibility of smoke entering the problem are not present in Florida in the months when these symptoms are present. This leaves only the neurogenic, psychic or emotional field unexplored.

I spent hours with these patients and I heard many stories of strain, fear, frustration and disappointment which were engendered by their school work. Most of these complaints were, of course, unjustified but nervous trouble does not depend upon true facts or conditions. If the patient thinks they are true the effect is the same as though the fact really existed.

What were some of these findings? At least 80% of these school children stated that "examinations" were approached with fear and trembling, sweating of the palms of the hands, axillary sweat, trembling of the hands and headaches were frequent before, during and after examinations.

A large number of these patients admitted a fear of the consequences and criticisms from their parents, their teachers or their companions if they did not pass or make the honor roll. The fear that they could not enter certain colleges if their grades were not all above 90% was expressed by 21 patients, mostly high school students. Specific instances of clashes of personalities between pupils and certain teachers was another factor, the telling of which was accompanied frequently with tears. Too much homework, too many extra curricular activities such as music, dancing, dramatic courses in addition to school work were frequently causes of the sense of pressure or of being "too pushed for time." The failure to make a club or sorority caused many deep hurts and even went to the extent, in 4 cases, of causing withdrawal from contact with all companions.

In some of these cases attempts were made at readjustments and here are a few examples:

One child had a definite antipathy toward her English teacher and a few of her classmates. She was transferred to another teacher and another class. No other change was made. Her asthmatic seizures disappeared in three weeks.

Another girl in high school was treated unsuccessfully for asthma during two school terms. She broke down and cried because she "couldn't make the honor roll, got dizzy, trembly and wheezy before examinations." The parents were cautioned to reward her if her grades were good and to minimize the importance of the honor roll. Her teacher talked to her and minimized the importance of examinations. The girl's general health improved, her asthmatic attacks became much less severe and fewer in number, and her school grades also improved.

These cases are to me examples of what can be done by removing the emotional factor involved in the production of a spell of asthma or hay fever. I wish to repeat: These children were all in the atopic group under active treatment and I maintain that the maladjustments were not basic causes of the allergic manifestations but I do believe that they added to the sum total of these children's troubles to a point where without their removal results would not have been attained. I do not wish my remarks to be construed as a criticism of our educational system. I simply feel that the emotional element plays a part in the work of not only the gastro-enterologist, the surgeon and other specialists, but also the allergist.

The cases given here are typical examples of many hundreds of similar ones which I have in my files but of which space does not permit a detailed report. While there are exceptions in which psychoneurotic elements seem to *cause* allergic seizures the vast majority can be explained in my mind only on the basis I have mentioned.

It would appear that in certain allergic children, such as those who fall into the category of the 65% mentioned, there is a need for adjustment. Their capacity to meet situations should be studied and corrected, or they should be kept well within the limits of their lessened ability. If this were done, in many instances, their allergic manifestations could then be controlled.

The same holds true for adults. An allergist needs the help of surgeons, laryngologists and other specialists but in my opinion he needs a good psychiatrist's help more often than all the others combined.

Conclusion

The clinical picture presented by the allergic individual is clouded by psychoneurotic manifestations in a great number of patients. Many reactions from medicines and hyposensitization treatments are on a fear basis, and not an allergic one. Many allergic seizures which cannot be explained on a basis of increased exposure to allergens can be explained on the basis of a complicating emotional experience. A neurosis complicating allergy requires recognition and treatment.

TRAUMA AND SYMPTOM FORMATION

Max M. Stern, M.D.

Part I. The Trauma

In the evolution of psychoanalysis, emphasis has shifted from random, incidental events to typical and developmentally determined processes; the role of trauma has receded somewhat into the background. Whereas in Freud's concept the trauma always remained the decisive factor, its character underwent a similar evolution. Incidental traumatic events, such as accidents, seductions, etc., were replaced by rather typical and ubiquitous experiences, such as threat of castration, trauma of birth, etc. Defining a traumatic situation as "a state of overexcitation which cannot be mastered psychically." Freud saw in the traumatic situation at birth the prototype for the affect of anxiety. Primal anxiety, the reaction in a traumatic situation, he explained as a hysterical reminiscence, viz., a purposeless repetition of the physiological processes determined by the traumatic situation at birth. The observation that specific traumata, such as the castration trauma, were influential in the life history of any human being, independent of individual occurrences, led Freud to the hypothesis of the phylogenetic inheritance of typical traumata.

Recent biological investigations enable us to divest the trauma theory of its last vestige of the fortuitous, without the need to have recourse to such somewhat involved concepts.

In a previous study I presented a new concept of trauma following Selye's investigation into the biological reactions in a situation of stress. According to Selye two systemic reactions occur as the result of stress. The first, the shock phase, leads to disorganization, to a failure of vital functions of circulation, respiration and the central nervous system. These *catabiotic processes,* as I have called them, may terminate in primary shock and death. In the stress reaction they are opposed by regulative (countershock) processes, designed to counteract such a failure of vital functions, which I termed "*anabiotic processes.*" Paralleling the concepts of primary (automatic) anxiety and psychic anxiety, I defined *primary trauma as a physiological condition characterized by a failure of homeostasis in a situation of stress: a predominance of catabiotic processes—due to a deficiency of anabiotic (countershock) processes—leads to failures of vital functions.*

Psychic trauma I defined as any experience which elicits an anticipatory repetition of previously experienced primary trauma.

Consequently, the primary trauma must no longer be traced back to birth alone: ". . . it is a danger situation in its own right because of the mechanism of shock which becomes operative throughout life, whenever excessive quantities of stimuli cause a disturbance of the homeostatic equilibrium which cannot be corrected by the usual mechanism."

The prototype of the primary trauma is fleeting shock reactions of the post-natal phase, which includes the first three months of life. These *post-natal primary traumata* are the consequence of a clash between an immature infantile organism and the demands of the external world, which it is not yet biologically equipped to meet. There is an inability to maintain homeostasis; signal processes are deficient.

In the primary traumata of the post-natal phase the deficiency of the homeostatic regulation is compensated by automatic responses of the whole organism; they form the core of the primary defences. The *primary defences* include increase of *motility*—mass movement, crying, as well as relief functions like defecation, urination—and phenomena pertaining to *perception,* such as identification, hallucination, projection, introjection, primary repression. The increase of motility is the basis for the developing aggressive trends. There occurs a *libidinization of primary defences* originating in the libidinization of body functions by the post-natal trauma. In the post-natal phase the primary defences are complemented by libidinal gratification through mothering. Severer frustrations in this phase are answered successively by *agitation* and *catatonoid reaction*, which are morbid primary defences: *agitation* consists of a pathologic increase of primary defences. *The catatonoid reaction,* the last line of defence against shock, is characterized by a generalized slowing down of vital functions, rigidity of musculature, stupor (often alternating with a break-through of agitation-impulses), indicating the larger participation of catabiotic reaction in the defence processes.

The vulnerability of the infantile organism, its tendency toward shock reaction, continues to a lesser extent into the second year of life. During this period of relative immaturity —especially in the later part—sexual overstimulation seems to reproduce the economic constellation of the post-natal trauma: the infantile organism is overwhelmed by sexual excitations which cannot find discharge in an adequate reaction, that is, in full orgasm. Clinical material justifies the assumption that in this phase instinctual over-stimulation during sleep or half-sleep leads to *pavor nocturnus* attacks, which are catatonoid reactions under the condition of sleep. They represent the *infantile trauma*.

Trauma, Mastery and Reparative Mastery

According to the above presented conception, trauma is a regular and essential part of human development. Neurosis, then, is not the effect of these normally occurring traumata, but the result of a *failure of the defence* against them. Inciting an ever-growing urge towards *mastery of reality*, these ubiquitous traumata—*post-natal* as well as *infantile*—may even be regarded as responsible for the enormous development of functions specific to the human species, such as anticipation, learning, etc., which through *mastery of reality* serve to avert the repetition of catastrophic experiences. In addition to the *urge for mastery,* they generate the *urge for belated mastery* of experienced traumata (reparative mastery). *Reparative mastery*—originating in the learning process—is an attempt at retroactive, magic correction, of traumatic experiences which could not be averted. Obviously the anticipatory function—which consists of a projection into the future of an attenuated whole recall of past experiences—would be seriously impaired in its task to prepare for action, if it were to include too many or too severe traumatic memories. Traumata have to be averted even in the attenuated form in which they occur in anticipation. Reparative mastery magically substitutes for the reality of the experienced trauma an imagined reality, in which the trauma is denied or mastered. This mechanism is especially effective in individuals or circumstances in which the process of thinking is either genuinely or regressively magic, as in the play of children, in dreams and fantasies, in rituals, in artistic creations, and finally in neurotic or psychotic disorders. Obviously the exuberant growth of anticipation in man leads to paradoxical effects. Originally generated to avert traumata, anticipation by repeating the traumata, although in an attenuated way, conjures up the danger from which it is supposed to protect.* The anticipatory process represents at once the blessing and the curse of human thinking. It perpetuates mastery and failure. It seems to be responsible for neurosis and psychosis.

A patient who had the fear of becoming insane swung steadily back and forth from the compulsion to conquer this danger through the magic use of the word "crazy" to the fear that just this word would call forth the danger. The double meaning of the word "to conjure" (beschwoeren) mirrors this paradox.

Reparative mastery seems to play a much greater part in the formation of the psychic structure than has hitherto been assumed.

---

* This constitutes the mechanism of "the return of the repressed."

In this paper I wish to show that the failure of reparative mastery of the infantile trauma is one of the determining factors in the formation of dreams and symptoms. In order to present such a concept which tries to clarify the intricate process involved in the genesis of neurosis, it is unavoidable to simplify by telescoping into single dramatic events developmental processes which, stretching over a long period of many years, and leaning on biological and psychological maturation (Hartman, *et al.*), oscillate between progressions and regressions, between phases of break-through of instinctual impulses and defence against them.

The outline of this presentation may be sketched as follows: (1) The infantile trauma is a primary traumatic reaction during sleep or half-sleep due to instinctual overexcitation which cannot be mastered. It can be conceived of as a *primary pavor nocturnus* and represents the *basic infantile trauma*. (2) The attempt at reparative mastery of this trauma seems to be an important function of the dream. (3) *Pavor nocturnus attacks proper* are failures of attempts at reparative mastery of the basic infantile trauma (primal scene) leading to its more or less attenuated repetition. (4) The *infantile trauma* reflected in primal scene and *pavor nocturnus* incites the formation of the castration complex, the extension of which is determined by the *pretraumatic disposition*. (5) *Neurosis* seems to be a consequence of the *failure of reparative mastery* of the infantile trauma; this failure leads to the breakthrough of the repressed, to a recall of the trauma. The ensuing anxiety has to be bound by symptom formation.

The Basic Infantile Trauma (Primal Scene)

Freud stated that "the oldest experiences of childhood are no longer to be obtained as such, but will be replaced in the analysis by 'transference and dreams.'" The primary trauma, viz., shock, is the experience *par excellence* that cannot "be obtained as such," owing to the blocking of registration (primary repression). It can be disclosed only through the above described signs of shock processes. Generally we may say that *signs of physiological shock in psychic phenomena, such as dreams or symptoms, etc., reveal these phenomena as reminiscence of previously experienced primary traumata.*

Now, clinical material shows that when signs referring to shock appear in a dream, reminiscences of *the primal scene* often appear also.

The following dream occurred after a patient had overheard sounds from an adjacent room where his friend (John) and the latter's girl-friend were sleeping:

"I am in a room with John. Then I am with his sister in the room next door. It is a kitchen. There is a 'Primus' stove. The head of the Primus is glowing, red, burning hot. It glows more and more. A terrific heat. I have *difficulty in breathing* and *feel black before my eyes*. Then the Primus blows up. I am *falling, stumbling*. I want to reach the door. I can't. Finally I succeed in breaking the window, at the last moment, and wake up." (A "Primus" meant also the third inhabitant in the room of a married couple.) The associations to "sister," "kitchen," Primus = penis, blowing up = orgasm, led to the oedipal situation and primal scene.

While *going under ether* a woman had the following hallucination: "The first sensation was enormous terror, a feeling of being violated. Then there came a kind of dream, as though I were climbing a mountain. Then I saw from each side of the mountain a sun rising; the two suns came closer and closer to each other, finally they met at the top and collided." She explained: "Two sexes met." Here we have the reverse: the anæsthesia revived a primal scene experience.

In both dreams the difficulties of breathing, the falling, the blacking-out, etc., which we recognize as shock symptoms, are connected with reminiscences of the primal scene. Are we allowed to assume that the child undergoes the primal-scene experience in a shock-like state?

In his *History of an Infantile Neuroses* Freud traces the *pavor nocturnus* dream about the wolves to the patient's witnessing a coitus between the parents at the age of one and a half. The child, Freud surmises, had finally interrupted the parents' intercourse; it had reacted to the traumatic experience by crying and defecation. Now, little is known about such immediate demonstrative reaction of children to the intercourse of parents. On the other hand, analytic experience seems to confirm over and over again Freud's concept of the link between the primal scene and *pavor nocturnus*. Our assumption that *the child undergoes the primal scene experience in a shock-like state, a state of catatonoid paralysis,* would solve the difficulty.

In his interpretation of the "Wolf Man" dream, Freud shifts the *attentive staring of the white wolves* sitting on the tree, through reversal, onto the sleeping child. The child "awoke and looked with *strained attention at the parents' intercourse."* I think that similarly we are allowed to shift the *motionlessness of the wolves,* which is especially emphasized by the patient, onto the child: *the child witnessed the primal scene in a state of immobility, overwhelmed by a paralysing fright reaction, in a catatonoid reaction.* Associations of dying reinforce this interpretation; they refer to the white colour of the wolves, leading to memories of the sick and dying white sheep, which, through identification, express the child's fear of death.

There have been various explanations for the effect of the "primal scene" upon the child. The concept of the sadistic misunderstanding is well known. We cannot deal extensively here with the problem of the primal scene on the basis of clinical material. Whether the "primal scene" is an actual occurrence, or a belated elaboration of sexual experiences in fantasies or in dreams, or a conglomeration of all these, can perhaps never be fully cleared up. In many cases, the striking role of noises, which during sleep penetrate through to the child's mind, points to a participation of at least some real happenings during the night.

The core of the primal scene is the oedipal situation, in which the child inevitably is *the excluded third part.* Being restricted to the role of passionate watching, the child's urge for sexual gratification is shifted to scoptophilia and identification. Infantile masturbation becomes the executive of the ensuing oedipal fantasies. However, owing to its unsatisfying character as well as to prohibitive measures (threats), masturbation must create additional tensions. I think we have not always considered the full import of the fact that the infantile organism is not able adequately to discharge sexual excitation; the child is not capable of full orgasm. Freud states that in infantile masturbation "*something is always lacking for full discharge* and gratification . . . and *this thing which is lacking, the reaction of orgasm,* finds equivalent expressions in other fields."

The Infantile Orgasm

Dealing with the problem of infantile orgasm Kinsey differentiates correctly between the *orgastic reflex* and the *orgastic pleasure sensation.* Orgastic reflexes prior to sexual maturity have been observed in a number of individuals. "Orgasm has been observed in boys of every age from five months to adolescence." If we evaluate the statistics critically (excluding e.g. the prepuberty age), then the number of observed orgastic reactions appears to be much slighter. Often, especially in younger children, the orgastic reflex reactions seem to be accompanied by marked signs of displeasure (weeping, abundance of tears 'especially among younger children').

It is difficult to determine exactly how the orgastic reflex discharges differ between infantile and mature individuals; it seems to me that the former is most often rather incomplete. But the most striking difference lies in the overpowering character of the *orgastic pleasure sensations* in mature orgasm, amounting to a complete extinction of the ego. Individuals who had masturbated before reaching sexual maturity clearly describe the break-through of mature orgasm, which occurred with the first seminal ejaculation, as something utterly different from their pre-adolescent orgastic experiences.

One patient, who since his eighth year had masturbated with a kind of orgastic climax, fought strenuously against his impulse, until he was overwhelmed by a full orgasm upon his first ejaculation. Under the impact of this experience, he abandoned his struggle for some time and masturbated daily.

Infantile orgasm, where it occurs, seems to be merely an abortive form of mature orgasm; it may suitably be described as *"orgasmoid."* In younger children it often involves such manifestations as sobbing or hysterical laughter, violent movements of arms and legs, sadistic and masochistic reactions, collapse, fainting, etc., indicating that pre-infantile orgasm is frequently connected with defensive reactions against shock.

Evidently the infantile orgasm is biologically incapable of sustaining the powerful excitation of the full orgastic pleasure sensation. In the waking state, the mechanisms of defence and discharge into motility as well as inhibition may prove effective in warding off excessive sexual excitation. However, they appear to be inadequate under the conditions of sleep: owing to the regressive, narcissistic body cathexis during sleep, there is in sleep a short circuit between ideation and body functions manifested in such phenomena as enuresis and nocturnal emissions (wet dreams).

Thus at night the child is unprotected against the breakthrough of over-strong sexual excitation, which throws it into a shock-like state.*

It seems very significant that the fear of orgasm is most often expressed in terms of shock sensations: *suffocating, falling, fainting, fading into nothingness,* etc., which explains the frequently quoted similarity between orgasm and dying. To neurotics the orgastic experience is more or less a threat; their sexual function is characterized by rather orgasmoid discharges.

We conclude: what is called "primal scene" is a primary traumatic situation in sleep or half-sleep, due to sexual overexcitation; it is a *primary pavor nocturnus* and represents the *basic infantile trauma*. The witnessing of the parents' intercourse seems to be only a partial factor in what constitutes the basic infantile trauma. Its typical occurrence is due to a pre-

---

* This hypothesis is confirmed by the observation that periods of infantile *pavor nocturnus* are often replaced by enuresis.

cocious libidinal development, a result of the precocious libidinization through the post-natal trauma.

In addition to sexual immaturity experience and environment play their part in the genesis of the infantile trauma. They create the *pretraumatic disposition* which will be discussed later.

Since object-conditioned sexual excitations begin as early as the end of the first year of life, we can safely place the occurrence of the *basic infantile trauma* within the period of relative shock-sensitivity, which extends to the end of the second year.

These considerations may explain why pathogenic excitations invariably seem to arise from the instincts of sexual life; they might fill the "gap in our theory," thus confirming Freud's opinion that "it is not psychology, but biology which is responsible for this gap."

Pavor Nocturnus and Infantile Trauma

Freud stated that the dreams which bring back a recollection of the psychic traumata of childhood do not permit a classification under the category of wish fulfilment. Actually they fulfil another function of the mental apparatus: namely, the attempt to master experienced traumata.

In view of the close connection between the basic infantile trauma (primal scene) and *pavor nocturnus,* it appears likely that the latter denotes a failure to achieve, in dreams, a reparative mastery of the basic trauma. The failure leads to a repetition of the original trauma, similar to the dreams of a traumatic neurosis. Fully developed *pavor nocturnus* attacks (nightmares) have to be understood as *repetition of the basic infantile trauma,* due to a failure of its reparative mastery. In children, this failure is due to relative immaturity; in adults, passive feminine or masochistic trends seem to be responsible for it.

Actually the manifold phenomena of fully developed *pavor nocturnus* attacks (nightmare), such as the inability to breathe, the feeling of oppression in the chest, the feeling of having an iron band around the head, of the shrinking of the body, withering, becoming rigid like stone or wood, sensations of depersonalization, of fainting, falling, etc., can be traced back to the somatic manifestations of the shock mechanism. They clearly point to a *progressive paralysis* affecting motility as well as the vital functions of circulation and respiration, denoting the failure of reparative mastery and the recurrence of the reactions of the basic infantile trauma. *Pavor nocturnus* may therefore be said to encompass all dreams in which the actual occurrence of shock reaction—especially the motor-paralysis reflected in the ability to move, to cry—indicate a relative failure of the attempt at reparative mastery.

Pavor Nocturnus Dreams

The *paralysis of motility* in *pavor nocturnus* dreams, i.e., the inability to move or scream, is so well known that it requires no special illustration. The successive phases of defences against shock mentioned above—namely, the phases of agitation and of the catatonoid reaction—are reflected in the dreams in which *increased motility,* such as running, climbing, etc., is followed by *paralysis,* as for instance in the typical persecution dreams. The dreamer is persecuted; he runs, but his movements are slow, inhibited; finally he is glued to the spot. The following dream presents an interesting variation:

"I came down a long *stairway*. Beneath the stairway I saw a *corpse,* straightened out, completely *flattened* as if by a barrel, the *toes sticking up* into the air. A *big black dog* wanted to jump at me, to *eat me*. I *ran away* and *leaped* through the front door with the dog after me, but I *remained hanging in mid-air*. I *couldn't move*. Suddenly I fell and awoke in terror."

Here we have a number of typical elements of *pavor nocturnus*. The catatonoid paralysis is *projected* into the *flattened corpse,* reminiscent of the flattened body in Tausk's "Influencing Machine"; the dog represents the *anxiety animal,* into which the threat from the sexual excitation is projected; the toe sticking up represents *denial of castration;* and finally, there is the *oral fear* of *being bitten*.

In Freud's "Staircase Dream," in which incompletely dressed he *jumps with ease* up a *flight of stairs* and is then *glued to the steps*, the *circulatory* and *respiratory* difficulties of the shock complex (which appear with the *inhibition of motility*) are, through reversal into the opposite, represented by the ease in *mounting the stairs;* the real meaning is revealed through the associations: *bronchial coughing—cardiac trouble*—sad thoughts about *death* which are connected with masturbation fears, viz., with the punishment for the uncontrollable, dirty vice of smoking, a substitute for masturbation.

A functional determinant of inhibited motility in dreams seems to be the frustrated wish to wake up, to escape the danger, the paralysis of motility thus reflecting the paralysis of the awakening function.*

Phenomena such as falling, sliding, gliding, fainting, fading away, sensations of a ring pressing upon the head, being anæsthetized, drowning, point to reactions of the *central nervous system*. Narcosis not infrequently revives the infantile sexual trauma. The disturbances of the vestibular functions are especially important. They involve disturbances of equilibrium, dizziness, changes of space perception, of body feelings and of the body image, such as enlargement, shrinking, impairment and fragmentation of the body, etc. In psychoanalytic practice, we are in the habit of stating, when sensations of this kind come up, such as unclear rotating objects, rhythmically approaching and receding objects, that *primal scene* material is approaching. The hypnagogic phenomena described by Isakower, as well as other hypnagogic phenomena, such as the sensations of falling, the rotating screen described by Lewin, etc., also seem to belong in this category. These vestibular sen-

---

* In passing, I would like to mention symbols in mythology which mirror the motor inhibition in *pavor nocturnus*, pointing up its connection with the primal scene: the Medusa, the sight of which turns the beholder into stone; Lot's wife, petrified by looking at the forbidden scene; the youth fainting away as he lifts the veil from the image of Sais; the tale of Bluebeard, and many others. The meaning of these symbols is: the primal scene turns the onlooker into stone or kills him.

sations, referring to changes of body feeling and body image (shrinking, swelling, fragmentation, etc.), play an important part in the formation of the castration complex, in line with the well-known equation: body equals phallus. We shall deal with it later.

Through the mechanism of projection, the body sensations during sleep are treated as though they were of external origin. *The threat from the paralysis of vital functions in pavor nocturnus is experienced as an external threat:* as a vampire sitting on the sleeper's chest, etc.; sensations such as fainting and withering are experienced as a crumbling of houses or of walls, or as earthquakes, etc.

In the dream: "I was attacked by a man; I shot at him, but the bullet came out very slowly and slowly trickled down to the ground," the inhibition of motility is projected onto the bullet. In the *pavor nocturnus* dream reported by Helene Deutsch, the terrifying, soft crumbling-away of the wall which separates the sleeper's room from that of his parents represents a condensation of shock sensations with the primal scene. We might apply the same interpretation to Freud's dream about "the men with the sparrow-hawk beaks carrying the dying mother"; the mother's *comatose condition* reflects the sleeper's reaction to the primal scene.

Of the many threatening objects in *pavor nocturnus,* like shadows, ghosts, demons, etc., the anxiety animals deserve special mention. Horses, bulls, dogs, wolves are well known as such, but anxiety animals also include spiders, octopuses, snakes, scorpions, bugs and bats, cockroaches, etc. For the latter, a patient gave the significant association: "They catch you unaware"—expressing the helplessness of being unprepared for the overwhelming shock, and also the uncanniness of the whole *pavor nocturnus* experience. In some cases the crawling of the bugs stood for the unpleasantness of sexual stimulation of skin and mucosa (tickling). Here we have the origin of manifold phobias, phobias of dogs, horses, wolves, spiders, ants, etc.

The anxiety in *pavor nocturnus* is almost invariably linked up with oral trends: being devoured, bitten by wolves, dogs, or swallowed by spiders, by octopuses, etc. These trends are due to a regression to oral sadistic defences against the threat; they indicate the revival of postnatal, traumatic experiences in *pavor nocturnus,* and point to the role of the *predisposition* in the formation of the oedipal trauma. It goes without saying that in addition to reparative mastery the factors which produced the basic trauma (instinctual wish fulfilment under the conditions of sleep, pretraumatic disposition, etc.) are likewise influential in the genesis of *pavor nocturnus.*

Pretraumatic Disposition

As mentioned above, experiential and environmental factors play a very important part in the genesis of the infantile trauma. Earlier shock experiences (post-natal shock), resulting in over-libidinization of body functions and increased libidinal dependence, previous frustrations of instinctual satisfaction and relief (oral, anal-urethral), aggressions, seduction, as well as prohibitions and threats from parents or parental figures, castration threats, nonsexual traumata such as accidents and operations and last but not least preceding basic traumata—all these anxiety-producing factors not only increase tension, but, through the sexual stimulation generated by fear, they add to the sexual excitation in the traumatic situation. I should like to define the role of the described pretraumatic experiences by saying that they create the *predisposition* determining the impact of the infantile trauma on the child. Neurosis, which seems to be due to a failure to cope with the normally occurring oedipal traumata, might then be explained in terms of the predisposition for the oedipal trauma.

Aggression against a parent, which figures most prominently in the majority of interpretations of *pavor nocturnus,* seems to be determined—apart from pre-oedipal and para-oedipal factors—by the child's desperate defence against the threat of being overwhelmed by shock which is projected onto the parent.

Conclusion

We have defined the primal scene dream as the basic infantile trauma (primary *pavor nocturnus*). *Pavor nocturnus* attacks were understood to be due to a failure of reparative mastery of the basic infantile trauma. This certainly is an abstraction which necessarily does not reflect the real sequence of events in childhood, about the details of which we have as yet no precise insight and which suggest a dialectic rather than a straightforward progression. We might be dealing with phases of libidinal activity followed by a series of defensive phases. One or more primal-scene experiences may be followed by a phase of defensive latency, later to be succeeded by a renewed libidinal break-through leading to *pavor nocturnus* attacks (cf. the Wolf Man dream). It appears—this might be said with all caution—that an initial onset of a *pavor nocturnus* phase occurs around the beginning of the second year, possibly terminating the period of early infantile sexuality and initiating a reinforcement of anal-sadistic mastery. This seems to be followed by a second onset at the age of three or four, based on renewed libidinal activity due to endocrine intensification comparable to the break-through of infantile sexuality in puberty. As with the onset of neurosis, the onset of a *pavor nocturnus* phase may be precipitated by specific experiences: e.g. operations, dreams, frustrations, sexual excitations, etc.

Effects of the Infantile Trauma

The recurrence of the previous primary basic trauma in *pavor nocturnus* turns the *infantile pavor nocturnus* into a more or less self-perpetuating trauma. With regard to its genetic effect, *pavor nocturnus* for many reasons takes over the pathogenic impact of the primal scene. For the purpose of this presentation we therefore hardly go far wrong if we simplify in subsuming both occurrences under the term of *infantile pavor nocturnus*, regarding the latter as the representative of the infantile trauma.

In order to evaluate the far-reaching effects of the infantile trauma, we have to take into consideration the fact that the hallucinations in *pavor nocturnus* assume an immeasurably stronger reality character than do ordinary dream hallucinations, partly because they correspond to *realistic, i.e. somatic sensations,* and, further, because *during the stage of awakening, a realistic character is imparted to the hallucinations by the only gradually reviving function of reality. Thus, like real occurrences, the hallucinations in infantile pavor nocturnus exert a formative influence throughout life*—which is of basic importance for the understanding of the origin of neurosis in general and of the formation of the castration complex in particular.

Pavor Nocturnus and Castration Complex

We ascribe the origin of castration anxiety, which, strangely enough, exists in equal strength in both sexes, to threats of castration, the sight of female genitals, sadistic misunderstanding, masturbation fears, etc. But it requires *an actual experience of real and severe danger* to give effective power to these fears and fantasies. This happens when the child is brought close to shock as a consequence of genital stimulation. The genital stimulation in *pavor nocturnus* is turned into a threat to the genitals which—through projection—is experienced as coming from parental figures, who actually incited the dangerous stimulation. They appear as castrating figures, as anxiety animals, burglars, ghosts, etc.

A patient dreamt: "I was asleep. I woke up, *obviously in sleep,* and discovered a man *sucking my penis with tremendous intensity.* I was conscious of the shape of his head and his hair. He pinned down my hips. I was struggling to get away from him. I was unable to move. I was pinned down."—This dream presents a condensation of catatonoid immobility with threatening genital stimulation.—In the following dream the castration anxiety appears undisguised: "A huge figure of a man coming from the right, *towering over* me with his big shoulder. I was paralysed, not able to move, to fight back; I was afraid of his coming closer and closer, of his hurting me. Suddenly his *right hand* reached out and *grabbed my genitals*. I jumped up, snapped into consciousness. I still felt rigid and frightened, and I was convinced that some one was in the room: *a burglar*."

Several patients who masturbated by tying a rope around the penis had fantasies of being strangled, choked to death, "as if someone ties a rope around your neck so that you choke, no circulation, and you die" (body-phallus) showing the connection between shock and castration. A girl was convinced that cutting the penis meant immediate death, through suffocation or heart failure.

I am inclined to see in the *infantile trauma represented in pavor nocturnus the ultimate origin of the castration trauma*, thus evaluating the hitherto accepted sources of castration anxiety as predisposing factors which determine its extent. Through the realistic body sensations and the reality quality of the hallucinations in *pavor nocturnus*, the fears of injury to the genitals acquire a power which remains effective throughout life. They keep the fear of death and of castration intimately connected.*

Part II. Infantile Trauma and Neurosis

In his important paper, "Fear, Guilt and Hate," Jones assumed that neurosis arises "out of the infant's response to the primal 'traumatic' situation and consequently to the oedipus danger that later developed out of it."

The symptom is a defence against castration anxiety. In view of the role of the infantile trauma in the formation of the castration complex, it is not surprising that the study of *pavor nocturnus* provides a rich store of information for the understanding of symptom formation. In many instances the causal connection between *pavor nocturnus* and specific symptoms is quite clearly apparent from the content of the latter. Often,

* One of the most archaic myths in the Bible points to *pavor nocturnus* as the origin of circumcision: Jahveh attacks Moses during the night, in order to kill him; the wife (or mother) saves him through performing the circumcision. Jacob's fight with the angel at night results in castration. (Hip literally means genital region.)

particularly in children, the beginning of a neurosis or psychosis is marked by an attack of *pavor nocturnus*. It is not unusual for patients to begin their stories with an account of nightmares; their earliest recollections seem to represent screen memories for infantile *pavor nocturnus* experiences.

The following examples demonstrate the import of the *pavor nocturnus* for the onset of neurosis, as well as for the content of symptoms, showing especially the significance of the confusion of dream hallucinations and reality, and the persistence of *pavor nocturnus* sensations in the manifest symptoms.

In the case of *Little Hans* the phobia began with a *pavor nocturnus* and was accompanied by anxiety attacks while going to sleep. The child's account of the anxiety dream—"I thought you were gone and I had no Mummy to coax with"—seems to represent merely this reaction to it; i.e. the cry for the mother. Later, the boy was afraid at night *that a horse would come into his room.*

In Freud's "History of an Infantile Neurosis," the manifest infantile neurosis starts with the dream of the wolves, a *pavor nocturnus* referring to the primal scene. This dream was the Leitmotif of the analysis extending over a number of years. The patient stated in a later letter published by Ferenczi: "The wolf-dream I told at the beginning of the treatment; the solution came only at the end of the treatment. The wolf-dream always seemed to be in the centre of my childhood dreams."— His screen memories—the governess saying: "Do look at my little tail"—obviously point to his *pavor nocturnus*.

In his paper on the *Schreber case,* Freud writes about the onset of the paranoic delusion: "One morning . . . while he was in a *state between sleeping and waking* the idea occurred to him, 'that after all it really must be very nice to be a woman submitting to the act of copulation.' "

Abraham traced back the onset of a phobia with hallucinations of animals to a *pavor nocturnus* attack following the witnessing of the parents' intercourse. The child, after having slept for a good hour, called for her mother with *screams of fear*. The girl could not distinguish between dream and reality. During the next days she had pronounced anxiety attacks in the evening, hallucinations of *animals,* marked astasia, abasia, and fear of falling.

In *Schnurmann's* case, a two-years-and-five-months-old girl "woke up screaming in the early evening shortly after falling asleep and insisted that a dog was in her bed . . . a few days later she started being afraid of dogs in the street, getting into a panic whenever she could discern a dog even at a great distance."

Brenner's interesting case of hallucinosis in a three-and-a-half-year-old child belongs in the same category. The number of examples quoted from the literature could be increased *ad libitum*.

Pavor Nocturnus and Symptom

In a *phobia of the dark,* the patient, a man of thirty-two, used to be seized at the onset of night by a panicky fear that he would fall, lose his head, that something like a polyp or an octopus would come out of the darkness and devour him. In his treatment actual *pavor nocturnus* attacks and childhood memories of night terrors played a great role. The analysis of a *pavor nocturnus* dream brought matters to a crisis. The associations led to the primal scene; the interpretation that the terrifying polyp meant the parents in the coital embrace brought on a panicky reaction: "I can't go on; my head, my head! Leave me alone, things are going black before my eyes." He struck wildly about him, sat up: "I am choking, I am choking!"—Violent anxiety attacks which followed could be worked through, whereupon the phobia of the dark diminished considerably and finally disappeared, except for some slight remnants.

A spider phobia of a girl of five started with a spider falling into her hair, and developed into a fear of touching a spider, and finally into an avoidance of touching the walls lest she touch a spider. This fear was a condensation of masturbation fears connected with various elements of *pavor nocturnus*. The spider and its web reminded her of sensations of *pavor nocturnus* "in which you are caught unawares, immobilized and swallowed up" (catatonoid reaction combined with oral fears). The gigantic eyes of the spider were a projection of her scoptophilia originating in the primal scene, combined with the fear of being watched in masturbation. The spider finally meant her genitals, and it reminded the girl of an operation upon her mother's genitals after which she saw the shaved-off pubic region (castration).

A fascinating example of the import of *pavor nocturnus* for the *onset* as well as for the *symptomatology* of a *psychosis* can be found in the autobiography of a schizophrenic girl (Sechehaye). Renée describes the onset of her psychosis at the age of five: "I remember very well when it happened. I was passing a school; I stopped to *listen* to a singing lesson, and at that instant a strange feeling came over me, a disturbing sense of *unreality*.— (It seems to me that I no longer recognized the school.)—The school had *become as large as a barracks;* the singing children were *prisoners* compelled to sing. At the same time my eye encountered a field of wheat *whose limits I could not see.* The yellow *vastness,* dazzling in the sun, bound up with the song of the children imprisoned in the school-barracks, filled me with such anxiety that I broke into sobs. . . . One day we were jumping rope at recess. When it came my turn and I saw my partner jump toward me where we were to meet and cross over, I was seized with *panic.* I *did not recognize* her. Standing at the other end of the rope, she had seemed smaller, but the nearer we approached each other, *the taller she grew, the more she swelled* in size. I cried out, 'Stop, Alice, you look like a lion; you frighten me!' " (italics mine).

Renée's report reveals distinctly sensations corresponding to those in *pavor nocturnus* (catatonoid reaction), as described above: it started with listening to noises; her body feelings were projected: the motor-paralysis appeared in the imprisoned children, the vestibular disturbances in the enlarged school, in the yellow, limitless vastness, and in the alarming swelling in size of the jumping schoolmates who are turned into anxiety animals; sensations accompanied by feelings of estrangement and overwhelming anxiety. We are tempted to assume that these attacks are attenuated repetitions of previous *pavor nocturnus* experiences.

Renée continues: "Suddenly I saw the resemblance of this phenomenon to my nightmare of 'the needle in the hay.' It was a dream that recurred often . . . and it caused me the most frightful anguish. *Later I always associated my unreal perceptions with the dream of the needle.*" (Italics mine.) Here is the dream: "A barn, brilliantly illuminated by electricity. The walls painted white, smooth—smooth and shining. In the *immensity,* a *needle*—fine, pointed, hard, glittering in the light. The *needle in the emptiness* filled me with *excruciating terror.* Then a haystack fills up the emptiness and *engulfs the needle.* The haystack, small at first, swells and swells; and in the centre the needle, endowed with tremendous electrical force, communicates its charge to the hay. The electrical current, the invasion by the hay, and the blinding light combine to augment the fear to a paroxysm of terror, and I woke up screaming, 'The needle, the needle!' What happened during the rope game was the same sort of thing: tension, something growing inordinately, and anxiety."

The needle, fine, pointed, hard, endowed with tremendous electrical force and lost in the immensity of unlimited space, represents the patient herself in the nightmare, and expresses the immobile rigidity and the overwhelming tension of the catatonoid state. In her subsequent psychotic seizures, Renée repeats over and over again her *pavor nocturnus* experience.

Renée's case is a striking illustration of the description of patients recovering from catatonia, who compared this condition with nightmares; they felt paralysed, and experienced this as being overwhelmed by external forces, such as hypnotic influences, electric currents, etc. There may be a causal connection between *pavor nocturnus* and the well-known paranoid hallucinations of machines, destroying the body by electric currents. (We encounter the sensations of electric current not infrequently in the *pavor nocturnus* attacks of our patients.) Renée writes: "I discovered that the persecutor was none other than the electric machine." Tausk's "influencing machine" appears to be a projection of a catatonoid *pavor nocturnus* state.

Again and again, in our clinical work as well as in literature, we come across phenomena which we are able to identify as originating from *pavor nocturnus,* if we are familiar with the described characteristic shock signs. It seems that the role of *pavor nocturnus* as a manifestation of the infantile trauma in symptom formation cannot be easily overestimated.

Reparative Mastery and Symptom Formation

It is not the purpose of this paper to describe the highly involved process of symptom formation in all its stages. Rather, it is intended to highlight one particular factor in this process; namely, the part which is played in it by reparative mastery of the infantile trauma.

Let us very briefly recapitulate Freud's ideas on symptom formation. Freud attributes the ultimate cause of neurosis to the process of repression; the infantile ego treats the majority of the sexual impulses as dangers and wards them off. The warded-off impulses continue to exist in the id as unconscious fantasies. Now, an unconscious fantasy "is actually identical with the fantasy which served the person in his sexual gratification during the period of masturbation." Under certain conditions—intensification of instinctual drives owing to the physical maturation during puberty, specific situations which re-activate repressed wishes—the unconscious fantasy is restimulated and will achieve expression of at least part of its content in the form of a morbid symptom. The symptom is "a sign of, and a substitute for, an instinctual gratification which has remained in abeyance."

According to Freud the repression occurred under the pressure of an external threat, imagined or real, viz. the castration, and was directed against the instinctual impulse bringing about the danger situation. Freud puts the question: why does this impulse—when restimulated at a more mature age—still continue to be warded off as a threat although the external *danger* situation no longer exists? He explained this as the consequence of the repression and the repetition compulsion of the id. Freud ascribes to the repetition compulsion an almost demonic power.

Since we conceive repression not merely as the reaction to an imagined threat (castration), but ultimately as the consequence of an actually experienced trauma (oedipal shock) through which alone the castration threat really becomes effective, we are able to formulate a hypothesis of symptom formation, while remaining within the frame of reparative mastery of a past trauma.

The most primitive way of reparative mastery seems to be active repetition of a passively experienced trauma.* Freud

---

* The urge to master the trauma which obeys the relief principle often overrides the pleasure principle, as e.g. in masochism. However, the pleasure principle comes again into its own in the libidinization of the reparative repetition.

states that to the Wolf Man the *repetition* of the trauma of the *primal scene* became the condition for his recovery. He writes: "... in this condition ('getting an enema from his servant') the patient was simply repeating the state of affairs at the time of the so-called primal scene. He remained fixed as though by a spell to the scene which had such decisive effect upon his sexual life, and *the return of which during the night of the dream brought the onset of his illness*." (Italics mine.)

The urge for reparative mastery seems to be ever present. It comes to the fore in dreams, fantasies and symptoms. It is especially strong when going to sleep, corresponding to the need for elimination of all unsettled wishes. This accounts for the widespread sleep-disturbing phenomena in childhood, such as fear of falling asleep, the Isakower phenomenon, insomnia, etc.

The Wolf Man writes in the above-mentioned report: "After ... (the wolf dream) ... I was afraid of similar dreams. As a preventive measure, I used, therefore, when going to sleep to imagine vividly all things I feared, and amidst them this dream."

The *phenomena associated with falling asleep,* as described by Isakower, are hallucinations containing rather successful reparative repetitions of *pavor nocturnus,* in which the reactivation of oral shock experiences is especially marked. Not even the waking up in fright is lacking. The patient's remark: "The condition brings about unpleasant tension with following release" points to the undoing of the trauma in the hallucination. The cloudy masses formed like a cylinder represented in my cases breast and penis, undoing the oral trauma as well as the castration. Often the patients purposely provoked the attack, or they tried to hold on to it deliberately, rationalizing that they want to recognize "what it's all about."

A patient reported: "After the *(pavor nocturnus)* attacks, I turned on this feeling at will by turning onto my back and tensing my muscles. I wanted to see whether I could move my jaw or tongue, but I couldn't." A patient with a phobia of scorpions reported that "scorpions always fascinated me. I had to look at them until I felt chilled unto my spine; then I yelled or ran away." The Little Hans' fear of horses became transformed more and more into an obsession for looking at them. Later, Hans tried to master the trauma in playing the falling horse.

In contradistinction to *pavor nocturnus* dreams or anxiety dreams, a great number of common dreams can easily be discerned as *successful* mastery of the infantile trauma. In the following dreams this meaning is quite obvious.

"I was falling, falling, and was deadly afraid of being killed when landing. Then I felt, 'I am indestructible.'"

"I was about to fall into an abyss; then I took a pill of bellacornal and dreamed that I went on sleeping." (On a certain occasion I had once advised this patient to take bellacornal.) In this dream, he takes refuge in a measure which in the oral phase protected him against shock.

The *flying dream* appears to be a successful elaboration of the falling dream. A variation of the flying dream is the diving dream of a patient: "I was in a large pool, bright, transparent, very clear, you could look through it. I was diving, moving around like a seal, effortlessly, with open eyes, a sensation like flying. A seal came, bumped into me. I grasped his fin and his tail. He pulled me along, up and down, he turned around and bit me in the way a puppy bites."—The reparative mastery is represented in the denial of the fear of being drowned or bitten, and in the playful character of the anxiety animal.

In other dreams the attempt at mastery of the trauma is less obvious. One example may serve for many: "I am quarrelling with a woman. She said, 'At last we will have a baby.' I, overjoyed, embraced her, put all my weight onto her and felt she wouldn't like that."—This dream was the patient's reaction to the news that his wife was pregnant, which threw him into anxiety about being tied down, crushed. A screen memory of the primal scene, frequently mentioned in his analysis, referred to his parents' "quarrelling in the other room." In the dream, the primal scene is reversed; he takes the place of the quarrelling father: not being pressed down, but pressing down in aggressive defence against the threat. The same patient dreamt: "I was in a church; medieval groups were quarrelling (the parents' primal scene). I *decided* to become one of the statues at the pillars." (Active decision replaces passive immobilization.)

This enlarges the scope of dream interpretation and enables us to identify such a considerable number of dreams as more or less strongly disguised elaborations of the infantile trauma, that we are inclined to recognize, with Freud, in the reparative mastery of trauma an important function of the dream. The dream repairs as well as perpetuates the trauma.

As to the unconscious fantasies—"the first preliminary stage in the mind of a symptom" which according to Freud originate from masturbation fantasies after the manipulative performance has been renounced—we are actually able to discern their content not only in dreams and hypnagogic phenomena but in the *play of children,* in *day-dreams,* and in the *fantasies* which accompany sexual activities. All these manifestations contain *attempts at reparative repetition of the infantile trauma.* This has been convincingly demonstrated by Freud, Melanie Klein, Erikson, Bornstein, and Anna Freud. The large role played by the anxiety-animals in children's fantasies and games points to the nature of the trauma: the animal which recalls the overwhelming anxiety of the *pavor nocturnus* is in the reparative fantasy turned into a protector against the threat.

The boy in Berta Bornstein's "Analysis of a Phobic Child," used to listen anxiously to the noises at night. In his fantasies he played the role of God and "made the analyst a frightened, sleeping child into whose ears God whispered dreams of wild colliding horses, of violent scenes in which 'Daddy throws Mummy out of the window. . . .' "

The reparative function of *the day-dreams* of adults—which are the successors of the child's play and which are reflected in poetic and other artistic creations—is elucidated in Freud's remark: "If at the end of one chapter the hero is left unconscious and bleeding from severe wounds, I am sure to find him at the beginning of the next being carefully tended and on the way to recovery."

In another paper, I have demonstrated that *free paintings* of adult neurotics (i.e. paintings which are produced by way of free associations) represent attempts at reparative mastery of infantile traumata, represented by the oedipal triad: primal scene, *pavor nocturnus* and masturbation.

It seems that the unconscious fantasies which repeat the

trauma find their expression in day-dreams, play, and action only if the revived trauma is altered in the sense of reparative mastery.

The Masturbation Fantasy

The *typical masturbation fantasy* into which, according to Anna Freud, "the whole past era of infantile sexuality and aggression has been compressed" and which is "the sole carrier of the child's sexuality" combines the gratification of the sexual impulse with attempts at reparative mastery of the infantile trauma connected with it.

In the above reported case of the *spider phobia,* the patient used to masturbate in adolescence while listening to the noises from her parents' bedroom, to the father's snoring, with the well-known masochistic fantasy of being a slave who was being tied to a tree (immobilized) and whipped. This masturbation fantasy developed from the infantile trauma via attempts at its reparative repetition.

She described her nightmare at the age of five: "I often woke up in the middle of the night from noises I had heard. I had had a terrible dream. I was not able to scream. I *could not move.* I petrified and felt that I was going to die. I did not have these nightmares when I was with my grandparents." Another time she reported: "In these years I couldn't go to sleep. I used to look at the *shadow on the walls* and to listen to the groaning-moaning *noises* father made in the other room. These noises sounded like dying, someone dying. Horrible thoughts went through my mind, of a *burglar* who would come through the window in the front of the house, or through the window of the kitchen. I asked myself through what window. I felt, now he is already in the house. He is coming into *my* room, because I am alone. *I let these images fill up my mind, until I couldn't stand it* any more. *It was like a nightmare, only that I was awake.* I knew it was silly, but finally I had to wake up my mother. I *whispered* until she came, and then I saw her alive she looked human, warm, like mother, not like shadows in the dark, which I saw in my fantasies, and which had no depth Later I felt more and more I shouldn't do it; it was lik *masturbation.* I was afraid that mother would known that had done it, that it was a kind of masturbation. They yelled a me, father hit me, I was ashamed, finally I stopped it." In the latency period—at the age of nine or ten—she developed a compulsive ritual. She reported: "When I went to bed and when I woke up in the night, which happened frequently, I had *to lie straight in the bed,* covered up tight way up to my neck; then I listened for *noises, without moving.* Next I *looked* from corner to corner, then from window to window, then to the door, while I remained *motionless* in the bed. *Next I sat up very quickly, perfectly straight, without making any noise, and looked out of the window.* This took away my anxiety; I lay down again and went to sleep."

Here we can follow the development from the libidinally cathected attempts at reparative repetition of the infantile trauma in the oedipal phase via the compulsive ritual of the latency to the masochistic masturbation fantasies of the adolescence. The attempts at reparative mastery had failed as a consequence of their libidinal cathexis; the failure provoked a breaking-through of the repressed, a repetition of the trauma. ("It was like a nightmare, only that I was awake.") The ritual represented a renewed attempt at magic undoing of the trauma; the act of quickly sitting up straight being a magic undoing of the motor paralysis in *pavor nocturnus,* the looking out of the window—proving to herself that there is nothing to be seen—a magic denial of both primal scene and castration, referring to an often repeated screen memory how as a child she had been awakened by the sounds of gardening shears beneath this window, when her mother clipped flowers and shrubs there early in the morning. The final masturbation fantasy of her adolescence contained a symbolic repetition of the infantile trauma.

Another patient had a *pavor nocturnus* dream that a man was standing on him and that sparks of fire dripping down upon him from this man ignited him. Later he masturbated with the masochistic fantasy that he was "a branded slave who holds his master's penis while the latter urinates." The above-mentioned dream of the patient in which he effortlessly dived and swam, being playfully pulled up and down by a seal who bit him "as puppies bite," was understood as a reparative repetition of a *pavor nocturnus.* He later masturbated by swimming with a naked penis and pulled-back foreskin.

Since the sexuality of the adult receives its specific character from the masturbation fantasies, the *amalgamation of libidinal gratification and reparative mastery in masturbation becomes henceforth the prototype for the future structure of his sexual relations.* That means that the gratification of sexual impulses can only be achieved on condition that the fantasies accompanying the gratification effect a magic reparation of the infantile trauma. This imparts to the sexual act more or less the function of undoing the oedipal trauma. The greater the impact of early traumata, the greater consequently is the degree to which the sexual act will become the executive of reparative mastery.

A patient in sexual intercourse used to suck forcefully at the nipples, feeling thereby an overpowering wish to eat them up. He combined sexual gratification with an acting out of oral sadistic defences against early frustration. Fear of retaliation (vagina dentata) led to premature ejaculation.

What characterizes the sexuality of the adult neurotic is the more or less dominant interference of reparative mastery with sexual gratification. This leads to fantasies of pervert character, masochistic, sadistic, homosexual, etc., and to more or less pronounced inhibition of orgastic gratification (orgasmoid); i.e. to frigidity and impotence; if magic thinking prevails, to acting out of these fantasies in *perversion*.

Failure of Reparative Mastery

The reported cases of the spider phobia and the phobia of the dark, Renée's seizures, the Isakower phenomenon, demonstrate a *failure of reparative mastery* inducing a more or less attenuated repetition of the original infantile trauma, a breakthrough of the repressed. This occurs under specific conditions like excessive strength of the original trauma, libidinization of reparative mastery, excessive stimulation or frustration, etc.

A female patient during the analytic session underwent an attenuated repetition of a *pavor nocturnus* attack while analyzing the masochistic fantasy of being chopped up in a bathtub. She suddenly became silent and finally said: "Now I had a strange feeling, as if I were here in a nightmare; it was like swimming in a sleep or in a dream." At the age of four, her older, very sadistic brother had thrown her fully dressed into a bathtub, and she had almost drowned. The associations led to reminiscences of the infantile trauma: primal scene and *pavor nocturnus* (being overwhelmed, drowning). She experienced a similar break-through during a sexual scene with her lover: "Yesterday when I was alone with Fred at home, I felt as if he were *a shadow*. I couldn't feel him, *I was dead*, I felt frozen, I imagined intercourse and I visualized him naked; then he became a monster and swelled up." Both incidents can be understood as break-throughs of the id into the ego, produced by an attenuated revival of *pavor nocturnus* experiences.

In his paper, "Hysterical Dreamstates," Abraham gives a fascinating description of the break-through of the primal trauma through the failure of reparative mastery. These breakthroughs which he called "twilight states" were usually induced by the patient in situations of sexual stimulation or frustration. They started with fantasies of grandeur, accompanied by ecstatic exaltation, but obviously represent the attempt at reparative mastery. This first phase rapidly merged into a second, with morbid anxiety, giddiness, distortions of space (persons in the vicinity appeared remarkably big), feelings that parts of the body had died off, sensations of immobility, falling, sinking down, feelings of vanishing and dying, associated with the most intense anxiety—phenomena which strikingly resemble the sensations in *pavor nocturnus* (catatonoid reaction). One of his patients used to start the "twilight state" by swift and energetic walking in the street, and regularly ended up with sensations of immobility, of inability to lift his legs; the "walking swiftly" in an elated state obviously represented an attempt at reparative mastery of the motor paralysis of *pavor nocturnus*. In another case, Abraham traces the break-through to a nightmare in which the patient was attacked by lions.

Katan's case illustrates a similar break-through: a sixteen-year-old girl in her first agoraphobic attack repeated an infantile *pavor nocturnus* attack in the street. She finally accosted a man whom she took for her father and asked him for help. In her *pavor nocturnus* attack she had called the father to her bed.

Other authors have described similar break-throughs.

In Renée's case the failure of reparative mastery acquires almost dramatic power. She describes how, time and again, listening to the noises of the wind provokes an attack, an outbreak of terror "mounting to a paroxysm." Nevertheless, she listens again and again. "At night I could not sleep, listening to the wind . . . my whole being attuned to it, palpitating, awaiting I know not what . . . I believed the wind blew from the North Pole . . . it was alive, monstrous, bending everything in its way. Then my room became enormous, disproportionate . . . the terror mounted to a paroxysm. . . . Fear, agonizing, boundless fear, overcame me . . . the frozen wind from the North Pole wanted to crush the earth, to destroy it. . . . Little by little I brought myself to confide to my friends that the world was about to be destroyed. . . ." It was her own anticipated collapse (shock), in which—through projection—she experienced the destruction of the world. I should not hesitate to consider this the meaning, in many instances, of the phenomenon of the "destruction-of-the-world."

My clinical material showed that in *agoraphobia* the temptation situation in the street elicits the *distortion of space sensation* (the "limitless vastness"); that in *claustrophobia* the feeling of being "closed in" is a revival of the *immobilization;* that *phobia of heights* originates in the *falling sensations* of the infantile traumatic situation; that *phobias of animals* originate in the recall of the *pavor nocturnus* trauma incited by the sight of the animal. In the case of Little Hans, the sight of the horses in the street elicited the recall of his *pavor nocturnus* anxiety

In compulsion neuroses and in so-called character neuroses the connection with *pavor nocturnus* seems to be less transparent. Here *pavor nocturnus* attacks or memories of them appear only when the treatment succeeds in "mobilizing the anxiety." We know that infantile anxiety hysteria is always at the base of adult neurosis.

Ego Regression and Symptom Formation

At this point, I would like to summarize briefly certain considerations concerning defences and regression, which I have discussed elsewhere in greater detail.

We have seen that the failure of reparative mastery induces an attenuated repetition of the infantile trauma, a break through of the repressed. This leads to an intrusion of the infantile ways of thinking—still active at the period of the infantile trauma—into the rational thought process. The very character of the revived trauma enhances this regression. Since the child endowed the hallucinations in *pavor nocturnus* with the quality of reality, its revival causes an invasion of the realistic thought process by the same primary process that prevailed in the original traumatic situation. The revived threat is projected on to objects and situations that facilitate this *transference,* and is responded to with regression to irrational *defensive* reactions, viz., a *regression to early infantile (primary) defences,* and a renewed *attempt at magic mastery.*

We described above *the primary defences* which in the early infantile period averted shock, and which are of a more physiological, automatic, compulsive character. They include mobilization of motility against shock, leading to aggression or flight: primitive relief reactions of anal-urethral character; early oral defences, such as oral gratification (oral dependency, clinging), and oral sadistic reactions against frustration, hallucination, projection, introjection, etc., as well as morbid primary defences, like agitation and catatonoid reaction. The stronger the break-through of the repressed, the more the repetition of the previous trauma takes on the character of an actual primary trauma, and the stronger will be the regression to primary defences and to magic mastery. Relatively trivial frustrations then provoke disproportionate and irrational defensive reactions. This regression is more or less *pathogenic* in character. It involves the threat of "loss of love," of being abandoned, which at that level means revival of the postnatal trauma and the loss of reality. The stirred up primary defences, therefore, have to be warded off by additional defences.

What had to be repressed in the phobia of both Little Hans and the Wolf Man were hostile aggressive impulses toward the father. Oral fears as a talionic punishment for oral aggression compelled both children to avoid the anxiety animals.

The manifest defences in neurosis are, therefore, principally directed against the regressions to pathogenic primary defences. These secondary defences, or defences proper, constitute, together with a renewed attempt at magic mastery, the specific form and function of the symptom.

The situation is further complicated through the libidinization of the reparative repetition of the oedipal trauma, due to the reaction in the latter as well as the libidinization of the primary defences originating in the libidinization of body functions by postnatal trauma.

The discussion of the correlation between regression to libidinized primary defences and the well-known concept of libido regression due to fixation must be deferred for future presentation. I believe that the concept of libido regression in many cases represents an oversimplification. A number of phenomena might perhaps be better explained as regressions to early, libidinized primary defences. The "reaching of the genital phase" in therapy, for example, may be understood as well as a liberation of the sexual function from an exaggerated urge for reparative mastery of the oedipal trauma.

SUMMARY

The basic infantile trauma usually designated as primal scene, which may be conceived of as a primary *pavor nocturnus* and which is reflected in the infantile *pavor nocturnus* attacks, instigates repression as well as attempts at reparative mastery. Later situations—such as reinforcement of libido in puberty, frustrations—resuscitate the threat from past traumata and the attempts at their mastery. Under certain conditions, like severity of the past traumata or their excessive libidinization, these attempts result in a repetition of the traumatic situation evoking a regression to pathogenic primary defences and renewed attempts at magic mastery (ego regression). This pathogenic regression has to be warded off by additional secondary defences. The symptom combines a counter-reaction against the primary defences incited by the break-through of the trauma with a renewed attempt at its magic mastery.

In *hysteria,* the somatic discharge of anxiety produced by the break-through of the repressed seems to be counteracting pathogenic primary defences as well as for a magic acting out of renewed reparative mastery. The somatic reactions may constitute the pathway to the conversion symptoms. In *phobia* a specific situation which restimulates an infantile impulse and thus revives the infantile trauma initiates an attempt at reparative mastery. Its failure provokes *anxiety* and pathogenic defences. The specific situation acquires the quality of danger and has to be avoided. *Compulsion neurosis* is characterized by the greater strength of pathogenic regressive defences of greater automatic (compulsive) character as a consequence of a more traumatic background. They become the main threat and are warded off by reaction formations and magic counteractions, undoing, isolation, etc. The stronger the underlying trauma, the more extensive the ego regression, which explains the successively growing *prevalence of magic thinking,* and of acting out. In *perversion* the revival of the infantile trauma seems to be responded to by the magic acting out of libidinized primary defences together with magic acting out of reparative mastery. In *psychosis,* the alarming character of the infantile trauma is due to the morbidity of the underlying anxiety process (insufficiency of anabiotic defences). In this case the reparative repetition of the trauma represents an exorbitant threat and elicits extreme irrational responses involving an extensive invasion by the primary process; on the one hand, there are incessant attempts at reparative magic mastery with hallucinations, identification, projection, introjection, repression, denial, etc., and on the other, there is a desperate acting out of all available defences, discharge reactions and counter-reactions, such as clinging, perversion, agitation, catatonoid reaction, depersonalization, depression, etc., including the whole gamut of the various forms of symptom formation.

Since we ascribe the function of mastery and reparative

mastery to the ego, we might define this presentation as a—rather fragmentary—attempt to describe an ego aspect of symptom formation. Paradoxically, the perpetuation of the trauma as well as the invasion by the primary process is caused by the very mechanism of anticipation which developed as protection against trauma, and which for this purpose incited realistic thinking.

Only passing reference can be made to the surprising wealth of material to be found in rituals, mythology, religion, folklore, literature, art, etc., revealing their meaning as magic reparation of trauma. Works of art seem to be a result of and a symbol for the symbiosis of libidinal gratification and reparative mastery, the latter being represented by the form aspect. Form, through introducing rule and proportion, symbolizes constancy and perpetual existence. Thus it magically masters death (shock) and destruction, which in the feeling of mankind are associated with orgasm.

COEXISTING ORGAN NEUROSES

A Clinical Study

Peter L. Giovacchini, M.D.

Modern dynamic psychiatry began with the study of somatic responses, those seen in conversion hysteria. Breuer and Freud, in arriving at theoretical formulations and conclusions, provided numerous interesting clinical examples, and since their time psychiatric investigators have reported many cases in which psychogenically induced somatic disturbances are conspicuous. It has been learned that not all these physical disturbances can be grouped nosologically with hysteria. This group also includes certain entities known today as psychosomatic disorders or organ neuroses.

I shall not attempt to review the extensive literature on this subject, since it has been ably reviewed elsewhere. I should like, however, to point out a major difference between the psychiatric and medical literature on psychosomatic disturbances. Whereas in the psychiatric literature all varieties of cases are discussed in terms of character structure, dynamics, and phenomenology, very rarely can examples of multiple psychosomatic entities in the same person be found. Referring to the psychiatric reports exclusively would give the reader the impression that such cases simply do not exist, or that at most they are rare enough to be considered oddities. Review of the medical literature, however, gives an entirely different picture. Studies of 50 or 100 cases of peptic ulcer and hypertension, or hypertension and asthma, or peptic ulcer and diabetes, or practically any other combination are not uncommon.

My experience has confirmed the impression gained from the medical literature. In a routine study of peptic ulcer patients admitted to the University of Chicago Clinics for vagotomy, many were found in whom one or even two other diseases that have been considered from the psychosomatic approach coexisted.

In this paper 2 such cases, which were studied more intensively than the others, will be discussed. Each of these 2 patients was seen for periods totaling 25 hours. During this time the histories were reconstructed and I was able to come to certain psychoanalytic conclusions concerning the conflict situations and character structures of the patients. The material collected is of such quantity that not all of the clinical details will be presented. A summary of the anamneses will be given, followed by a speculative formulation.

Case 1

The patient was a 50-year-old, unmarried crane operator of Yugoslavian descent who came to the University of Chicago Clinics in 1950 because of gastrointestinal symptoms. The symptoms had been present intermittently since 1922, and he had had many previous hospitalizations. The diagnosis of ulcer was well established. The patient enjoyed his hospitalization and derived some gratification from the attention that was paid his diet, he himself being extremely careful about indiscretions. His bowel habits were regular, and the only bowel disturbance was a tendency toward constipation; there was no history of diarrhea.

History

In 1942 the patient was drafted into the army, but he was constantly on sick call and was discharged after six months. During his military duty his symptoms had become more frequent and more severe. At home his distress continued, though improving somewhat as a result of his amateurish manipulation of his diet.

In October, 1947, a routine urine examination at his place of employment revealed glycosuria, and a diagnosis of diabetes mellitus was made. He became diligent about testing his urine and adjusting his insulin dosage, but the diabetic diet increased his ulcer pains and caused him to begin vomiting. Five or six weeks prior to hospitalization, the pain became so intense that he could not sleep. He stated that it frequently caused him to "cry like a baby." Otherwise his health was good and he was not aware of any other disabilities.

A summary of the history revealed that the patient had been born in Yugoslavia. He had had a sister who had died before his birth. His mother died when he was 3 months old, and his father, he believed, was killed by the Germans during World War II, although he was not certain of this point. He described his father as kind hearted but hot tempered, a man who was generous and emotional but who had to have his own way in all matters. The father remarried shortly after the mother's death, and the patient hated his stepmother. He was not able to get along with her in any area, but he found her most irritating quality to be her depreciation of him to his father, whose anger would be stimulated and who would then beat the son violently.

At the age of 15 the patient came to America, where he believed he would find riches and luxury. However, his life consisted of hard work in coal mines, on the railroad, and as a crane operator. His first seven years in the United States were spent with relatives or friends of the family, but because of various situational circumstances he had to give up this family existence and live more or less on his own. Thereafter he moved around frequently, living in hotels and boarding houses most of the time. It was at this time that his ulcer symptoms began, and he attributed them to the fact that he had to eat in restaurants.

Description

The patient claimed to have had many sexual contacts, and even at the time of this study felt that sexual intercourse was his greatest pleasure. He had been married three times, the wife on two occasions having been selected by elderly women friends. The first marriage was dissolved because his wife was unfaithful, had venereal disease, and "did not take care of him" properly. The patient stressed the last point, together with the fact that he could not get along with his father-in-law. The second marriage was broken up because his wife was an alcoholic and always treated him in a hostile, belligerent fashion. He claimed also to have been the active one in obtaining the divorce from his third wife. In this case, he attributed the difficulty to the fact that in-laws were always telling his wife what to do and that she in turn would nag him. He resented it to the point that he finally effected a legal separation. At the time of admission, he was again living alone.

The patient was a large, heavy man with good muscular development. He spoke English with a foreign accent. The only significant physical finding was a blood pressure of 160/110. He was mild in manner, compliant, and generally cooperative. He tended to boast a good deal of his sexual prowess. Much of his demeanor was reminiscent of that of an adolescent schoolboy, although he attempted to show himself as a generous, affable person. He seemed to have very definite limitations in the social, cultural, and intellectual spheres, but relative to his social milieu there were no gross abnormalities. His behavior with the nurses tended to be flirtatious and sometimes demanding. He was chiefly preoccupied with various fleeting symptoms and with the fact that his food intake had to be restricted because of the vagotomy. He was much concerned over the latter point.

This patient showed himself to be intensely concerned with matters relating to food, eating, and being taken care of. He had all the traits of a markedly dependent person who, from the viewpoint of the libido theory, could be described as orally fixated. His overt behavior seemed to have been designed to obtain gratification of extreme oral dependent needs. The patient had actively sought satisfaction of his need "to be taken care of." Like a nomad, he seemed to have wandered from one dependent relationship to another.

The ulcer symptoms developed at a time when the environment made it impossible for the patient to obtain as much dependent gratification as his unconscious, and to a large extent his conscious, personality demanded. His dependent demands seemed to show themselves directly; instead of developing systematic defenses against them, he acted them out. His conflict began then when his sources of oral gratification were cut off for external reasons; it was not denied because of internal guilt.

This constellation of factors fits in well with the conflict situation that has been postulated for peptic ulcer by Alexander and his coworkers, even though most of their patients had defenses against recognition of their dependent needs. The patient's unconscious wish to be fed had become part of his character structure, and derivatives of this instinctual impulse were being acted out in an ego-syntonic fashion.

In spite of the deprivation this patient had experienced in his object relationships, his attitude was still one of naive, childish optimism. Whereas Alexander's patients denied their dependency needs, this patient's defense was to deny that he was not going to be taken care of and gratified orally. Obviously such a defense is a poor one. To continue to deny that one is not being fed and to believe that one's hunger is being satisfied when such is not the case can work only until the physiological needs will no longer accept such fantasied substitutive rewards. Fenichel noted this same defensive feature in some of his patients and called it the "optimism of the oral character."

Concerning the patient's hypertension, there were some interesting features in the family constellation which have been considered characteristic for many such patients. His father was a strict, authoritative, dominating, and fearsome figure. During the course of several interviews, it became apparent that the patient harbored intense but chronically inhibited hostile feelings toward him. At no time was he ever able to express them overtly. The fact that anger could be dangerous had been impressed upon him in two ways: First, he feared that his hostile wishes could actually cause the destruction of the object toward whom they were directed, his fantasies and associations bearing this out. Second, he was fearful for his own safety, since he knew his father was capable of extremely violent retaliation, as evidenced by the particularly brutal beatings he had suffered. These are not unusual attitudes about hostile feelings. When these exists the additional factor of loss of dependency if destructive wishes are found out, the patient is even more apt to suppress or repress such instinctual impulses. This state of inhibition is one of conflict, and is believed by Alexander and Saul to be characteristic of the hypertensive patient.

Case 2

The patient was a 52-year-old toolmaker who was found to have both hypertension and duodenal ulcer. His gastrointestinal symptoms had been present for approximately 36 years. They began with abdominal cramps and "heartburn," when he was in high school in 1914. In 1918 he was inducted into the army, and his disturbance became more intense; however, no positive diagnosis was reached. The symptom complex continued until 1935 when he suffered a perforation. Emergency surgery was performed and a dietary regimen instituted. He was then fairly well until 1945, when the ulcer symptoms returned with greater intensity than previously. From that time on, he was on a series of diets; eventually vagotomy was performed, the year before this study took place.

History

The patient was the oldest of four children and was in constant rivalry with his next brother, who was 1½ years younger. He stated that they were always fighting, but that when it came to blame or punishment it was he who received the censure of his parents. He described his father's attitude as inconsistent. The father seemed to be a mild-mannered person with a jovial, likable nature. However, on occasion he would become strict and punitive, and the patient remembered his spankings as having been extremely severe. He would frequently run to his mother for protection. The mother's pattern was more uniform, and the patient felt definitely that he loved her more than he did his father. She, too, was said to have had a harsh temper, but he did not feel it to be so dangerous as that of his father. Still, he believed that the mother could have given him more and that she had shown favoritism toward his next sibling.

In spite of the fact that he was dissatisfied with the home situation, he remained with his parents until he was 26 years old, even though he had been married at the age of 24. He felt that his marital life had been reasonably harmonious except for quarrels over his alcoholism. He drank heavily up until 1935 when his ulcer perforated, but after that he was afraid to drink. He stated that he had never derived much pleasure from sexual intercourse, had very few contacts, and that for some time he had been continent because his ulcer pain interfered with his enjoyment of the sexual act.

The patient had never formed any lasting or warm interpersonal relationships. He had no real friends, nor had he even been able to maintain much contact with his family, which at this time consisted of his mother and siblings; his father had died two years previously after an alcoholic episode. Although his mother was strict and prohibitive toward both drinking and smoking, she was not able to prevent either the patient or the youngest brother from drinking. His wife had the same attitude as his mother toward both the patient and their children, who were at this period in their twenties. The patient stated that he himself had been stern with his children and that he did not have any particular bond with them.

Description

During the interviews, the patient presented a hard, immobile facial expression. He was courteous but indicated that he was a man with definitely set ideas who was "not going to stand being pushed around." He showed little emotion when discussing the various events of his life except occasionally to betray hostile attitudes toward the significant persons in both the present and the past. He felt that life had not treated him well and that, because of his efforts at hard work, he deserved much more than he had actually received. It was fairly obvious that his adjustment socially, domestically, vocationally, and sexually had been poor.

Physical examination of this patient was for the most part noncontributory. He was a man of average height, somewhat asthenic, but apparently wiry. He found it difficult to relax throughout the examination. His tendon reflexes seemed to be somewhat exaggerated, though not to the point of spasticity. The only abnormal finding was a blood pressure of 168/110.

The patient emphasized the point that he had always worked hard and been able to make his own way, although it was fairly obvious from the history that he was a dependent person. His verbalizations were intended to give the examiner the impression that he was dealing with a very resourceful, autonomous man, and he emphasized the fact that he had always been able to get along on his own and that no one every gave him any "handouts." He impressed the examiner with the aggressive elements of his behavior.

The hostile elements did not seem to be so deeply hidden in this patient's personality as they were in that of the first patient. On the other hand, the very obvious clinging, demanding dependency of the first patient was not overtly manifested here. This patient presented an autonomous and belligerently self-assertive front, this being the more typical of the classic ulcer patient. However, all the material indicated that his self-assertiveness was defensive, an overcompensatory attitude designed to keep his intense dependent strivings in a state of repression. There were indications from the interviews as to why he was so ashamed and afraid of recognizing his orality consciously, but this will not be discussed here inasmuch as in this respect the patient did not differ appreciably from others whose cases have been published previously. His ego, therefore, used the defensive mechanism of reaction formation, which became fused with extremely hostile feelings.

It is true that in the history there was evidence of acting out of oral dependent needs, as in alcoholism. The patient's ulcer symptoms, however, became more definitely established when he gave up drinking and other such acting-out manifestations. Even though there remained many direct representations of dependent needs in his everyday behavior, the ulcer seemed to be kept active chiefly by the tension resulting from internalization of oral demands.

Discussion

One of the noteworthy points in these two cases is the widely different character structures of the patients.

The first patient showed his dependent needs openly, denying only the fact that they were not being gratified. In spite of this denial, however, there was real frustration at the environmental level, and the pain of this was correlated with the beginning of his ulcer. Hostility, on the other hand, had been maintained in a state of repression and certainly was far from obvious, in contrast to his dependent orientation, when his personality is considered in terms of ego operations.

The second patient presented an entirely different picture. This patient's belligerent self-assertiveness was his most obvious feature. The main axis of all his object relationships was hostility, which was most definitely manifested from the point of view of ego functioning. He expressed his hostility in his attitudes and behavior, but because of it he also set up visceral tensions that led to hypertension. His dependent needs were internalized. In both these patients, whether the instinctual forces were kept in a state of repression by the ego's defenses or whether they were diffusely incorporated into the character structure, becoming ego-syntonic and then coming into conflict with reality, tension was created which had its effect upon visceral functions.

Frustration can lead to similar responses in persons with widely different character structures. In our studies of vagotomized patients at the University of Chicago Clinics we observed a large number of patients, all of whom had peptic ulcer but in whom, psychiatrically, the character structure ranged from neurotic to severely psychotic. In this instance we consider ulcer as the similar response.

Each mode of response or the conflict per se must in turn contribute certain finite qualities to the personality structure. In some cases it would seem likely that a certain emotional constellation would be incompatible with a given ego structure. The physiological counterpart of such an incompatibility is seen where one disease causes amelioration of another, as in the case of hypothyroidism and cardiac disease. In the cases presented here, the ulcer and hypertensive conflict situation are compatible with each other, as evidenced by the fact that they do exist side by side. It is conceivable, however, that in another person, because of a different characterological makeup and genetic development, such coexistence would not be possible.

The ego has a variety of defense mechanisms at its disposal.

The soma can be thought of as having the same capacity for flexibility. The tension resulting from a particular conflict may express itself through more than one organ system. It may for a time under certain stresses and unique circumstances satisfy itself with one particular part of the body, and then for imperfectly understood reasons revert to a different organ system. These reasons may be changes in external relationships, childhood training, or perhaps even organic sensitization.

Alexander, by utilizing the psychoanalytic approach to the problems of psychosomatic medicine, postulated that, when a feeling cannot be expressed semantically or through the action of higher mentational or integrative centers, tension is created which activates the visceral components of such feelings. The chronic influence of such tension can lead to actual pathological changes such as those noted in peptic ulcer, hypertension, asthma, and other entities which have been so studied. In both peptic ulcer and hypertension a characteristic conflict situation was found to be typical of the patients examined or analyzed. In the patients discussed here, where ulcer and hypertension coexist, the same conflicts are seen and, even in combination with each other, maintain their specificity.

Little mention is made regarding diabetes because this metabolic disturbance is imperfectly understood from a psychosomatic point of view. Studies by various observers reveal the difficulty in evaluating the etiological significance of the psychodynamic features in this disease. The fact that the physiology of diabetes is also imperfectly understood complicates the problem.

In summary, the psychosomatic "fomulas" that have been postulated by the Chicago Institute for Psychoanalysis seem to apply to the cases reported in this study, even though the entities were found in combination with each other.

SOME SYMPTOMS AND SIGNS OF ANXIETY STATES

Ovid O. Meyer, M.D.

To almost every physician it has become quite evident that the problems of anxiety and tension are extremely common, either as the sole explanation for the patient coming to the doctor, or in association with organic disease. Since this appears to be the fact, it behooves the general practitioner, internist and pediatrist to be aware of the symptoms that indicate the correct diagnosis. Actually, every type of specialist should be cognizant of indications that the patient's complaints are not based upon organic disease primarily, in order to avoid unfortunate mistakes and needless operations.

The majority of these patients can be adequately treated by the doctor not a specialist in mental diseases, once an alertness to the problems and a moderate amount of experience are attained. Further, he can usually separate the mild from the severe cases. The former he can manage successfully himself, the latter, a minority, he can and should refer to a psychiatrist.

Some doctors are prone to overlook many of the symptoms and signs of functional disease and see only the organic condition, feeling insecure in their appraisal of non-organic disease. This insecurity probably is due to a certain vagueness in much that is said and written about these problems. This is written with the attempt to be as explicit as possible and to indicate that there are many specific signs that properly lead to the correct diagnosis of functional disease. What is submitted here is largely based upon experience as an internist without any special training in nervous disease, but with a deep interest in these worthy, unhappy people.

The following list of symptoms and signs include those that are so common that the doctor is promptly alerted to the true situation and the diagnosis is readily made. Others are less well known but equally important in suggesting the proper diagnosis of an anxiety tension state. In this listing, no attempt is made to give the differential diagnosis to be considered for each symptom. The purpose is rather to record the symptoms and signs that should make one consider the possibility or probability of non-organic disease.

Categories

It must be appreciated that for every patient three possible categories must be considered under which the case may fit.

Overlay. In nearly every patient with organic disease, there is some functional overlay of varying intensity. The sick patient, whether his illness be acute, subacute, or chronic, has mental and personality changes of such a nature that he is not himself while he is ill and usually not for some time after the illness. This is widely recognized and accepted by nearly all physicians.

Associated disease. A second category includes those cases in which functional disease is primary, possibly due to maladaptation to environment in any of many ways, with associated or perhaps resultant organic disease such as peptic ulcer, ulcerative colitis, dermatitis, or hypertension.

No organic relation. A third group is comprised of patients with functional disease which exists without evident organic disease; or, if organic disease exists, it is not responsible for the symptoms. Often in the patients of this group there is a physiologic disturbance such as irritability of the colon, tachycardia, or excessive perspiration.

Symptoms

(a) *Headache.* This very common symptom is most often localized in the back of the head and neck, although it may be frontal. If the pain is on top of the head, it usually suggests a severe, often hysterical type of psychoneurotic disorder.

(b) *Inability to read or think.* These symptoms indicate the patients' inability to concentrate on anything but themselves and their problems. In moderately severe or severe cases, these are usually present.

(b_1) *Insomnia.* A symptom that is often on the same basis as (b). Some have trouble getting to sleep; others develop the pattern of awakening early without the ability to fall asleep again—a very suggestive symptom of an emotional disorder.

(c) *Dizziness.* This is frequently a symptom resulting from hyperventilation inadvertently carried on, which may be a conditioned reaction to stress.

(d) *Palpitation and tachycardia.* These are common signs of anxiety frequently associated with (c), (e), and (f)—as resultants of persistent hyperventilation.

(e) *Faintness.* This is also common with hyperventilation of tension states and an important cause of fear.

(f) *Sense of tightness in the chest.* A symptom that is usually associated with hyperventilation and awesome for the patient, but less common than the other symptoms listed.

(g) *Anorexia.* This is a very common symptom which frequently occurs for brief periods, with the recurrent episodes of anxiety and excessive emotional tension experienced by most individuals at one time or another. However, chronic anorexia with resultant weight loss or failure to gain weight is often due to fatigue which develops because of persistent emotional stress and overactivity with wasted purposeful or purposeless muscle activity.

(h), (i), (j), *Nausea, Emesis, Diarrhea.* These occur with further aggravation commonly reflecting sustained repressed resentment. Little or no anxiety may be existent.

(k) *Aerophagia.* Swallowing of air and then belching occurs perhaps more frequently in the somewhat debilitated tense person and is likely to be habitual. It is relatively common after an operation or after a prolonged or serious illness, especially in a tense, high-strung individual.

(*l*) *Abdominal pain.* Pain of the spastic colon, which is commonly present in anxiety-tension states, is usually present throughout the abdomen or is variable in location, more often on the left, and is *relieved by defecation.*

(*m*) *Backache.* In my experience, this is an occasional symptom. Coccydynia is nearly always a symptom of psychoneurosis and, as a consequence, surgical measures such as amputation of the coccyx are usually very disappointing in their results.

(*n*) *Pain and stiffness in the shoulder region.* Lorenz and Musser have recently called attention to the importance and frequency of this symptom in psychoneurotics, often seriously ill psychoneurotics. The left shoulder was involved twice as often as the right. The symptom may be very persistent and lead to many extensive negative roentgenographic examinations, spinal puncture and even a myelogram amongst other tests.

Commonly several of the symptoms listed here may exist in the same individual. However, one symptom is likely to predominate, although a subsequent shift to another predominating symptom is not unusual. Characteristically, even with a multiplicity of complaints, a certain vagueness is common in the patient's description of his symptoms.

The type of person who comes to the doctor with a list of complaints on a piece of paper is very well known to all physicians. The diagnosis of psychoneurosis can usually be made readily. What is more, the psychoneurosis is usually of long standing, and the patient is insecure—"I might forget something."

Any of these symptoms or symptom complexes should alert the physician. Sometimes the first impression gained from the history suggesting organic disease may be altered when a careful social history is taken and it is found that the husband is a ruffian, the supervisor of the job is difficult, there exists an unhappy love affair or parent-child relationship, or some other

SOME SYMPTOMS AND SIGNS OF ANXIETY STATES

situation of stress in the patient's everyday life. Obviously, circumstances such as these may readily account for many psychic and somatic complaints. The social history is extremely important. It is very distressing to see how often it is haphazardly and inadequately recorded. To obtain it properly, the inquirer must be passive and objective, neither facetious nor scolding, neither critical nor too aggressively sleuthing. Slowly, if the approach is proper, the story will come out, and the diagnosis will be made possible.

The past medical history may also be significant. Unnecessarily prolonged illnesses, multiple operations, or obscure and mild illnesses are often suggestive.

In addition, the family history may be vital in establishing the diagnosis. The patient may think that he has cancer or heart disease, and may present a good symptomatic pattern because of knowledge of the complaints of some relative or acquaintance ill or recently deceased because of one of these conditions.

After the history, a complete and careful physical examination should be done to reassure the patient as to one's thoroughness and to have a firm foundation upon which to build the psychotherapy that is to follow. The examination can do harm and make the patient needlessly apprehensive, however, if it is overdone in certain details. For example, if too much attention is directed to the heart, or if the blood pressure is checked at the time of each visit, anxiety on the part of the patient may result. The complete examination should be done with finality, and, unless new indications arise, it should not be checked in detail for weeks or months. One must realize, of course, that sooner or later the neurotic does develop serious organic disease as do all of us. The physician may be sadly awakened if he forgets this fact.

SIGNS

The specific physical signs that should immediately suggest an anxiety tension state may be listed as follows:

(a) *Sighing.* The patient who, while sitting beside your desk giving the history, sighs frequently, is nearly always fatigued and fatigued because of a state of emotional unrest and tension of considerable duration. That patient is hyperventilating and, hence, is likely to have the symptoms of hyperventilation—i.e., dizziness, lightheadedness, palpitation, a sense of tightness in the chest, and possibly precordial pain.

(b) *Tinted glasses.* Whenever a patient wears tinted glasses, one can suspect an anxiety tension state. This is not invariably so, not everyone who wears tinted glasses has psychoneurosis, but it is very commonly true that tinted glasses have this significance. I have confirmed this observation hundreds of times. Our residents are usually skeptical when first introduced to this sign, but are readily converted after one or two months of looking for its significance and observing the type of individuals who demonstrate it. The tinted glasses have two purposes: First, they serve as a shield from the world; and, secondly, because these patients are uneasy and secrete an excess of adrenalin, their pupils are often widely dilated, so that bright light is distressing.

(c) *Bitten fingernails.* Bitten fingernails almost invariably indicate that the person, adult or child, is a nervous, emotionally unstable person. I have seen several hundred patients with hyperthyroidism, and they are nervous emotional people, too, but I can remember no more than four of these who bit the fingernails.

(d) *Axillary perspiration.* In the tense person, excessive axillary perspiration will often be present and will drip to the examining table. If the patient is recumbent for some minutes, two round spots of perspiration will be present on the sheet after he gets up from the table. I have observed this sign more often in men. It is a specific sign of tension, which may exist only because of being in the doctor's office and may not be primarily indicative of a psychoneurosis, although neurotics commonly exhibit it. Patients with hypermetabolism also, of course, demonstrate this excessive perspiration.

Jitteriness and restlessness, as observed when one talks to and examines the patient, need not in themselves indicate that a significant emotional disorder exists. It often does, but there is the "go-getter" type who is often jittery although in no sense neurotic.

With these hints from history of the illness and physical examination and from carefully obtained social, past medical, and family histories, one can usually arrive at the correct diagnosis. It is wrong, very wrong, to make a diagnosis of functional disease only by exclusion of organic disease, for organic disease may exist—gallstones, for example, or cardiac disease—without being cause of the symptomatology. The approach must be a positive one, and it can be if some of these symptoms and signs are kept in mind.

And then, having made the diagnosis, one should carefully offer the patient an explanation for his complaints, step by step. Harm may be done if the physician is too precipitous or brusque in his approach. The patient will usually require repeated conferences and reassuring supervision. Temporarily, mild sedation may be helpful, but this therapy should, ordinarily, be of short duration. The physician, contrary to frequent practice, should neither ignore the patient, promptly refer him to someone else, unless it appears that the illness is so serious that a psychiatrist is needed for treatment, nor treat him for long periods with sedatives, merely because he feels unsure of himself in management of these cases.

Understanding discussions between physician and patient are of great benefit, and are very worth while. I have seen ambulance-transported patients enter the hospital and, after two or three weeks of treatment composed largely of interviews, be well and able to walk out of the hospital. It is true that relapses occur, but during remissions the patient may be a functionally 100 per cent individual, whereas the cardiac patient, for example, who has regained compensation may be but 50 per cent of normal, functionally. Time spent with the patient who has psychosomatic disease is generally time well spent and extremely worth while. These individuals are usually very interesting and very grateful patients. And, as Dale Groom has said, "A patient's mind can be as interesting as his colon." Finally, we must remember that we all have a threshold for indefinite anxieties, pains, and bodily complaints, It is just that some have higher thresholds than others.

EXPERIMENTAL STUDIES ON ANXIETY REACTIONS

Thomas H. Holmes, M.D. and
Herbert S. Ripley, M.D.

Introduction

This report deals with observations of man's attempts at adaptation in experimentally induced and naturally occurring situations, with particular emphasis on stress-induced anxiety. The following definition of the term "anxiety" is used: a feeling of apprehension in response to danger which threatens the integrity of the individual. This state is accompanied by alterations in one or more physiologic variables, which may differ in degree, integration, and duration among individuals and in the same person from time to time.

In this study techniques from the physiologic, psychologic, and sociologic disciplines have been employed. No uniform method has been applied to all observations. Rather, each experimental situation was evaluated in context by the method or combination of methods deemed most likely to yield information pertaining to the question asked. No attempt has been made to include illustrative examples of all the psychophysiologic and psychosocial correlates of anxiety. Rather, selected data have been organized into a frame of reference designed to emphasize the relevance of anxiety to man's attempt at the maintenance of homeostasis and the natural history of illness.

Anxiety, Sustained Muscle Contraction and Back Pain

The importance of the role of the autonomic nervous system in anxiety reactions previously has been reported. It should

A 32-year-old white Roman Catholic housewife and part-time nurse of German extraction complained of pain of 5 years' duration in the lumbosacral region. Action potentials were recorded from the back muscles as the subject discussed her unhappy childhood. She lay rigid and motionless on the table, giving free expression to her intense anxiety commingled with feelings of resentment, humiliation, and guilt. When increased electrical activity had been sustained for 6 minutes, the subject noted the onset of a backache which persisted for 30 minutes. The conversation was directed to neutral topics and the patient immediately became relaxed and at ease. The pain promptly disappeared as the increased electrical activity and muscle tension subsided. Eight and a half minutes later the conversation about personal problems was resumed. Both sustained muscle tension and increased electrical activity reappeared, and one and a half minutes later the patient again complained of back pain. She was then diverted and reassured and once again she became relaxed. The muscle tension and electrical activity from the muscles subsided, and the pain disappeared.

Comment.—The genesis of the pain in this anxious subject is dependent on the circulatory and metabolic dynamics of skeletal muscle activity. The actual process of contraction, by obstructing mechanically the arterioles supplying the muscles with blood, renders the muscle relatively ischemic for the duration of the contraction. The degree of ischemia is roughly proportional to the contraction strength, a strongly contracting muscle being almost completely ischemic. Thus, depending on the form, duration, and intensity of motor activity, the muscle may be relatively ischemic over a long time interval. This prolonged state of anaerobic activity allows for the accumulation in the tissues of metabolic products which would otherwise have been dissipated in the presence of adequate blood flow. These noxious metabolites constitute the critical stimulus for the pain in the backache syndrome. The available evidence indicates that muscle potassium is the pain factor or one of its important components.

Urinary 17-Ketosteroid Excretion During Period of Acute Anxiety

The subject was a tense, anxious, and insecure 29-year-old white male physician. Comparison is made between 2 days, of what were for him a period of relative comfort and productivity, and one day of intense anxiety with grossly impaired productivity. On December 8 and 14, the days of relative security, the subject's 24-hour excretion of 17-ketosteroids was 43.05 mg. and 43.83 mg. respectively. The fractional values for December 8 were: morning, 2.39 mg./hr., afternoon 1.907 mg./hr., evening 1.59 mg./hr., night 1.62 mg./hr.; and for December 14: morning 2.60 mg./hr., afternoon 2.26 mg./hr., evening 1.48 mg./hr., and night 1.47 mg./hr.

On the day of stress the subject found himself confronted with an overwhelming work schedule. He was anxious, tired, irritable, and preoccupied with personal conflicts evolving from the current phase of his psychoanalysis. He was tense and restless and noted a persistent twitch involving the left eyelid. He felt dissatisfied, and his difficulty in concentration was associated with low productivity. Despite his mounting fatigue and poor effectiveness he drove himself at his work until midnight. Sleep was punctuated with frequent anxiety dreams. Total 17-ketosteroid excretion for this day was 87.25 mg. Fractional values were uniformly elevated over comparable times on the control days, with the night sample containing the greatest amounts: morning 3.24 mg./hr., afternoon 3.54 mg./hr., evening 2.54 mg./hr. and night 4.66 mg./hr.

Comment.—In general, variations in urinary excretion of 17-ketosteroids observed in a variety of experimental situations appeared to be directly related to the need of mobilization of bodily resources for action.

It is postulated that: (1) the alterations in the excretion of 17-ketosteroids observed were an index of the amount of adrenocortical hormone produced; (2) during action, tissue utilization of adrenocortical hormones occurs in skeletal muscles and is roughly proportional to the form, intensity, and duration of the activity.

In settings of security, taking action was associated with a moderate decrease in excretion of 17-ketosteroids. In settings of competitive reactions or intense feelings of anxiety, tension, or hostility, taking action was associated with sustained or slightly elevated 17-ketosteroid excretion. If, in such a setting, action was not taken, there occurred marked elevations in excretion of 17-ketosteroids. Exhausting action (heavy exercise) regardless of affect or life setting was invariably associated with a profound decrease in excretion of 17-ketosteroids followed by a marked rise during the recovery period. When taking action did not appear to be required by the threatening situation and the ensuing inactivity was not accompanied by overt anxiety and tension, there was a decrease in excretion of 17-ketosteroids.

Nasal and Gastric Function During Anxiety

The following observation made on an adult male subject with a large gastric fistula documents alterations in 2 physiologic systems participating simultaneously in anxiety states. It is also illustrative of variations in function of the same system at different times. As will be noted, the way in which the subject perceives the stimulus situation, and reacts to it are different for each occasion.

The subject was obliged to remove from a laboratory cage a rat that had been dead for some hours. In the cage were a number of living rats who had macerated the cadaver. He was obliged to put his unprotected hand into the cage, and in spite of his experience he had fears of rat bites and their implications. Furthermore, the cannibalism of the rats and the decayed condition of the malodorous cadaver gave rise to nausea. He experienced intense apprehension and disgust. Both his gastric and nasal mucosae became pale and stayed so for several hours.

At the time of the next observation, the subject's wife was about to visit the hospital because of troublesome varicose veins. His concern about hospitals and sickness and his dependence upon his wife for the proper conduct of the home engendered conflict with feelings of anxiety and resentment. Hyperemia and engorgement were noted in both the gastric and nasal mucosae.

Early Conditioning Experiences and the Genesis of Anxiety

Infants with excessive crying during the first 3 months were investigated and compared with noncrying infants. The babies with excessive crying had anxious, unsmiling facial expressions and during crying displayed considerably more frenzied motor activity, wheezing, and sweating than did the noncrying group. Regurgitation and passage of flatus often occurred toward the end of a period of excessive crying.

Upper gastrointestinal roentgenograms were done at 5 to 7 weeks of age. In all instances the films of the crying children revealed excessive gas and more rapid stomach emptying than occurred in the noncrying group. The crying infants showed wide fluctuations in absolute eosinophil counts ranging from 0 to 1442/cu. mm., while counts in the noncrying babies were stable within the normal range. Elevations of eosinophil levels occurred within 15 minutes after beginning of crying, and persisted, with the excessive crying, for as long as 2 weeks. Hyperemia, hypersecretion, and swelling of the nasal mucous membranes appeared earlier and were sustained at greater magnitude in the infants with excessive crying. The crying babies had increased muscle tension when awake. As determined by the Wetzel Grid growth rate increased during the 3-month crying period. The excessively crying babies had significantly more illness than did the noncrying infants. These included upper respiratory infections, skin rashes, diarrhea alternating with constipation, regurgitation and accidents.

Excessive crying most commonly occurred in settings of domestic conflict and tension arising from the parents' attitudes toward their infant and problems in social and interpersonal relations. In the earliest neonatal relationships the parents of the crying babies were insecure, anxious, tense, and unable to achieve satisfaction from their performance. The mothers were strikingly inconsistent in the frequency, duration, quantity, and quality of handling and feeding, and in the length of time allowed to elapse before responding to the infant's cries. These mothers were unable to make discriminating judgments concerning their infant's communication and their attempts at child care were often unrelated to the child's needs. The crying, by provoking or increasing the mothers' anxiety, tended to establish a vicious circle, the parents' behavior becoming more inappropriate and the infant's crying more aggravated. It was in such settings that the physiologic variables of the infants showed fluctuations of the greatest magnitude and duration and that illness was most apt to occur. By contrast, the parents of the noncrying babies were consistent in the application of their techniques of child care and their assessment of the infant's communication.

Comment.—In the first month of life crying in both groups of babies persisted until individual needs were satisfied. After about 6 weeks of age the 2 groups were distinct. The noncrying infants were relaxed and happy. Crying, when it did occur stopped promptly with the presence of a parent or other adult. The success of this adaptive behavior appears related to the regular and appropriate need satisfaction which characterized the previous experience of the noncrying infants. Infants in the high crying group at the same age were tense, restless, and irritable. The presence of a parent or adult commonly initiated or enhanced the crying. It appears that because of their early conditioning experiences these infants failed to associate mother's presence with satisfaction and security. Rather, the parents' communication actually connoted danger, frustration, or deprivation to the baby and provoked a reaction of anxiety manifested as crying with its physiologic concomitants. These inferences are in agreement with those of Benedek and Freud.

Anxiety States and Disease

The evidence thus far adduced indicates that threats of danger due to stressful life situations may become important in the genesis of illness. Often the discomfort and tissue damage evoked by symbols are indistinguishable from that produced by physical and chemical agents or infectious microorganisms. It, therefore, appears relevant to an understanding of the natural history of disease to consider the effects on bodily integrity of the interaction of multiple noxious stimuli applied simultaneously.

Effects of Anxiety-Provoking Stimuli Introduced During Exposure of Hay Fever Patient to Pollen

A 57-year-old housewife born in the British West Indies of mixed Negro and white stock complained of "hay fever" of 5 years' duration and had a strongly positive ragweed skin test.

The experiment was performed during the hay fever season while the subject was feeling calm, secure, and relaxed. She was free of hay fever symptoms, and her nasal mucous membranes appeared moderately red with small amounts of secretion and swelling apparent. She was then exposed in the experimental pollen room for 109 minutes. Mild symptoms of rhinitis and low grade nasal hyperfunction ensued within 30 minutes. These symptoms subsided after 8 minutes and aside from some nasal obstruction the patient remained comfortable for the next 10 minutes.

At this point an interview was begun which the patient quickly directed toward the unsatisfactory relationship which existed between her husband and her second daughter. As she discussed this she became tense and anxious and her voice became whining and petulant. Examination revealed a marked increase in the nasal hyperfunction. At the same time, increased symptoms of rhinitis recurred.

After this problem had been discussed for 33 minutes she was diverted to neutral topics and felt much reassured. Gradually over the next 28 minutes she regained her feelings of well-being, and despite the fact that she was still being exposed to pollen in the pollen room, nasal hyperfunction subsided, symptoms disappeared and she remained comfortable for the duration of the experiment.

Comment.—It has been demonstrated repeatedly that the alterations in nasal function accompanying conflictual settings are often sufficient to produce troublesome nasal symptoms and pathologic tissue changes. Also from a study of the histories of patients exhibiting common nasal disorders and from observations on individuals followed over long periods, it has been possible to establish a correlation between a setting of conflict with anxiety and nasal hyperfunction and an exacerbation of nasal disease. Further, since conflicts evolving from difficulties in interpersonal and social adjustments often remain unresolved for long periods, the accompanying anxiety and nasal hyperfunction may become both intense and sustained. In such a setting the nasal tissues become unable to tolerate the additional alterations in nasal function engendered by new threats or assaults on bodily integrity. Thus, the nasal hyperfunction appearing as a part of an individual's response to a threatening life situation causing conflict and anxiety may constitute a major etiologic factor in nasal dysfunction. When combined with other environmental stimuli capable of producing nasal hyperfunction, it becomes relevant to the genesis of many common acute and chronic disorders of the nasal and paranasal spaces.

Anxiety and Pre-existing Disease

Regardless of the nature of the etiologic factors, a disease process, once established, constitutes a new stimulus situation, which in turn may initiate inappropriate and costly reactions. In the following observation an attempt has been made to explore the significance of anxiety appearing during the course of a well-established disease process.

The subject was a 55-year-old Greek male who had been admitted to the hospital 3 months previously complaining of left lower quadrant pain. The extensive diagnostic procedures carried out during the interim had failed to reveal the cause of the pain. The patient became progressively discouraged and anxious and, as his discomfort increased, he complained bitterly about "being neglected" and was continually concerned with "what was going to happen" to him. At the time of the following experiment he appeared chronically ill and had a decubitus ulcer on the right hip. His communication was that of anxiety and depression, and he complained freely of generalized abdominal and back pain of steady, dull, and aching quality. Examination revealed considerable muscle spasm of the abdomen and the strip muscles of the back. The abdomen was tender throughout but more so on the left side. Tenderness of the back muscles was striking, being most prominent in the left lumbar region. Firm pressure over these "trigger areas" not only increased the pain in the back but also in the left lower quadrant of the abdomen.

At this point, as the examiner reassured him, the patient was given 0.25 gm. of sodium amytal intravenously. He promptly became relaxed and calm and the pain completely subsided. Examination revealed the muscles of the back and abdomen to be relaxed with only moderate tenderness to pressure. Pressure over the tender areas in the back caused no radiation of pain into the abdomen. Palpation of the relaxed abdomen revealed a moderate sized mass in the left upper quadrant, found at operation to be a hypernephroma. Manipulation of the mass caused intense pain to which the patient reacted with overt anxiety and agitation. He was again reassured and gradually the pain subsided.

Comment.—It is apparent from this observation that the tumor involving pain-sensitive structures was not the only source of discomfort. The complete subsidence of pain following the dissipation of anxiety and skeletal muscle tension by the sodium amytal indicates that the skeletal muscles were a major source as well. On the other hand, pressure or displacement of the abdominal mass was necessary for the production of noxious sensations from the pain-sensitive structures involved by the new growth.

The following rationale for these observations is offered. As a result of the barrage of impulses arising from the pain-sensitive structures in the new growth, 3 reactions were set in motion: local spinal cord reflexes leading to segmental skeletal muscle spasm, the genesis of secondary hyperalgesia involving segmentally both superficial and deep pain-sensitive tissues, and the genesis of anxiety as part of the patient's total reaction to a threatening situation of which pain was only one component. The additional skeletal muscle tension caused by the anxiety became the secondary pain source. The pain from the sustained skeletal muscle spasm, by perpetuating the anxiety, initiated a vicious cycle which also perpetuated the discomfort even in the absence of constant pain from the hypernephroma.

ANXIETY, DISEASE, AND SOCIAL PERSPECTIVE

Cultural Conflict and Tuberculosis

Psychosocial data have been obtained from a representative sample of approximately 1,000 patients with tuberculosis drawn from the metropolitan area of Seattle, Washington. The subjects were 70% male, 22% nonwhite, and 61% unmarried. The median age was 41 years with 64% older than age 35. When compared with the 1950 United States census figures for Seattle (50.1% male, 5.9% nonwhite, 34.8% unmarried, median age 34.4 years, 55.4% age 35 and over), the tuberculosis group represents a marked variation in character of population. Income and education also deviated from the urban median and was more like that of the rural population of the state. Only 11.5% of the patients earned $4,000 per year or more compared with 43.8% in Seattle and 15.9% for the state. The median level of education for patients was 10.9 years. For Seattle's population the median educational level was 12.1 years, for rural nonfarm it was 10.2 years, and for rural farm 9.2 years. The white patients tended to be first or second generation Americans and hence originated from divergent cultural backgrounds to a greater extent than the majority of the population of the city. Over half of the patients had migrated to the city from rural areas. High frequencies of residential and occupational mobility and social isolation completed the pattern of nomadism for the males. The females had almost invariably engaged in productive work and 75% were employed at the time the disease was discovered.

Additional social perspective was provided by ecologic studies on all the 481 newly detected cases of active tuberculosis in Seattle in 1952: 269 white males, 88 white females, 88 nonwhite males, and 36 nonwhite females. Utilizing census tract data, the city was divided into 4 relatively distinct socio-economic residential areas: Area I included the city center and Seattle's

"Skid Road" population, Area II the "working class" population of the city, Area III the typically "middle-class" population, and Area IV included Seattle's "well-to-do" population. Tuberculosis rates per 100,000 population were analyzed by area of residence, age, sex, and race (see Tables 1 and 2).

TABLE 1

TUBERCULOSIS ATTACK RATES PER 100,000 BY SEX AND AGE, FOR SEATTLE AREAS, 1952

	Male To age 29	Male 30 and over	Female To age 29	Female 30 and over
I	188	616	239	159
II	73	297	56	85
III	41	176	40	41
IV	27	114	33	39
Total	150		53	

Rates ranged from significantly high in Area I to significantly low at the periphery (Area IV), irrespective of age or sex. The nonwhite rate, however, was highest in the better socio-economic area at the city periphery. Diagnostically, far-advanced tuberculosis was the mode for Area I, moderately advanced disease for Area II, and minimal tuberculosis for Areas III and IV.

TABLE 2

TUBERCULOSIS ATTACK RATES PER 100,000 BY AGE AND BY ETHNIC-SEX CATEGORY. SEATTLE AREAS, 1952

	Age Range Under age 30	Age Range 30 and over	White Male	White Female	Non-White Male	Non-White Female
I	189	457	482	140	762	535
II	53	196	166	49	481	275
III	39	105	91	29	468	276
IV	28	71	57	32	1,137	569
Total	44	146	83		347	

Life history data revealed the tuberculosis subjects to be sensitive, anxious, rigid, and emotionally labile. These patients, when compared with the cultural norms, were marginal people at the time of onset of tuberculosis. They started life with an unfavorable social status and grew up in an environment that was for them crippling. They were, in essence, strangers attempting to find a place for themselves in the contemporary American scene. As perceived by the individuals with tuberculosis, the poorly understood world in which they lived was a source of perennial danger and the threat of being "walled off" and rendered "helpless" was always imminent. The nature of their attitudes and life experiences made it unusually difficult for them to decide what was expected of them or what they expected of themselves. As a consequence their attempts at adjustment were characterized by unrealistic striving which was not only unrewarding but also productive of cumulative conflict, anxiety, and depression.

Disintegration of the patient's precarious psychosocial adjustment almost invariably occurred in the 2-year period preceding the onset or relapse of disease. The manifestations of the life crisis that ensued included high frequencies of broken marriages and changes in residential and occupational status. Alcoholism, frequent and persistent psychosomatic disorders, and mental illness were common. It was in this setting of increasing life stress acting on individuals whose limited capacities were no longer adequate for resolving problems or achieving satisfaction that tuberculosis apparently developed.

Comment.—In keeping with other investigations of the relationship of the social process to illness, these psychosocial data indicate that cultural conflict and anxiety contribute significantly to the natural history of tuberculosis. The consequences of ethnic, racial, and economic minority status and the processes of urbanization and industrialism are clearly evident.

Psychophysiologic Reactions and Tuberculosis

Since it has been demonstrated that adrenal hormones influence resistance in tuberculosis, the relationship of life stress and adrenocortical function in these patients was investigated. Patients with pulmonary tuberculosis exhibited widely fluctuating 17-ketosteroid excretion patterns ranging from 2.0 mg./24 hrs. to 30 mg./24 hrs. A majority of the patients demonstrated excretion levels below the normal expected for their age and sex.

Chest X-rays revealed that patients with reduced 17-ketosteroid output had extensive and exudative tuberculosis. Patients with elevated 17-ketosteroids in the urine exhibited well-localized, fibrotic or nodular tuberculosis. There were exceptions to this general relationship suggesting that factors other than severity of disease were influencing adrenocortical function.

It was observed that 17-ketosteroid excretion appeared to be consistently related to the emotional state of the patient (see case of male physician above). Patients with very low levels of excretion were overtly depressed, apathetic, and withdrawn. Patients with normal values were reasonably comfortable in their adjustment. Those with above normal output were tense, conflict-ridden, and exhibited the well-known clinical signs of anxiety, such as restlessness, irritability, insomnia, tachycardia, labile blood pressure and palmar sweating.

Rapid and profound changes in 17-ketosteroid excretion were observed to accompany changes in emotional states resulting from acute or chronic stress situations arising during the course of hospitalization. These alterations in adrenocortical function persisted for the duration of the emotional response.

Despite standard antimicrobial therapy, distinct trends in the course of the disease were evident. Patients whose 17-ketosteroid output remained stationary near the normal level showed satisfactory improvement in their disease as did those whose level of output was changing toward normal from above or below. In contrast, patients with a stationary excretion level at some distance above or below normal improved slowly or not at all. The degree of improvement was related to the proximity of the excretion to the normal level. The patients whose disease became worse and those who died exhibited progressive depression and low or declining excretion.

Comment.—The 17-ketosteroid excretion observed in these cases indicating significant alteration of adrenocortical activity in tuberculosis is in agreement with the findings of others. The fact that alterations in 17-ketosteroid excretion parallel changes in the course of tuberculosis suggests that endogenous adrenocortical homones influence resistance to tuberculosis. From these observations it is suggested that adrenocortical activity plays a role in resistance to tuberculosis and that the effects of life stress upon the course of tuberculosis, in part, may be mediated via the adrenal gland.

Formulation

In daily living, the relationship of tribal man to his environment is constantly influenced by stimuli of widely varying origin, character, and significance. Alterations in behavior occur only in response to certain of these stimuli. Further, the degree to which afferent impulses evoked by a given stimulus are consciously perceived and evaluated is variable and may or may not be relevant to the ensuing reaction. The character and significance of such changes in behavior as do occur will be largely determined by the stimulus situation, the individual's biologic endowment, and his past experience. Viewed from a biologic perspective these modifications in behavior appear to be adaptive and protective.

In response to life stress, patterns of adaptive and protective behavior may be relatively free from anxiety. These include phobic, amnesic, compulsive, obsessive, hypochondriacal, and conversion hysterical reactions. Closely allied are the processes of repression and rationalization. Although these reactions may be due directly to frustration, deprivation, and symbols of danger, they often represent the techniques utilized for attempting to re-establish homeostasis after the threat has been acknowledged and anxiety and tension have occurred. Although these methods for dealing with problems may be more or less successful, they seriously impair performance and restrict capacities for flexibility and maturity. In addition, these patterns of behavior may themselves contribute to the genesis of anxiety.

The occurrence of anxiety as the only emotion present has seldom been encountered in these psychophysiologic studies. Rather, the response of which anxiety is a part is composed of a medley of feeling states of various combinations and intensities: guilt, anger, hostility, resentment, humiliation, euphoria, depression, etc. Functional alterations of the biochemical and physiologic systems of the body invariably accompany these emotional states and are mediated by neurohumeral mechanisms. Important to the specificity and character of integration of these psychophysiologic components of behavior is the way in which the individual perceives his relationship to a given situation and what if anything he does or feels like doing about it. The effectiveness of these adaptive and protective patterns of behavior depends on their pertinence to the stimulus, their magnitude and duration. The mobilization of bodily resources when appropriate in context may facilitate the resolution of danger and conflict at little cost to the individual. When inappropriate, these functional alterations in homeostatic mechanisms become sustained and productive of discomfort and tissue destruction. Not only do they fail to achieve their purpose, but actually are responsible for the genesis of additional danger and threat to security.

A concept long recognized by students of human behavior is that early conditioning experiences play an important role in determining the character of an individual's behavior and adjustment in later life. It has been emphasized further that these early experiences are significant factors in many psychiatric illnesses, often through the activation of anxiety. More recently in investigations of the natural history of a host of "psychosomatic disorders," much speculative emphasis has been placed on the importance of these early life situations to the evolution of specific patterns of psychophysiologic responses which may be productive of selective organ dysfunction and symptoms in later life. The observations on infants reported here documents the origin of some of the psychophysiologic reactions which may contribute to the evolution of specific and repetitive anxiety reactions and disease.

Considered in social context, man's concept of himself and his conformance with what is expected of him results in large part from the cultural milieu in which he lives. The evolution of attitudes, values, aspirations, and techniques for achieving goals which approximate the tribal norms is essential to homeostasis, productivity and satisfaction. The success of this process of cultural conditioning depends in part on the nature of the individual, the nature of social pressures and the effectiveness of methods available for dealing with them. Stable civilizations provide a milieu in which the individual can usually define his status with relative ease. In such a way of life the possibilities for culture conflict are minimized and the techniques for resolving tensions are reasonably effective. By contrast, in societies undergoing rapid change, as in the United States, the individual often experiences considerable difficulty in finding his place and making accurate discriminations concerning what is and what is not dangerous. The possibilities for culture conflict abound and the techniques for dealing with ensuing difficulties become attenuated. As a further consequence the individual's knowledge concerning the availability and applicability of these methods is often faulty or incomplete. Therefore, anxiety, discomfort, tissue damage, and impairment of performance, which occur as by-products of attempts at adaptation, become inextricably linked to cultural conflict.

Summary

Inherent in man's biologic endowment is the need for homeostasis and the equipment for its maintenance. Assaults upon and threats to his physical and emotional integrity which upset this homeostasis provoke adaptive reactions intended to restore the equilibrium within the internal milieu of the body, and between the body's internal and external environment. Such reactions to life stress usually are manifested as alterations in behavior which may vary widely in degree, content, duration, and effectiveness. When sustained these reactions may be productive of discomfort and impairment of tissue integrity. Many of the illnesses experienced by man, then, may occur in large part as a by-product of his attempts at adaptation.

COMPULSION NEUROSIS WITH CACHEXIA (ANOREXIA NERVOSA)

Franklin S. Du Bois, M.D.

Historical

It has long been known that disorders of appetite may originate in the psyche. Classical literature is replete with examples of hyperorexia and anorexia and their relation to mental status or personality type. Medical literature, though lagging behind lay expression, offered its first report on the topic in 1694 when Morton referred to "consumption of mental origin." However, it remained for Sir William W. Gull, in an address before the British Medical Association at Oxford in 1868 to mention "young women emaciated to the last degree through hysteric apepsia." Slightly later, the same author presented his classic description of "anorexia nervosa" and since then little has been added to his admirable and astute observations. He described "a peculiar form of disease occurring mostly in young women," characterized by repugnance to food, extreme emaciation, amenorrhea, and personality changes. About the same time, Lasègue gave an account of the illness under the title "hysterical anorexia" but Gull's term, anorexia nervosa, was more widely accepted and has remained so until the present day. More dramatically perhaps than any other clinical entity this disease demonstrates the inseparability of mind and body. It vividly illustrates the effect of emotions on bodily functions and, conversely, the result of a malfunctioning body on the personality. Accordingly, the question early arose as to how the ailment originated. From the time of Gull until 1914 it was generally accepted that the primary lesion was in the psychological rather than in the physiological structure. However, when Simmonds reported the syndrome of hypophyseal cachexia, the possibility of destruction of the pituitary gland as an etiologic factor was introduced. Confusion followed, and for a time all extreme cases of emaciation, both recovered and fatal, were ascribed to a pituitary dysfunction. But, with more careful study and the accumulation of autopsy material, it became apparent that Simmonds' disease presented many distinguishing characteristics clinically as well as a regularly present destruction of the anterior lobe of the hypophysis not found in anorexia nervosa. As a result, the pendulum has once again swung in the direction of a psychogenic origin for the latter. Although there is some support for the view that the disease is a functional dyspituitarism and an infrequent recent proposal that somatic factors contribute to its cause, prevailing opinion holds that anorexia nervosa is a graphic illustration of the influence of emotions on bodily functions, primarily a psychologic and secondarily a physiologic disturbance.

If this contemporary conclusion is correct, what are the powerful psychodynamic forces that lead to virtual starvation, extreme emaciation, and sometimes death? It is inconceivable that a well-integrated personality could foster such unusual behavior. What, then, is the nature of the personality disorder and, more specifically, in what nosological category of present-day psychiatry should the ailment be placed? As indicated by the title of this paper, it is the author's opinion that anorexia nervosa is fundamentally a compulsion neurosis, with cachexia as a leading symptom.

Validating facts are difficult to present in any psychiatric problem, and support of the above interpretation with conclusive data is no exception. The most frequent method employed is to offer a group of typical clinical histories; however, no individual histories are being submitted in this report although the study is based on 10 cases. Such inclusions are laborious and ill-rewarding since it can always be said that the histories are prepared from a prejudiced opinion. Consequently, the 10 cases will be described collectively and then, from this formulation, it will be demonstrated that anorexia nervosa can appropriately be termed a compulsion neurosis with cachexia.

CLINICAL PICTURE

The term, clinical picture, does not refer to a description of anorexia nervosa as a fully developed disease, such as may be found in any one of many authoritative text books of medicine or psychiatry, but rather to a description of the patient and her personality. Such an approach requires that both a physical and a psychological profile be drawn.

A. Physical Profile

The patient, usually an unmarried female* between the ages of 18 and 25, is brought to the physician by her parents who are troubled by her emaciation and inadequate eating. Upon examination cachexia is found to be extreme. The skin is dry, frequently covered with excess hair (hypertrichosis) and occasionally scaling. The extremities are cold and blue-white. Amenorrhea and constipation are regularly present as are slow pulse (50-65), low body temperature (95-98 F) and hypotension (blood pressure ranging from 85 to 95 systolic and 50 to 60 diastolic). Cheilitis, glossy tongue, gingivitis and carious teeth are frequently seen. Aside from low basal metabolic rate (—20% to —40%), electroencephalogram that records abnormal waves,** vaginal smear of the atrophic type, and flat glucose tolerance curve, all laboratory studies are within normal limits. These include red, white, and differential blood

---

* It is said that the disease may very rarely be seen in the male, but there has been no such occurrence in the present series.

** Electroencephalographic studies were made on 3 patients (Dr. B. L. Pacella, electrocephalographer). Irregular mixtures of low to moderate voltage 12 to 16 cycles per second activity characterized the tracings. Occasional random and short series of 8 to 11 cycles per second potentials exhibiting distorted contours were noted. Hyperventilation resulted in a few 7 to 8 cycles per second potentials. Dr. Pacella interpreted these tracings as abnormal and suggested that they were indicative of cerebral dysfunction of a physiologic type very likely based on malnutrition.

counts, urinalysis, Wassermann, blood chemical studies (including fasting blood sugar and blood cholesterol) and x-rays of the skull. In spite of her obvious general ill health, the patient is remarkably active, demonstrating physical energy in a way that is entirely out of keeping with her marked state of malnutrition. Family and friends assert that she never seems to tire, and the physician notes that she is virtually anæsthetic to feelings of fatigue.

Only one disorder, Simmonds' disease, presents a similar clinical picture and this can readily be differentiated. Although it likewise occurs chiefly in women, it is more frequently seen in middle age and is usually precipitated by a physical illness. Weight loss at first is not great but is dramatic and profound in later stages. Premature aging, wrinkling of the skin, deciduation of pubic and axillary hair, loss of sexual desire (previously present), and atrophy of the sexual organs are prominent. Amenorrhea is present in only about one-half of the cases. Lassitude and weakness are conspicuous. Low basal metabolic rate, vaginal smear of atrophic type, and disturbed glucose tolerance curve are present.

B. *Psychological Profile*

A psychological profile of a disease is only of value if drawn from both horizontal and cross-sectional prespectives, the former as it depicts the development of the ailment and the latter as it pictures the disorder at any stage of its evolution. For the present inquiry, a total horizontal and a single cross-sectional study will be made. The horizontal profile will illustrate the developing personality of the patient with anorexia nervosa and the cross-sectional profile the personality in its definitive form.

1. *In horizontal section*

The child who later develops anorexia nervosa is a good little girl. More likely than not, she is the product of unstable parents and has collaterals in which neurosis or psychosis is frequently encountered. Usually the mother is too wrapped up in the child. The youngster has difficulty fitting into the family constellation and does not make friends easily. She is described by her parents as having been a lonely, somewhat seclusive, fanciful little girl with a vivid imagination. Fairly regularly the father or the mother is interested in food, cooking, calories, diets, and the like and, as a result, the child's eating is very early under close surveillance. In the pre-adolescent years she is apt to be a chubby, intelligent, energetic, and obedient girl. With the advent of the menarche, irritability and aloofness increase and there may be open discord between her and one parent, more frequently the mother. In spite of this conflict she is dependent upon home and leans more and more on family supports. And then school friends or members of the family begin to tease her about her "double chin" or "piano legs" or call her "fatty." Very soon a reaction is precipitated. She begins to diet, usually rigorously and remorselessly and in the face of a lusty appetite. Anorexia comes later, and with it a more rapid diminution of food consumption. Contemporaries begin to be interested in boys and enjoy dates but not the girl who is destined for a full-blown anorexia nervosa. True, she may go to dancing school and be with boys but she is not genuinely interested. Concurrently, it is noticed that she becomes busier, is constantly on the go, has many irons in the fire, and complains of so little time. She always feels pushed. Conscientious in the extreme, she devotes long hours to her studies, makes good marks, and is perfection in decorum. As a result she may become "teacher's pet" and be held up to other members of her class as a shining example of rectitude. Only rarely is she active in competitive sports. Mood swings begin to be apparent and with these come periods of irritability and increasing stubbornness. Following graduation from secondary school, the young lady may attempt college or marriage, either of which is generally a failure, and at this juncture family pressure force treatment.

2. In cross section

The young woman afflicted with anorexia nervosa has certain distinguishing personality qualities.* She is a tense, hyperactive, alert, rigid person. Usually she walks, talks, and thinks rapidly. She is inordinately ambitious, drives herself hard, is markedly sensitive, and obviously feels insecure. An immature and severe conscience guides her actions and she is said to be hyperconscientious. Neatness, meticulosity, and a mulish stubbornness not amenable to reason make her a rank perfectionist. Usually she is introverted, serious, self-willed, and lacking in the warmth and spontaneity that are consistent with her years. She is a "little old lady" or the puritanical "old maid," yet respected and admired by her female contemporaries. Boys, however, pay little attention to her and she has no genuine interest in them. If, because of social or family pressure, she has married, sexual adjustment is unsatisfactory with repugnance for coitus a prominent feature. Furthermore, masturbation is vigorously denied and homosexual attachment unknown.

The patient with anorexia nervosa is moody, weeps easily, may complain of being nervous, and almost always feels that that she is not wanted and has been a failure. And these attitudes toward self exist in spite of superior performance. Usually she is proud of her emaciation and what it represents in terms of accomplishment—her ability to diet better than other girls—and has a fear of gaining weight and a horror of becoming fat. With it all, the patient is quite dependent, desirous of attention, and fearful of giving her confidence to anyone.

---

* Clinical psychological studies were carried out on 4 patients (Gladys Tallman, M.A., psychologist). The Wechsler-Bellevue battery regularly demonstrated intelligence in the high average or superior range while the Goodenough and the Rorschach tests equally consistently showed a neurotic pattern laden with anxiety associated with a sexual problem. The sexual problem in every instance seemed to revolve around fear of the opposite sex and sexual relationships. Interestingly, of the 4 subjects were converted sinistrals.

Compulsion Neurosis With Cachexia (Anorexia Nervosa)

Anorexia nervosa has long been considered a visceral symptom of hysterical origin. Dejerine termed it "primary mental anorexia" and believed it to be on an emotional base. Subsequent authors regularly termed it "hysterical anorexia." Only recently has it been suggested that the disease is a type of compulsion neurosis. Palmer (April, 1939) first made the proposal. Shortly therafter (July, 1939), Rahman, Richardson, and Ripley noted that the ailment is a neurosis with "compulsive obsessive, anxious, and depressive features." Likewise, Waller, Kaufman, and Deutsch observed obsessive-compulsive elements in the personality of the patients they studied. The present group of patients and those reviewed in the literature demonstrate features highly consistent with the accepted description of the obsessive individual. Further, if one compares the delineation of the definitive anorexic personality, as outlined in the previous section, with that of Freud's "anal-erotic character" he finds much in common. From early childhood both have been aggressive, perfectionistic, punctilious types of individuals with a marked sensitivity to sex and an unusual interest in body function and form. Orderliness, meticulosity, parsimony, and stubbornness, amounting to obstinancy, are characteristic. The imperative, regularly recurring, and persistent thoughts of food conform with the typical pattern of obsessive thinking in the same way that the imperative urges to avoid food in a repetitive, illogical, and uncontrolled way conform with the typical pattern of compulsive acting. The continual reflections upon food and dietary problems, both in self and in others, furnish the ruminative component, while the highly characteristic and obvious tension and tension activity complete the links in the formulation of an obsessive–compulsive–ruminative–tension state (Meyer). This combination of forces leads to cachexia; hence, the term compulsion neurosis with cachexia seems justified. Lastly, it should be added, as was emphasized by Pardee, that "actual loss of appetite is a rare occurrence." The patient do not eat because of lack of appetite, but because they are afraid to eat, thus the term anorexia is inappropriate.

Etiology

There seems little doubt that compulsion neurosis with cachexia originates early in life and slowly evolves into the clinical syndrome that becomes manifest at puberty or in the early postpubertal period. This suggests that a constitutional factor may be of considerable importance. Some support for this assumption is offered by Sheldon and Richardson, who point out that endocrine involvement, as evidenced by disturbance in the menstrual cycle, regularly precedes loss of weight. Richardson further proposes more specifically that the constitutional defect may be in the nature of an endocrine deficiency. The fact that the histories of such patients are replete with familial psychopathy might also be interpreted as supportive evidence of an inherent predilection for neurotic illness. It seems unlikely, however, in the light of accumulated clinical data, that constitutional predisposition is the most significant factor in bringing about compulsion neurosis with cachexia.

Since the time of Gull, a morbid mental state has been considered a component of the illness. Even so, it is not yet known what part of the psychopathology is of causative significance and what part is the result of the disease process. It is apparent, however, that the patient's major problem is a disturbance of her interpersonal relationships: quite significantly in society as a whole, more sharply with her female contemporaries, very severely within the family constellation and to the point of repulsion in associations with the opposite sex. Therefore, it can be said that the more intimate the relationship with other human beings, the more repugnant and threatening it is to the patient. How does she defend herself from the seeming menace of these associations? The patient defends herself by not eating.

Various theories have been offered as to the primary gains

achieved by the rejection of food. *First,* is that suggested by Brown, who emphasized how inanition prevented the individual from maturing and facing adult responsibilities. He concluded that the disorder is a problem in growing up. Wilson *et al.* likewise stressed that the Rorschach indicated immaturity above everything else.

Second, is the more generally accepted thesis that there is a correlation between appetite for food and appetite for sex. Thus, thwarting and ultimately eliminating the desire for food brings about a state of malnutrition that keeps all biological processes at a low level and ultimately eliminates sexual desire. In this way the timid individual is relieved of the responsibility of dealing with her strong erotic impulses. As a corollary of this mechanism, it is a noteworthy fact that in all patients reticence in discussion of sexual topics is extreme and conscious sexual thoughts and sensations are denied. Unquestionably there is suppression and repression of sexual material.

Third, Waller, Kaufman, and Deutsch have emphasized that the neurosis is a symbolization of pregnancy fantasies through the gastrointestinal tract. They believe that the symptoms are an elaboration and acting out in the somatic sphere of a specific type of wish. According to them a desire for oral impregnation leads to compulsive eating and obesity in the earlier years. Rejection of food and malnutrition appear later as a ritualistic cleansing due to feelings of guilt. They believe that the menses are suppressed as a direct denial of genital sexuality and that the constipation symbolizes the child in the abdomen.

Fourth, Ryle has suggested that the precipitating factors emanate from emotional conflict centering in the home, while Pardee has gone a step further and said that the most uniform single factor is a conflict between the patient and her parents. He believes that an ambivalence, close dependence upon and antagonism toward the mother, and a great admiration of the father due to an unresolved Oedipus situation bring about violent conflict and subsequent attempts to establish independence from the parents who represent an intolerable psychological situation. Because of parental oversolicitude and subjugation, efforts to achieve independence are unsuccessful and the patient develops extremely aggressive thoughts toward her parents. Strong feelings of guilt result. Rejection of food is a masochistic device of atonement for this guilt. Palmer also has stressed the unhappy home relations with spoiling and overindulgence on the part of one parent and hate and hostility directed toward the other. It was his belief that the intense repression of these hostile instinctual impulses motivated the self-punitive and expiatory symptoms.

Fifth, Pardee has also mentioned the significance of poor training. He stated that these young women could not grow up because they were neither trained to do so nor allowed to do so by indulgent, apprehensive, and neurotic fathers or mothers. He found the mother more frequently at fault. In this connection, it should be added that the mechanism of contagion may also play a significant rôle, inasmuch as several of the present group of patients have mirrored their mothers in physical appearance, ideas, neurotic attitudes, methods of speech, and mannerisms. They are indeed "chips off the old block."

Lastly, it has been pointed out frequently that schizophrenic features are prominent in many cases of compulsion neurosis with cachexia. Langdon-Brown thought that dementia præcox was in the background. Brill stated that many were truly schizophrenic. Nicolle also discussed the illness as possibly belonging in the class of latent schizophrenia. More recently Smalldon has concluded that the disease is not a neurosis but a sweeping total personality disorder. In this connection it is to be remembered that Stanley Cobb placed compulsion neurosis just above schizophrenia in his graded classification of mental disease.

The secondary gains achieved by rejection of food are rather obvious. Inadequate eating brings about great solicitude, attention, and spoiling from the parents and enables the patient to regress to infantile reactions and dominate her restricted environment. Furthermore, the resultant emaciation constitutes an excellent defense against establishing a love relationship, because a gaunt, haggard female is extremely unattractive to the male. It is perhaps for these reasons that the patient demonstrates a definite element of gratification in her behavior. There is no doubt that she takes pride in her unique accomplishment and repugnant appearance.

In addition to these psychologic mechanisms which are significant factors in the production of the behavior disturbance described, one must also consider the effects of inanition on the thought processes. Surprisingly, this important physiologic causative agent is not mentioned by a single author in the literature reviewed pertaining to anorexia nervosa. Psychiatrists have long been aware that changes in the internal environment of the individual may produce deviations in thought and action; as exemplified by toxic deliria or personality reactions of the organic type. Similarly, starvation or semistarvation results in behavior disturbances. Schiele and Brozek, by semistarvation under controlled conditions, produced a neurosis characterized by "intense preoccupation with thoughts of food, emotional change tending toward irritability and depression, decrease in self-initiated activity, loss of sexual drive, and social introversion." These experimentally determined personality deviations have a close parallel in natural starvation, and likewise fairly closely approximate the characteristic symptoms observed in compulsion neurosis with cachexia. In addition, a critical study of Schiele and Brozek's report reveals specific obsessions and compulsions as a feature in several cases. Accordingly, it would seem safe to conclude that a certain part of the behavioral changes in this disorder are the direct result of improperly functioning ill-nourished organs.

From the material here submitted and from the cited authors' interpretations one is brought to the inescapable conclusion that this form of cachexia represents a severe derangement of the entire biologic organism. "The behavioral, emotional, and social manifestations of starvation may be looked upon as psychosomatic phenomena in a broad sense, that is, they are the results of a complex interaction between anatomic, physiologic, individual-psychologic, and social-psychologic factors." On the basis of evidence available it seems likely that constitutional predisposition makes a fertile soil for the formation of this deep and sweeping personality disorder. Compulsion neurosis with cachexia becomes a manifest illness at the pubertal period as the child apparently tries desperately to reject her sexuality and the physical and emotional responsibilities related thereto. Specifically why this is true is at present unknown. But whatever may be the dynamic psychological factors, it is apparent that intense, inhibited, and poorly directed emotional forces bring about a pattern of thought, feeling, and action more nearly consonant with obsessive-compulsive neurosis than any other known clinical entity. It would further seem evident that the illness is fostered and perpetuated by profound secondary malnutrition.

Prognosis and Treatment

Prognosis and treatment go hand in hand because the ultimate outlook for the patient suffering from compulsion neurosis with cachexia depends in large measure on the methods of therapy employed. No doubt many mild cases recover spontaneously, a not unreasonable assumption in the light of the importance of growing up and the resolution of parental ties as curative agents, two events that usually occur with the progression of years. Such patients never reach the physician and their frequency and clinical course are unknown. However, very likely such a group exists, because the incidence of menstrual disturbances and dietary problems in adolescent girls is high. Perhaps many of these minor illnesses fall into the category of mild compulsion neurosis with cachexia. But when the disorder is fully developed and of a severity such as has been described in this paper, it, like all obsessive-compulsive reactions, is difficult to treat, not only from day to day but also on a long-term basis so as to achieve recovery and to avoid relapse. Magendantz and Proger support this view and hold that the possibility of satisfactory treatment is remote and that permanent recovery is improbable. On the other hand, Ross reported 16 out of 19 cases absolutely well following a Weir-Mitchell regime of bed rest, isolation, high caloric diet, and a superficial discussion of problems. Of the 10 cases included in this report, 5 achieved socially satisfactory though emotionally limited adjustments. All held to their personality qualities of introspection, stubbornness, and lack of warmth, and all but one continued to have difficulty adjusting to the opposite sex. Regularly, after attaining proper weights, they later dropped to lower levels and remained thin, though not cachectic, individuals. Two patients, after satisfactory initial gains, discontinued treatment. One is known to have relapsed and the other could not be followed up. Three patients are still under treatment, two progressing satisfactorily and one unsatisfactorily.

Described methods of treatment are quite variable. Certain authors recommend superficial reassurance and forced feeding while others stress the essentiality of deep psychotherapy and the relative unimportance of physical measures. Likewise there is no unanimity as to the most helpful attitude of the physician. For example, Venables asserts that the doctor must take a very firm position and "be prepared to fight for every mouthful" of food the patient takes. Similarly, Ryle says that the patient must be dominated by her physician and her nurse. On the other hand, Palmer states that efforts of exhortation, persuasion, and coaxing are to be strictly avoided, and Richardson holds that such coercive measures are positively dangerous inasmuch as they may precipitate suicidal attempts.

The author's method of treatment has consisted of a coordinated program of psychotherapeutic and somatotherapeutic procedures. It has been learned that even though the major treatment is psychological it must be correlated with adequate physical measures, if satisfactory results are to be achieved. Furthermore, active treatment and long-term follow-up must be carried out over a substantial period of time, occasionally years, in order to effect cure and minimize relapse.

The first requirement is that the patient be removed from her home and placed on a definite regime in a sanitarium, nursing home, or hospital. This accomplishes the dual purpose of freeing the patient from neurotic parental influence and offering a setting where her total behavior can be guided 24 hours a day. More frequently than not special nursing is required to guide dietary requirements, to prevent the frequent hiding or vomiting of food, and to control the prominent symptoms of hyperactivity and waste of precious energy. The program starts at bed rest or on a semiambulatory basis and consists of 6 modest feedings with low bulk and a value of approximately 1,500 calories per day. Vitamins orally and parenterally, together with intramuscular injections of liver once or twice each week, a high fluid intake, and mild cathartics, complete the initial physical regime. Should gentle purgatives prove ineffective in the control of the constipation that is so persistent during the early stages of treatment, a simple soapsuds enema is administered every other day, as may be necessary. During the initial period the patient may be quite uncomfortable with abdominal distension, eructation, and moderately severe bowel cramps. Because her previous diet has been quantitatively negligible, virtually each mouthful of food creates discomfort. Hence, repeated reassurance and explanation of causes of discomfort must be given by both physician and nurse. With abundant praise, reassurance, and encouragement these first difficulties are surmounted so that both caloric content and bulk of diet can be increased gradually. After 2 to 3 weeks the program should be elevated to 3 regular meals and 3 intermediate nourishments with a total of 3,000 to 3,500 calories in 24 hours. Should the patient be unable to accept this volume of food, insulin in tonic doses (5 to 25 U) should be administered 45 to 60 minutes before each meal.* About

---

* Insulin as a stimulant to appetite in this type of case has been much discussed in the literature. By several, its use has been deplored because it was believed that the blood sugar is already at a low level. By others, insulin has been found to be an effectual adjunct to treatment, a conclusion with which the author concurs. Insulin, when administered prudently and in small dosage, car-

this time abdominal discomfort has largely disappeared and the physical regime of the patient can be increased. With greater activity, edema of the feet, ankles, and lower legs frequently appears and is an annoying though short-lived symptom. Presumably this extravasation of fluid into the tissues is due to stasis, since all evidence of swelling disappears within a few days. The cardiovascular apparatus rapidly adjusts itself to the new and increased load of work. By the end of the third week the patient should be able to cooperate in a program that includes one full hour of exercise and one full hour of occupational therapy twice each day in conjunction with an after-luncheon rest period and adequate time for reading and play.

Although necessary physical procedures in the care of the patient have been outlined in some detail, it is not to be forgotten that, as was pointed out by Evans, the fundamental purpose of treatment is to remove the psychological protest to food. It is the neurosis and not the appetite that must be the prime focus of attack by the physician. Therefore, psychotherapy is the major remedial agent. Little reference should be made to diet and the family and nursing personnel are instructed to avoid talking about food or the patient's dietary habits. During the early weeks of treatment psychotherapy consists of reassurance and explanation combined with general mental hygiene re-education.* From this training the patient receives a working

---

ries no risk and powerfully enhances food intake. In fact it may frequently prove to be a decisive factor in the early stages of treatment. In none of the present cases was insulin given as a shock procedure such as described by Wilson Rymarkiewiczowa, and White in their efforts to interrupt the habit of refusal of food.

In this connection it should also be added that other endocrine products (pituitary hormones, estrogenic substances, and thyroid extract), suggested by many authors, were not employed. There would seem to be no rationale for the use of pituitary materials or estrogens since menstrual function is resumed in due time without supplementary glandular therapy. Thyroid when administered in effective dosage causes weight loss. These findings support the observations of Pardee.

* The method of re-education employed is that of Doctor William B. Terhune, Medical Director of the Silver Hill Foundation, and consists of a series of booklets describing principles of adaptation, management of emotions, and technique

knowledge of the nervous system and the emotions, and the therapist is given opportunity to establish rapport and appraise his patient and her problems. At the end of approximately 3 weeks, therapy proceeds gradually to a deeper level. Most patients are intelligent and verbally cooperative and early demonstrate partial insight. But the therapist must not be deceived because, as was pointed out by Palmer, even though these patients profess to have no fear arising from internal sources, their actions belie their statements. They adhere desperately to the well-established patterns of behavior. Accordingly, one proceeds cautiously and slowly into a discussion of his patient's feelings of hostility toward her parents, her ambivalence, her fear of sex and its various connotations of intimate relationship, her feelings of guilt, and lastly, her refusal of food as a punitive and expiatory process. Somewhere along the way significant dynamic factors are encountered and when the related anxiety is eliminated by free and open discussion, tenseness and resistance begin to disappear. Finally, and of almost equal importance, the patient's general maladjustment is considered and efforts are directed toward total personality improvement. This includes discussions of maturity and immaturity, the hedonistic principle of conduct, and the necessity of establishing purposes and goals in life. Without exception, it has been necessary to help the patient plan for the future and evolve a setting for living and working outside of the home that will in due time bring independence and a sense of belonging. It is these latter goals that demand long-term follow-up and guidance. In subsequent interviews, at first weekly and then in decreasing frequency, practical problems of everyday living and human relationships are discussed, dynamic factors previously considered are reviewed, and new and better habit patterns are encouraged and reinforced. Active therapy lasts approximately 3 months

---

of living. The patient reads and discusses these booklets with the physician and then is taught to apply the newly acquired information to her own difficulties. All patients in the present series were treated in collaboration with Doctor Terhune.

while subsequent follow-up continues for as long as 3 years. In spite of these methods, tendency to relapse is marked and occasionally it is necessary for the patient to come into sanitarium residence for short periods in order to regain lost ground. The treatment of compulsion neurosis with cachexia is always a sustained challenge to the therapist.

Summary and Conclusion

Anorexia nervosa dramatically demonstrates the inseparability of mind and body and is a classic example of a psychosomatic disorder. It is primarily a psychic and secondarily a somatic disturbance. Inasmuch as the personality reaction of the individual suffering from anorexia nervosa more nearly conforms to compulsion neurosis than that of any other psychiatric disorder and, in addition, has cachexia rather than anorexia as a leading symptom, it is suggested that the illness would be more accurately termed compulsion neurosis with cachexia. Although definitive data as to etiology are not available, evidence presented indicates that constitutional defect probably predisposes to the illness, which becomes manifest at puberty or shortly thereafter because of severe and deep psychological conflicts centering in the family constellation. The dynamics of these conflicts are discussed and the conclusion drawn that the patient's basic difficulty lies in her more intimate interpersonal relationships. Adequate physiological and psychological treatment, described in detail, offers a reasonably good prognosis, although the tendency to relapse is great.

DIAGNOSIS AND TREATMENT OF THE PHOBIC REACTION

Walter I. Tucker, M.D.

One of the commonest neuroses seen in clinic practice is marked by severe phobic reactions with varying degrees of anxiety, somatic symptoms, and hysterical and obsessive-compulsive tendencies. This type of neurotic reaction has previously been called anxiety hysteria, and it occurs when the external life stress becomes sufficiently severe in individuals who have a dependent type of personality disorder.

It occurs most frequently in young wives and mothers, is more frequent in married than in single women, and more frequent in women than in men. The vital statistics of 100 patients seen over the course of about 1 year is presented in Table 1.

The only complete study of this syndrome was by Terhune in 1949. Otherwise the literature abounds in theories of phobias, which have been summarized by Terhune, and analytic studies of specific phobias on a few patients. Terhune emphasized the immaturity of these patients, their inability to adjust to responsibility and stress, and the need for directive rather than nondirective treatment. These principles are supported by the present study, but there are other factors which are important to emphasize in the diagnosis and treatment of this disease. The fact that Terhune's patients were, for the most part, hospitalized patients from financially privileged families, and that most of those reported here were clinic outpatients from all financial levels, may account for some differences in the findings emphasized.

TABLE 1
Phobic Reaction—Age and Sex Distribution

	Under 20	20-29	30-39	40-49	Total
Female					
Married	0	21	33	12	66
Single	3	17	2	1	23
Total	3	38	35	13	89
Male					
Married	0	3	3	2	8
Single	0	2	1	0	3
Total	0	5	4	2	11
Grand Total	3	43	39	15	100

The following case report will serve to identify this type of disorder.

Mrs. M.D., age 23, has been married for 2 years and had a son, age 15 months. After the birth of her baby she had increasing tension, fatigue, indigestion, palpitation and insomina. She began to have episodes of extreme anxiety with tremulousness, weakness, dizziness, and numbness with crying. She called these episodes nervous hunger and said they were relieved by eating. She sighed frequently and complained of difficulty in getting her breath. She had phobias of going out alone, of crowds, of dying, and of insanity, and was unable to do any of her housework.

Hyperventilation produced all the symptoms of which she complained during an episode. She had a spell during the glucose tolerance test (which was normal), and was relieved by reassurance. A complete physical examination was made, including routine blood and urine examinations and stomach roentgenograms, all of which were normal.

Authoritative and detailed reassurance, explanation of her symptoms with the correction of misconceptions, the advice to avoid hyperventilation, symptomatic medication, and encouragement concerning activity resulted in immediate improvement in the acute symptoms. The solution of a religious conflict over pregnancy by the acceptance of "rhythm" after a talk with her priest helped her further. However, she continued to have the same symptoms to a lesser and variable extent.

Her mother had died in childbirth and she had been brought up by her grandmother who continually insisted that her father was a terrible man and was responsible for her mother's death. She had been sickly as a child and her grandmother had restricted her activity for the reason that "she almost died once." The grandmother still telephoned her every day, she still saw the grandmother frequently, and was still seeking her affection and approval which she had never had.

Although this patient originally seemed an extremely immature personality, she undertook the responsibility for better understanding herself and was able to follow directions for the improvement of her adjustments in spite of symptomatic distress. Remissions and exacerbations of her symptoms occurred over a period of 8 months, but she finally achieved a fairly stable condition with rare symptoms and good functional capacity. She developed fair insight, was able to emancipate herself from her grandmother's influence and modify some of her attitudes, resulting in a better acceptance of the female role and a better adjustment to her husband and child.

Differential Diagnosis

This condition must be differentiated from physical as well as other neurotic disorders. The somatic complaints may be treated as an organic disease, which only fixes the symptoms, or the patient may be dismissed as being "just nervous," without being convinced of the absence of organic disease and without advice as to what to do about it. The patient will "go the rounds" from one doctor to another, getting conflicting opinions and advice which serve to increase and fix the anxiety and confusion.

A previous paper pointed out how the hyperventilation syndrome can be confused with various organic conditions such as epilepsy, pheochromocytoma, brain tumor, hypoglycemia, cardiac and gastrointestinal disorders. Lewis recently has written on the importance of hyperventilation. Inasmuch as hyperventilation tendencies are present to some extent in almost every case, the same difficulties in differential diagnosis may exist.

The first necessity, then, is to institute studies sufficient to convince not only the physician, but also the patient, as to the absence of organic disease. In addition to a complete physical examination there may be need for roentgenograms, an electrocardiogram, gastrointestinal studies, an electroencephalogram or a glucose tolerance test.

It is also important to differentiate this syndrome from the obsessive-compulsive neurosis, which is much less amenable to treatment and has a much poorer prognosis. The patients who are suffering from the phobic reaction may have some obsessive-compulsive tendencies which are not outstanding or disabling, and the development of the phobic reaction can be attributed to some acute or cumulative life stress. The obsessive-compulsive neurotic with phobias usually has a long history of such symptoms of varying severity not necessarily attributable to any specific stress.

Hyperventilation

A tendency to hyperventilate often occurs in association with the acute anxiety or phobic episodes. This is usually the reaction to a feeling of oppression in the chest or of acute suffocation and air hunger. There may be only an increase in sighing respirations, but at times there may be an acute hysterical reaction with gasping for breath, crying, and screaming, which alarms not only the patient but the family as well. Often the patient is not aware of overbreathing, but the husband or others can usually verify this. Symptoms complained of most commonly are fear, weakness, palpitation, tremulousness, sweating, faintness, and numbness of the extremities and the face. Actual fainting may occur (which is an hysterical reaction), or cardiac or gastrointestinal reactions may be prominent, making differential diagnosis a problem. Crying may follow a short period of hyperventilation.

It is important to have the patient voluntarily hyperventilate, to aid both diagnosis and treatment. The response helps to differentiate the symptoms from other disorders. As an entering wedge for treatment it is of great help to be able to demonstrate to the patient how symptoms similar to the attacks can be produced by voluntarily overbreathing. This helps her to realize that her own actions and reactions can have a bearing on the production of symptoms. She is advised to try to avoid hyperventilation with any subsequent attack, and thus is supplied with a task to perform to help herself rather than to continue feeling completely helpless and succumbing to fear and panic.

Phobias

The patient is full of fears. There are almost always fears of some serious organic disease such as cancer, brain tumor, or heart disease, and almost always a fear of insanity or "cracking up." It is necessary to determine what fears exist in order to institute specific studies to try to relieve the patient. Fears regarding health are often irrational or morbid and remain in spite of reasonable reassurance, and thus constitute phobias.

Many other phobias commonly are present. A phobia of going out alone may cause the patient to restrict herself entirely to the home, not daring to leave the premises alone. She is afraid that she will have an attack, will faint, have a stroke, die, or that she will "crack up." In spite of the fact that none of these things has ever occurred and she is reassured that they will not, the phobia remains. If she attempts to go out alone, an acute anxiety reaction occurs and starts the train of events leading to hyperventilation, secondary fears, and hysterical reactions. There may commonly be phobias of crowds, of going to the theater or to church, to a restaurant or on a subway, and the same fears of what may happen exist. There may be a phobia of high places with a fear that she may jump off, or that she may otherwise injure or kill herself. This is sometimes interpreted as a suicidal tendency; however, it is really not a desire or impulse to self-destruction but only a fear of it. There is a vast difference, and I have never known such a patient to do anything to harm herself in these instances. Another common phobia is a fear of harming the children or others, so that the sight of knives or other weapons produces an anxiety reaction. This likewise is not a conscious impulse to harm anyone, but only a fear that such may occur, nor have I ever known such a patient to harm anyone.

Dynamics

The primary difficulty, an immaturity in personality development, with a dependent relationship to the parents, was apparent in 77 of the 100 patients. The overt neurotic reactions develop when the strain of adjustment to responsibilities becomes too great. This is, of course, a matter of degree. There may be relatively slight personality difficulty, but a great deal of strain, such as the problem of an alcoholic husband, financial insecurity, annual pregnancies, and the influence of a neurotic mother. Or there may be a marked personality defect with overt neurotic symptoms from an early age and very little environmental strain. However, a problem almost always exists in the relationship with the parents, usually the mother, and the relationship is ambivalent. There is unhealthy dependence on the mother, which ranges from complete dependence on a completely dominant mother, to a fear of doing anything of which the mother does not approve—a dependence on the mother's approval. At the same time, there is usually some degree of resentment and rebellion in the relationship with the mother. The background is that of insecurity in childhood as a result of parental strife, lack of parental affection, overprotection and overcriticism by parents. The result is an adult patient still seeking approval and affection from the parents, which will never be given. There is also frequently an acquisition of unhealthy marital attitudes from the mother, such as rejection of sexual activity, fear of childbirth, the martyr attitude toward the role of a wife and mother, and resentment toward men for placing her in such a role. The husband may be identified with the father, with resentments and hostility transferred to him, and demands made on him to treat her as a child and give her what she had always hoped to get from her father. The patient often enters marriage with motivations of immature romantic love, or with the object of security and being cared for, or to get away from an unpleasant home situation. There is little wonder that such a person has difficulty in adjusting to the duties and responsibilities of a wife and mother. Furthermore, it is usually not long until the conflict of loyalties arises—loyalty to the husband and children or loyalty to the parents. Many such patients are sensitive and given to excessive worry and tend to hold in their feelings in the attempt to keep peace at any price. If such is the case, the patient finds herself "in the middle" between her husband and her parents, attempting to please everyone. Further problems and strains arise with the arrival of children and there is often conflict over pregnancy, particularly that based on religious beliefs. Symptoms develop, and more anxiety, insecurity and confusion arise when the cause is not found.

Treatment

The first requisite of treatment is the establishment of the diagnosis, and sufficient explanation and reassurance. The patient has a great many fears and much confusion about her physical condition, and there must be authoritative reassurance on all points. There is often resistance to accepting the diagnosis of a nervous disorder as responsible for all the trouble. This is partly due to misconceptions about nervous disorders, such as the implication that nervous symptoms are imaginary and should be overcome by an effort of the will. It is often a great help in this explanation to have the patient demonstrate to herself that severe symptoms can be produced by hyperventilation. This aids her to understand that certain symptoms which are by no means imaginary can be produced by her own actions, and that she can assume some responsibility for averting symptoms by modifying her actions. The phobias particularly need to be explained, and specific reassurance given that the feared events will not take place. The patient can be reassured that she will not faint or have a heart attack or die when the acute anxiety attacks occur. The almost universal fear of "cracking up" or "going insane" can be partly assuaged by stating that this is not the type of nervous disorder that leads to insanity. The phobia of harming self or others is often the most distressing reaction. It is of help to explain to the patient that this is not an impulse to such action but only a fear that such an action may occur. She can be assured that such an action never does occur in such conditions, and that these phobias seem to have no specific meaning in themselves but are only an expression of underlying insecurity. The explanations do not prevent the phobias, but they do help the patient to live with them with less severe anxiety. The effectiveness of reassurance depends on the timing, on the thoroughness with which it is done, and on the confidence in the physician. It usually has to be repeated several times. It is not effective if undertaken before a thorough study is made and all fears and misconceptions are considered.

The patient may be in such a condition that she is severely disabled and unable to carry out the responsibilities of the care of the home and children. The acute symptoms occur when the strain and conflict have become too great, so that often arrangements have to be made to relieve the patient partially, or perhaps wholly, of such responsibilities for the time being. Sometimes it is necessary to get her completely away from the home and preferably into a neutral environment. The cooperation and understanding of the husband must be enlisted, if possible. He also may be anxious and uncertain about the physical condition; or on the other hand, may have no sympathy or patience whatsoever and tells his wife "it is all in your head," and that she can overcome it herself. It is necessary to help him to understand that the physical condition is normal, but that she is sick and that the symptoms are just as real and disabling even though they are of nervous origin.

The patient should be urged to increase her activities gradually in spite of phobias; to learn that she can take the action associated with a phobic reaction, go forward in spite of some anxiety, and thereby gain confidence to go farther the next time.

There may be a particular conflict over whether to have another baby and the patient may have been told by others that she ought to have one as this would help or cure her. There may be a religious conflict over this, with the teachings of the church conflicting with her fear of pregnancy. Pregnancy is usually contraindicated at the time, as the patient has already passed her limit of adjustment, and the cooperation of the husband is necessary in accepting this advice.

When this much is accomplished, there is usually a marked improvement, with reduction of acute anxiety, phobias, and other symptoms. Then the real work begins, and the chances of further help depend on the modifiability of the environment, and the attitude and resources of the patient. If the patient is willing to accept some responsibility for her own health, and willing to undergo some distress and work hard, progress can be made toward a more mature and healthier adjustment. In many cases, however, such a favorable set of circumstances does not exist, and then the outlook for any permanent help is poor. Mother is often living in the same house, or nearby, or the patient has to see her every day or talk to her on the telephone several times a day, which exerts considerable influence. Sometimes it is possible to arrange for the patient to separate herself from the mother's undue influence by moving to a different location, or by voluntarily reducing the personal contacts with the mother. Such a separation is possible only if the patient has some degree of independence and ability to direct her own life. Be it gradually or precipitously, however, she must learn about her unhealthy relationships with the mother and strive to modify them. She must learn to become less dependent on the mother's approval by finding approval elsewhere. She must learn to place herself and her own family's needs ahead of her need to please the mother. And finally, she needs to learn to disagree with the mother without a feeling of guilt or fear. The possibility of accomplishing these aims depends on many factors, not the least of which are the personality and circumstances of the mother. The mother frequently is neurotic also and likely to be demanding, critical, or overprotective, thus tending to produce insecurity and immaturity in the children. In fact, the mother may have been at one time very like the patient and many of my patients say, "I swore I would be different from my mother, but now I find myself doing the same thing to my children."

The personality and influence of the father also contribute to the problem, particularly if he is overprotective or overpunitive, and there may be a problem in the patient's relationship to both parents. However, the father is more frequently a passive individual who plays a relatively minor role in influence on the patient.

When this type of phobic reaction occurs in men, the dynamics are similar, in that there is usually a problem in the relationship to the parents, principally the mother.

When the modification of the unhealthy relationship with the parents is achieved, it is then possible to arrive at a healthier and more satisfying relationship with others, particularly the husband. The course of progress must be directed toward greater security and maturity, which is a slow process, and the degree of progress made along this path varies with the environmental obstacles along the way and the resources of the patient. A great deal of progress can often be made, however, which is satisfying to the patient as well as the physician, with continued reassurance, support, and encouragement.

It should be emphasized that the treatment needs to be strongly supportive and directive in patients of this type, and I believe that a nondirective analytic approach is ineffective. Some of my patients had previously been treated by other psychiatrists, using the nondirective analytic method. These patients were not helped and often became more confused and disturbed.

Results

Although the results of psychotherapy are notoriously difficult to evaluate. I believe that some report of results is essential in evaluating any type of treatment, and psychotherapy should not be excluded from this test.

The results are shown in Table 2. Of the 100 patients, 28 were seen only once for diagnosis, and many of the other patients did not or could not continue with treatment until dis-

TABLE 2
Phobic Reaction—Results of Treatment

	Diagnosis only	Unchanged	Improved	Recovered	Total
Female					
Married	22	11	21	12	66
Single	2	2	13	6	23
Male					
Married	3	1	2	2	8
Single	1	0	2	0	3
Grand Total	28	14	38	20	100

charged. Of the 72 patients seen more than once, the number of visits ranged from 2 to 33, with an average of 7. Patients were considered "recovered" if they were relieved of all symptoms, were functioning without handicap, and had made a sufficient gain in maturity and independence. They were considered "improved" if they were significantly relieved of phobias and able to carry out their responsibilities.

The effectiveness of treatment depended not so much on the number of visits as on the attitude and resources of the patient, and the modifiability of the environment. It is seen that the percentage of improvement and recovery was greater in the single girls, which is due to the fact that both the patient and the environment were more susceptible to change.

Summary

The clinical features of this type of phobic reaction are chronic and acute anxiety with various somatic symptoms and with phobias as a prominent part of the picture.

It is a commonly seen neurotic reaction and occurs most frequently in young wives and mothers, yet it is often misdiagnosed and mismanaged by physicians in all fields of medical practice.

The differential diagnosis is discussed with reference to the necessity of ruling out organic disease to the satisfaction of both physician and patient, and distinguishing the phobic reaction from more chronic phobic obsessive states.

Hyperventilation occurs frequently in association with anxiety attacks. The importance is stressed of recognizing this and demonstrating it to the patient.

Phobias are discussed with particular reference to explanation and reassurance.

The dynamics are presented as the reaction of a dependent type of personality subjected to stress in adjustment.

Treatment is discussed with emphasis on preliminary management and the necessity for directive rather than nondirective treatment.

The results of treatment in 100 patients are reported.

SEPARATION REACTION IN PSYCHOSOMATIC DISEASE AND NEUROSIS

Henry H. Brewster, M.D.

The reaction of grief, defined as the normal response of an individual to bereavement, has been discussed by Freud, Melanie Klein and Abraham, who have given a dynamic formulation to grief and, in particular, have pointed out the relation of mourning to the depressive psychoses. Helene Deutsch has described special instances when grief is unexpectedly absent, while Lindemann has demonstrated that following a bereavement a patient may develop a neurotic symptom or signs of a psychosomatic disease instead of grief.

In a psychiatric study of ulcerative colitis, Lindemann found that a close time relation existed between the death of a person important to the patient and the onset of colitis. Cobb, Bauer, and Whiting noted that 7 of 50 patients with rheumatoid arthritis had lost a parent or spouse prior to the exacerbation of symptoms. Lidz observed the importance of the death of the mother in patients with hyperthyroidism.

While grief, or a substitute for it, appears to be the expected response to bereavement, a reaction resembling grief can occur after the temporary separation of one person from another. Rosenbaum and Bond have documented the reaction to such a separation in a family when one member left for service in the Army, and they found signs of grief in the various members of the family. Felix Deutsch has recently presented clinical examples of "separation neurosis."

The purpose of the present study was to observe the effect of separation, to compare this effect insofar as possible with that of bereavement, and to compare the significance of separation in a neurosis and in a psychosomatic illness. To this end, 6 patients were subjected to separation from their psychotherapist, who was the author in each case. Three of the patients had a psychosomatic disease. By way of contrast, 3 patients were selected who had a neurosis. The diagnoses of the 6 were: psychogenic vomiting, reactive depression, phobia, ulcerative colitis (in 2 patients), and rheumatoid arthritis. During the initial period of psychotherapy of each patient, special attention was given to the nature of the patient's dependency upon the therapist. Then the therapist left for a month's vacation. In the course of psychotherapy which followed, observations were made of the nature of the patient's reaction to this separation.

A 13-year-old boy, the son of a teacher, was brought for treatment by his mother, a stiff, quiet, rigorously neat woman of 50. He had been vomiting frequently since he was 4. Examinations showed no evidence of organic disease.

He made a singular appearance at the first interview. His gait was like that of a girl. He spoke quietly and with restraint, lowering his eyes when facing the therapist. His voice was high-pitched and whining. He was shy and appeared scared, guarding his remarks as if to avoid risking the disapproval of the therapist. He sat motionless in a chair, and answered questions asked him.

In the initial interview he indicated that his mother was a methodical and strict taskmaster, whom he and his father feared to cross. She punished him for getting less than B at school, and especially if he vomited his breakfast. He felt helpless to combat her, even when she allocated all his spare time to music lessons.

After two months of weekly interviews, his behavior changed. He walked like a man. He talked vigorously about his vacation plans to go fishing, blew bubble gum, whistled. His mother had been scolding him but he didn't mind. His vomiting had stopped. He was now thinking of the therapist as "an awfully good friend."

Then came the separation of a month from the therapist. Next seen, his behavior had reverted to its original form and he was vomiting. He had been discouraged, sad, and lonely,

SEPARATION REACTION

often angry. He considered running away from home. Often he thought of the therapist, especially when his mother scolded him for not eating. Yet within two weeks of the resumption of treatment, he had regained the state of improvement which had existed prior to the separation.

It is evident that this passive, effeminate boy found in the therapist a more useful model of imitation than in his father. With it, he was able in the course of two months to give up his neurotic symptom of vomiting and to tolerate the aggressive demands of his mother. In that it led to a recurrence of his presenting symptoms, the reaction to separation demonstrated the boy's need to depend upon the therapist. The fact that the boy was angry and sad when he thought of the missing therapist indicates that he felt rejected by the therapist in the same sense as a person in mourning. It should be noted that where it took two months for the original symptom to disappear, the reaction to separation was over within two weeks of the resumption of treatment.

An attractive, 26-year-old housewife came for treatment because, since her marriage of a year's duration, she had been subject to crying spells, sleeplessness, and fears of pregnancy. Her marriage had meant that she move a great distance from her parents' home and live in squalid circumstances.

During a month of weekly interviews, she was much concerned with affectionate memories of her father, an itinerant minister. Her husband seemed unintelligent and unsympathetic by comparison. But she took to working as a mother's helper and she no longer was sleepless or given to crying spells.

After a month of separation from the therapist, she cancelled her appointment in order to go home and visit her parents. At the next appointment she was acid and provocative. She had felt "every way there was to feel, from the highest to the lowest." She sat behind the therapist, announced that she was not sure she could continue with therapy. She opened a camera, snapped a picture, then stated she had no film in the camera. Subsequently, she was able to express her anger at the interruption of therapy. Within three weeks, there was no more evidence of depression of provocative behavior, and she and her husband had moved from the squalid apartment into the home of a psychiatrist, who was the son of a minister.

This young housewife, the daughter of a minister, finding difficulty in adjusting to her marriage, became depressed over her separation from home, especially from her father. She obtained relief from these depressive feelings during a month and a half of therapy, in which the therapist became a substitute for her father. In response to the month of separation from the therapist, during which depressive feelings recurred, she returned home to her father. When psychotherapy was resumed, the therapist met only a display of anger in the form of bitter remarks and provocative behavior. Her response to separation appeared to be a reenactment of her sense of being rejected by her father. After another month of therapy, she was no longer depressed and had found a substitute for both her father and the therapist; i.e., employment in the home of a psychiatrist whose father was a minister.

A 30-year-old, single woman complained of being anxious, restless, afraid to be in a crowd, fearful of harming others, apprehensive she was going insane. Objectively, her body was in perpetual movement: with her hands she would tear paper into small bits; her abdomen contracted convulsively; her face twitched.

From the age of 5, when her father left the home, she lived under the close supervision of her mother. She shared the same bed as mother and she reported all her social activities to her mother. After her father's death (when she was 17), she developed the above symptoms. But when her mother died (when she was 20), these symptoms promptly disappeared and she assumed her mother's job as stenographer to a judge. Subsequently, she moved away to make her home with the family of her mother's sister. The marriage of her niece and the simultaneous loss of her employer, an older man, caused the recurrence of her symptoms. Her aunt, meanwhile, became an obligatory companion for her. Whenever the aunt would leave the house, she would become either furious or apprehensive that disaster would occur.

During two months of interviews on alternate days, her symptoms in large part subsided. Though she anticipated the interviews with pleasure, she appeared to cling to them with a desperate tenacity. Of her father, she could recall little except that he left the home. She compared the therapist to her former employer, an older man for whom she was a stenographer and with whom she talked intimately every day (as she had to her mother). Of her mother, she felt: "I was inside of her. I had no personality of my own. I started to live after her death. I was reborn."

Warned of the approaching month's separation from the therapist, she was promptly reminded of her father's leaving home, grew angry, demanded sedation. The therapist now looked to her like her father; she realized they both had the same first names. She became dejected and the twitching movements reappeared. During the month of separation she was subject to bouts of crying. Several times she smashed the contents of her room. It was finally necessary to admit her to the hospital. Next seen by the therapist, all of her original symptoms had recurred. In addition, she was furious at all doctors, fearful she would die, and obsessed with the thoughts she might choke people. Within three weeks of resuming therapy she was again as she had been before being warned of the month of separation.

This girl's neurosis centered around an ambivalent attachment to her mother. Her human relationships, whether to men or women, were all cut after this pattern. The nature of her life with her mother between the ages of 5 and 20 illustrates the infantile character of such a relationship. At first she was able to tolerate the death of her mother by literally filling her mother's shoes (i.e., incorporating the image of the mother). But it became necesary to find substitutes for the original obligatory companion, first in an employer, then her aunt, and finally the therapist. That the attachment to her mother and mother-substitutes was ambivalent is demonstrated by the fury aroused in her by any separation, no matter how temporary, from her aunt.

During the actual month of separation from the therapist, her neurotic symptoms returned with a vengeance, together with intense loneliness and incapacitating anger with the therapist. The separation, therefore, served not only as a signal that she had been abandoned, but as a trigger for the ambivalent feelings inherent in her attachment to the therapist. Within three weeks of the resumption of interviews after the separation, the storm which had been precipitated by the mention of the therapist's vacation had cleared.

A 33-year-old man, married and a university graduate student, came for psychiatric treatment of diarrhea. He was having 20-40 stools daily, with tenesmus, anorexia, and great fatigue. Medical examination demonstrated the diagnosis of ulcerative colitis.

He had always been a shy and solitary individual, though a successful student. Subject to inconsolable weeping spells in youth, he felt that his mother was unable to show affection. His father, a civil servant, had a strict code of conduct which he accepted tractably. The one person upon whom he found he could depend was the director of a laboratory, a man he met when he was 7 and for whom he worked when he was 28. It was after leaving this man's laboratory that he developed his first attack of ulcerative colitis. The second episode of colitis occurred two years later when his fiancée's father postponed his marriage. The colitis had recurred again a year before he came to treatment, when his professor told him that he had an undesirable personality.

His colitis stopped after two months of bi-weekly interviews. In the ensuing eight months, he found that he could concentrate on his work more successfully, though subject to depressions and obsessed by details. Meanwhile, he grew aware of a childlike dependency upon the therapist. At first, he took to reading psychiatric books. Then, he enjoyed the fantasy he was a psychiatrist. Finally, he thought of himself "like a leech without teeth, with a need for attachment to an object" and a desire to monopolize the life of the therapist.

As soon as he was informed of the approaching separation from the therapist, he found it difficult to concentrate upon his work, felt alone. Unable to sleep, he worked longer hours. "I feel I need warm milk to make myself feel right. . . . In my throat, I breathe quietly because I cannot yell. The times I used to cry unrestrainedly, Mother became upset." During the separation he sensed an unknown danger and he grew tense. Then it was as if he withdrew into his own body; nor could he

SEPARATION REACTION

work or speak to anyone. When psychotherapy resumed, he emerged gradually from this emotional state in the course of two months.

The relation of this patient to the therapist followed the pattern of all of his significant human relationships: i.e., infantile dependency. He described it in the terms of the dependent parasite sucking on its host, with the aggressive desire to monopolize the life of the therapist. For him, this state was vulnerable. The mere suggestion of separation from the therapist aroused a feeling "like an unwanted child against whom the mother had turned." Faced by the separation itself, he succeeded to a process resembling schizophrenic withdrawal, in which he felt totally isolated and unable to initiate useful action. It is significant that, severe as his response to separation appeared to be, it was possible for him to recover from this emotional state within two months of the resumption of therapy, and to realize that he had often experienced such feelings in the past.

A 40-year-old minister had had progressive rheumatoid arthritis over the course of eight years, involving his knees, hips, hands, and shoulders. He was referred for psychotherapy while under medical treatment in the hospital for pain, stiffness, and swelling of these joints.

He described his youth as a lonely one, lived on a farm with his stepfather and mother. His older sister, a business executive, left the home early due to disputes with the mother. His mother "didn't understand pleasure. Her life consisted of duties to be done and she expected that of me. No love was wasted between us. . . . She nagged my stepfather from morning to night. I felt sorry for him." He became a minister with a militant urge to erase sin and "drive the whole world to Christ." But when he tried to convert his sister, she was insulted and his arthritis commenced. When the sister later stopped communicating with him, he got married. His arthritis grew worse following the birth of a fourth child.

On the medical ward he soon became one to whom other male patients turned for advice. In interviews, despite a sense of sinfulness and a great fear of disapproval, he came to look forward to seeing the therapist. Warned of the approaching separation from the therapist, he grew irritable and aware of feelings of anger at his family, his parish, hospital personnel. He debated whether to go home for his wedding anniversary or to wait in the hospital for the therapist to return.

During the month of separation, his arthritis, which had become less painful, was intensified. He lay in bed rigidly, out of communication with the other patients, much of the time with his face to the wall. Next seen, he indicated that he had missed the therapist. However, he became quite depressed, his arthritis grew more painful, he dreamed of stuffing a dirty carpet into his mother's mouth, and he anticipated calamities happening to his children and himself. At the end of a month, these symptoms let up. Meanwhile, he succeeded in helping a depressed arthritic patient, who had consulted him and whom the therapist encouraged him to advise. To the therapist he commented: "The parent gives the child guiding principles. I was thinking of you in those terms." Subsequently, he felt in good spirits, stated that he believed he would recover from his arthritis, and became hopeful about his parish and children.

In the initial two months of weekly psychiatric interviews, the arthritic patient found narcissistic approval he had looked for from his parents in the past, and from Christ in the present. There was slight relief in his arthritic pain. With the threat of separation from the therapist, he grew sorrowful and angry. During the month of separation, he withdrew into a shell, physically and emotionally; he lay in bed, encased in a plaster cast, and failed to communicate with persons about him. With the resumption of interviews, he emerged from this shell gradually over the course of a month. During this emergence, it was evident that he regarded the therapist as a mother against whom he was impelled to vent his fury orally. This is illustrated by the dream in which he is lying naked on the floor, speaks harsh words to his mother, then stuffs a dirty rug into his mother's mouth. The dream was followed by severe joint pain and depression and the fear that he was losing control of his children and of his parish. But, at the end of a month, after the arthritic patient whom he had been counseling became well, he was in good spirits and he had no pain in his joints. Able to thus identify with the therapist, he then became aware that he had leaned heavily on his mother in childhood, as he now confessed to be doing with the therapist.

A 26-year-old, single girl, a college graduate, had had recurrent attacks of ulcerative colitis for two years. She came for psychotherapy the day after she arrived in this city in which she had no family or friends.

Socially a lone wolf, she had invariably alienated herself from her few friends by her own jealousy and the anticipation that she would be deserted, despite pre-eminence in studies and athletics at school and college.

During six months of psychotherapy, she worked as an editorial assistant, but spent much time by herself, preoccupied with the memory of an old girl friend. At church she would pray to be "kept a whole person." She anticipated many sorts of calamity happening to her, especially at the hands of a man. From a frequency of 8-10 times daily and nightly, her diarrhea dropped to 3-4 times without bleeding.

Toward the therapist she became aware of tender feelings, but of a tentative nature. Every night she would talk to him, calling him by his first name. He seemed to be inside of her. Then she would feel whole. But at interviews, he seemed different and she felt "broken up and crippled, my mind and part of my intestine."

In the month of separation she slept poorly, felt dejected, worked extra time, and saw little of her few acquaintances. "I felt as if I'd like to tear things apart and beat people up. I thought it would be nice to cry, but I couldn't." In a series of unmailed letters addressed to the therapist, she wrote about herself with an intimacy and tenderness seldom encountered in interviews.

When psychotherapy was resumed, she indicated that her diarrhea had grown more severe. She was disappointed that she could not talk to the therapist as well as to the doctor of her correspondence. She grew angry at the therapist for not understanding her. Subsequently, she grew abusive, accusing the therapist of feeding her only crumbs. Three months after the end of the month of separation, she left therapy precipitously to go to another city in order to find a woman therapist.

This girl with ulcerative colitis demonstrated the impoverished personality of a schizoid character. Upon the therapist she came to feel dependent, but in a bizarre way. In the manner of a schizophrenic, she split the therapist into two people. One was the person whom she felt was inside of her and whom she addressed tenderly at night when she felt whole. The other was the doctor whom she encountered in interviews, where she felt cold, broken, and crippled.

The month of separation served only to increase her fears of being harmed and rejected by the therapist of interviews. She became irritated, dejected, fatigued, and more lonely. The process of splitting the therapist she carried further. Toward the doctor of her night conversations she turned her whole attention and addressed letters of great warmth. Toward the doctor of interviews she felt increasing hostility until finally it was necessary for her to seek a woman (i.e., a mother towards whom she felt less hostile).

Discussion

The reaction of these patients to separation bears resemblances to the symptomatic picture of grief described by Lindemann. All the patients experienced a subjective sensation which they defined as missing the therapist. Often striking was the patient's preoccupation with thoughts of or the image of the missing therapist. It was common for the patient to respond with irritability to other people. Finally, there were frequent alterations in the established patterns of the patient's behavior. For example, the two patients with ulcerative colitis lost so much enthusiasm for their work that activities which had been automatic for them were carried on with the greatest effort. The minister with arthritis slipped into complete social isolation by lying in bed with his face to the wall. In the reaction of the man with ulcerative colitis to separation, there was no external evidence of hostility. Instead, he showed a picture of withdrawal resembling schizophrenia, in which, unable to find help in the external world of reality, he retreated in fantasy to the interior of his own body where he could feel nothing except fatigue and the desire to sleep.

Dynamically, the nature of the reaction to separation varied with the nature of the patient's neurotic illness. Both the boy with vomiting and the girl with the reactive depression regarded the therapist as a necessary, paternal figure; the boy was still in need of an adequate "father" with whom to identify; the girl, of a "father" as an object of her instinctual heterosexual longings. Both of them were able to tolerate the month of separation with a modicum of discomfort and disappointment in these needs, but without total disorganization of their emotional lives. At the other extreme are the minister with arthritis and the man with ulcerative colitis, both narcissistic personalities whose instinctive drives are still expressed principally in oral terms. For them the therapist represented a guiding or nourishing mother. During separation they succumbed to a vegetative existence, having severed emotional relatedness to everyone about them. The same could be said for the girl with ulcerative colitis, for whom the separation served only to intensify her already hostile feelings for the therapist to such a point as to rupture therapy. The reaction of the girl with the phobia to the separation stands somewhere in between these two extremes. She responded as if she had lost an object of affection but also, as demonstrated by her impulse to be destructive, a target of extremely ambivalent feelings.

Each of these patients assigned feelings to the therapist characteristic of the patient's psychological needs and development. The separation was clearly an interruption of these transference feelings. Grief, too, is a response to an interruption of feelings. But while bereavement, of which grief is the expression, refers to a *permanent* cessation of an interpersonal relationship, separation is only a *temporary* interruption, having the promise of restoration. It is, therefore, not surprising that the recovery from the reaction to separation as described seemed more rapid than might be expected from grief. The reaction to separation resembled grief in that the more infantile and regressive was the expression of the patient's relationship to the therapist, the more severe was the reaction to separation.

Of the 6 patients studied the response to separation was far more severe in the 3 with ulcerative colitis and rheumatoid arthritis than in the 3 with neuroses. Likewise, the 3 patients with psychosomatic illness demonstrated a more defective psychological development; they were more narcissistic, more dependent, and prone to instinctual expression in oral-sadistic terms.

Separation has a practical significance that bereavement has not. The separation of one partner of a human relationship from another occurs frequently, whereas bereavement is a less common experience. If a patient can react as vigorously to such a temporary separation from a therapist as described, then any interruption of a physician's relationships to a patient can be looked upon as a stimulus to the development of a reaction to separation. Ferenczi has long since described the "Sunday neurosis," in which the patient developed depression on Sunday; i.e., a day on which the patient did not see the psychotherapist. The ending of the patient's therapeutic interviews with the doctor, or the referral of a patient from one doctor to another, may be in themselves provocative of a separation reaction. As such, these situations may well deserve further study and examination, especially if the clinical improvement by any type of medical therapy is not to be undone by the symptoms of a reaction to separation.

Summary

The reaction of 6 psychiatric patients to a month's separation from their common therapist is described. Three of the patients had a neurosis, 2 had ulcerative colitis, and 1 rheumatoid arthritis.

The reaction to separation of these patients bore symptomatic resemblance to the grief of normal individuals. It consisted of subjective feelings of loss, of irritability, of preoccupation with the image of the missing therapist, of inability to initiate and maintain useful conduct. There were instances of incapacitating hostility directed against specific persons and of schizophrenic-like withdrawal.

The reaction to separation was more severe in the 3 patients with psychosomatic illness than in the 3 patients with neuroses. Likewise, the 3 with psychosomatic illness showed signs of more defective psychological development; they were more narcissistic, more dependent; and more prone to infantile instinctual expression than the 3 with neuroses.

The separation was considered an interruption of transference feelings for the therapist. While grief refers to a permanent personal loss, the reaction of separation refers to a temporary interruption of an interpersonal relationship having the promise of restoration. The recovery from the reaction to separation was shorter than might be expected from grief.

Separation has the practical significance that it occurs more frequently than bereavement. Therefore, any interruption of the relationship to the patient, no matter how temporary, should be viewed as a potential stimulus to a reaction of separation and should be prepared for by the physician.

EMOTIONAL PROBLEMS OF THE MIDDLE-AGED MAN

Otto Billig, M.D., and Robert Adams, M.D.

In comparison with the amount of material written about the middle-aged woman, little attention is paid to this period of life in the male. Most published studies have been devoted to endocrinological data and symptomatology of the "male climacteric."

Heller and Myers postulated the concept of a "male climacteric" as an entity comparable to the menopause in women. Twenty-three of their cases had elevation of gonadotropic hormone excretion comparable to that in castrated males. These authors separated the male climacteric patients from psychoneurotic men with similar symptoms, by endocrine studies and by the response of these patients to replacement hormone therapy. They believed the syndrome of the male climacteric to be relatively rare.

Landrum pointed out the difficulties of quantitative determination of circulating androgens needed to prove decreased gonadal function. He could find only a "symptomatic but otherwise occult testicular deficiency." He agreed that the "male climacteric" syndrome was infrequent.

The symptomatology is adequately described by Werner in an article reporting 273 cases. All complained of "nervousness." The more common complaints were depression, irritability, decreased memory and concentration, crying, sleep disturbances, worry, loss of interest and self-confidence, headache. Circulatory complaints including sweating, vertigo, numbness and tingling, tachycardia and palpitation. "Hot flashes" were a complaint in

Werner's patients, though other authors did not find this. Other general symptoms included fatiguability and potency disturbances. Werner attributed the syndrome of the male climacteric to a decreased gonadal function resulting in a disturbance of the pituitary-gonad equilibrium. Since all of the symptoms described are seen in psychoneuroses, they are not specific for decreased testicular function. Bauer, in a criticism of the article by Heller and Myers, held that the term, male climacteric, should be used to designate the cessation of gonadal function at a definite period of life, with all symptoms a consequence of this alteration of the endocrine function. Lansing expressed similar views. Landrum held that the symptoms of the male climacteric were psychogenic and that the term should not be used.

The term, male climacteric, implies a physiological, inevitable major change in the life of every man, comparable to that occurring in women. There is no evidence at this time to support such a concept.

The term is being used, then, to cover a psychiatric syndrome occurring in the middle-aged man, rather than a relatively rare condition of testicular insufficiency. Prados and Ruddick reported 30 such cases. They postulated that glandular disturbances with attendant waning sexual powers threaten the man with loss of his love object, mobilizing and reactivating previous conflicts and anxieties. He is thus forced to regress to pregenital levels with symptoms reflecting passivity and dependence.

It may prove worth while to investigate the emotional meaning of middle age in our society. Dunn noted in a discussion of Werner's article that the "male climacteric" was important because it occurred usually in men with great responsibilities. The patients in Prados and Ruddick's series frequently gave a history of ambition and striving for achievement and success. A recent study described the dependency needs and depressive features of middle-aged miners as contrasted with anxiety neuroses in the younger generation. The cultural and economic factors were considered important contributing areas.

On becoming of middle age, the man of Western culture has reached another important period in his life. We have only to visualize his position within his own family and within his cultural group. Up to that time he has gathered new experiences which emphasized his need to prove himself and to gain recognition; to be successful, he had to struggle and to compete. He had to defend himself against competition—otherwise, he would have failed. Success in his job, social position and family were based on acceptance by his group—at first at home, then in school, and later in his job. As Margaret Mead points out, competition plays a basic dynamic role in the American family. The mother permits the child a great deal of freedom and shows considerable love, but it is conditioned on success—in play with other children, with rivals at school and in sports. Such conditional love is withdrawn—to a greater or lesser degree—when the child is unsuccessful. By this factor, anxieties and insecurities are produced: Lack of success may mean loss of love. The importance of leadership is emphasized from early childhood on. Knowledge and ability are not recognized on their own merit, but primarily for what they mean in relation to others. The parent, the teacher, and later the foreman are not satisfied with achievement, but with how the individual rates in his class-standing or in his production. The child learns to struggle for position and power. This conditional love makes him eager to outdo and displace his rival. He may not be able to accomplish this at the moment, but hopes to achieve it when he has gathered more strength and experience. The need for displacing the successful rival has found innumerable expressions in all Western literature. The dynamic struggle between the rivals has been primarily observed from the viewpoint of the one struggling for success or leadership—in the Oedipus myth from Oedipus' viewpoint. It seems that the older man's fear of his younger rival has not been sufficiently emphasized as a dynamic force. But in Sophocles' play it receives support in

Jocasta's words: ". . . that Laius should die—the dread thing which he feared—by his child's hand." And Laius was killed with "the silver just lightly strewn among his hair"—apparently at middle age. The prophecy of the oracle symbolizes the inherent struggle between generations.*

The father's unconscious hostility toward his unborn child is found in the custom of the couvade. Among some primitive tribes the "expectant father" must refrain from any activity. His actions are believed to bring death, injury or malformation to the child, the symbolism of activity betraying his hostile intents. ". . . the retaliative nature of the taboo [demands], that the father should suffer the same torture which he wished to inflict on his child. . . ." In some primitive societies the father sacrifices with gifts to the mother's brothers; in our society he passes out cigars when a son is born to him. Occasionally, the unacceptable birth intensifies his anxiety to the point of a frank psychosis.

Case 1

A 25-year-old high school teacher was admitted to the hospital with the complaint of, "I think I am going crazy." His symptoms developed rather acutely one month prior to admission with a typical anxiety attack during his wife's fifth month of pregnancy. Afterward he became fearful of having a brain tumor. Physical examinations by several doctors and specialists did not satisfy him. He became increasingly preoccupied with his symptoms, considering himself hopeless. He lost interest in his surroundings and appeared in a "daze." He complained of feeling unreal and showed moderate ideas of reference.

The patient is the youngest of six children. The mother was 10 years older than the father and was 49 years old when the patient was born. The father had desired an older wife, since "men die younger than their wives." Although neither parent had finished grammar school, they were extremely ambitious for their children. All the patient's siblings finished college, receiving either masters' or Ph.D. degrees. Little affection was shown at home. The father worked long hours, never having

* Parallel themes can be found from the myths of many people to modern plays such as *The Death of a Salesman*.

any spare time for the children. When at home, the children had to be quiet in order not to disturb him. The father was strict and emotionally unresponsive. During his childhood, the patient showed enuresis, nightmares, sleep walking. He appeared destructive and was described as a "dare-devil."

The patient married at the age of 22, his wife being a year older. She is a very controlling individual. About 18 months before his admission to the hospital, the patient's wife had a spontaneous abortion. It was a planned pregnancy, and the patient appeared very grieved immediately after the abortion. But he once mentioned later that he was not sorry that they had lost the first pregnancy. The onset of the patient's emotional disturbance was laid in the fifth month of the wife's second pregnancy. The patient hinted that he didn't want this child either. When his wife threatened to abort during the third and fourth month, he expressed hope for an abortion. Soon afterward, he began to appear moody and withdrawn, and developed the symptoms described.

Apparently, the dissociative episode was precipitated by the wife's pregnancy and threatened abortion. The patient was closely attached to his own mother and showed marked antagonism against a severe and unresponsive father figure. He felt powerless in expressing his hostile feelings when he was a child—repressions resulted. The pregnancy of his wife, the abortion and his ill-concealed wish for a second abortion created marked conflicts. His hostile desires against the unborn child reactivated his own unresolved Oedipal feelings and his awareness of his original hostility toward his own father. The resultant guilt led him to the role of Laius when the oracle predicted his death "by his child's hand." He then defended himself by displacing his repressed hostility from his father to his yet unborn child. But he developed the anxiety of Laius that his child would "kill" him when it reached maturity—that is, with "the silver just lightly strewn among his hair," his own middle age.*

Therefore, one can expect two vulnerable periods in the adult man who has not resolved his Oedipal conflict: (1) at the

---

* Reik calls attention to certain South American tribes who consider "the child [. . . as] the father of the man." The grandfather is called the *"little father."* Their rituals seeks protection from the fear that the grandfather will come to life in the grandchild. The Indian man fears that the hostility against his own father will be avenged by his child. A similar mechanism is pointed out by E. Jones in *The Phantasy on Reversal of Generations.*

birth of a child, particularly of the first male child; (2) at middle age when he fears that his real (or symbolic) son has grown sufficiently powerful to displace him.

Case 2

A small-town merchant, aged 54, has shown depressive and, alternating, elated moods for the last five years. The illness started shortly after an automobile accident to his only son. It was necessary for the patient to sign some insurance papers. Soon afterward he developed delusions of having done something wrong and that he would be sent to jail. The symptoms were intensified, and he became severely depressed.

The patient had grown up in a very rigid and narrowly religious home. The father was described as a domineering, unreasonably strict man who punished the patient severely with slight provocation. A poor provider, the father spent many months away from home looking for jobs. There was considerable tension, and the patient witnessed frequent quarrels. The mother was affectionate and kind, and the patient considered himself the mother's favorite. She was particularly attentive to him during the father's long absences; she allowed him to sleep in bed with her while the father was away. The patient looked forward to the father's trips and often wished that he would not return.

The patient is the youngest of seven siblings; he had five brothers and a sister. The oldest brother's personality is described as very much like the father's, an austere, emotionally cold and rigid person. This is in direct contrast to the patient who is well liked in the community, has many friends, was always "jolly" and very much interested in the welfare of others. At the age of 25, the patient planned to open a store with a friend but was encouraged by the family to go in busines with the oldest brother. The patient was controlled by the oldest brother, and all business policies were determined by this brother, who was extremely conservative, while the patient was full of new expansive ideas. The patient resented being restricted, but never felt able to assert himself. A few years ago he had tried to take his son into his business but the brother objected, believing that the patient wanted to push him, the brother, out. Following this the patient set his son up in busines alone, actually as a competitor to himself, and to his financial loss. The patient did this despite never having been close to his son.

In the beginning of his marriage the patient did not welcome the wife's pregnancy, since a child would be a "financial burden" at the time "I started out in business." He was also openly jealous of his wife's attention to the son and resented their discussing matters. It was the patient's impression that he was not welcome to participate in such discussions and felt "pushed out." He wanted the son to support him completely when he, himself, became depressed, just as his own father had demanded such support from his children. He resented the son's "spending money on his girl friend, buying a car and having a good time."

The cultural environment increased the emotional conflicts of the patient. The small southern town where he lived fostered definitely outlined traditions of comunity life. The family belonged to a rigid and strict church in which the oldest brother was a deacon. The patient's concept of God was that God could see everything and would punish all evil done. God was a stern and unforgiving figure.

To summarize: A male patient develops a severe depression at the age of 49, following an accident to his son. The patient had had a poor relationship with his own father, with ill-concealed death wishes against the father. He was strongly attached to a solicitous mother. The oldest brother continued in the role of the punitive father, maintaining similar hostile feelings in the patient. The cultural environment intensified the conflicts, contributing to the existing feelings of guilt. The patient felt threatened by the relationship between his son and his wife, creating a reactivation of his own earlier Oedipal feelings. The son's accident precipitated the clinical symptoms.

The "male climacteric" depressions have been more frequently recognized in "successful" men. Such men have been able to prove themselves in competition. As pointed out previously, this competition is built on a "conditioned" love. The threat of the loss of love lends itself to introjection of the conflict and subsequent depression.

In non-competitive (or better: low-competitive) social groups, love and approval are not conditioned on success. Existing unresolved Oedipal conflicts are expressed in conversion or anxiety reactions. About 150 patients (almost all males) of an industrial group were studied. They were admitted to Vanderbilt University Hospital with one or another form of persistent, handicapping illness. Over 75 per cent of these patients were between 35 and 55 years old; more than half of the middle-aged men had clear-cut emotional illnesses, primarily anxiety and conversion reactions, while an additional third had psychosomatic problems. Only about 15 per cent of all middle-aged patients proved to have definite organic diseases. The emotional reactions were precipitated by minor accidents or injuries in about 15 per cent while the reactions of an additional 10 per cent were preceded by some kind of physical difficulty. The patient group came from isolated mountain areas of a culturally-restricted environment of rigid standards. Its members had little contact with outside groups.

The case histories were of striking similarity, almost stereotyped: The father was usually strict, austere; he "made the children walk the chalk line." The mother often suffered from long-lasting neurotic complaints. Little outward affection was shown in the home; the family was often preoccupied with meeting the most immediate necessities of life. The country was barren and not sufficiently productive. There were usually several other children of the family; its members left the small country town rarely; they visited the larger cities only in cases of some emergency. Neuropathic traits of childhood such as enuresis, nail biting, nocturnal fears were frequent and were usually handled by shaming or other disciplinary measures. School attendance was poor, often considered as an unnecessary luxury interfering with supporting the family. The boys started to help the father, working on the farm or in the mines at an early age, not infrequently before being 10 years old. A boy, insecure in his relation to his strict father, was often afraid of him. The late 'teens were a difficult adjustment period characterized by various forms of rebellion. The early years of marriage were difficult; the young husband preferred "to run around with the boys," did heavy social drinking; the young wife nagged him to "settle down." Several children were born within a few years. In most cases, the young man became a steady worker giving up "the gang." He worked hard and long hours with little outside contacts. He belonged to a fundamentalist church. Approaching middle age he became increasingly concerned with his health. A minor illness, injury or accident might precipitate a several emotional reaction, either an anxiety or conversion reaction. Treatment usually proved difficult because of the educational and cultural limitations.

It seems also that in these cases the patient was unable to resolve his Oedipal feelings with a strict threatening father. He had to repress his hostile feelings against him at an early age, but rebelled against authoritarian figures during his adolescence and early adulthood. He had difficulties in assuming the marital role, both as husband and father, manifesting anxiety or conversion symptoms at middle age.

The man who has emotional disturbances during midlife is likely to be the man who has only partially resolved his own Oedipal conflicts. These conflicts do not always result in definite clinical syndromes but may become manifest in certain personality patterns leading gradually to a change in cultural attitudes. The unconscious hostility of the elder toward the younger is symbolized in the primitive customs of initiation ceremonies in which the young member of the tribe is "tested" by the witch doctor, the symbol of tribal authority. The youth has to undergo severe tests that are only manifestations of his elders' marked aggression toward him. The novice may die a symbolic death; when he is reborn as a full (adult) member he may not be permitted to mention the names of his family. This protective amnesia prevents him from contacts with his father and mother. The hazing performed by medieval labor guilds or modern fraternities probably could be traced back to similar mechanisms.

The unacceptance of the son who is a rival often results in a contempt for his activities. "The American father, brought up in the tradition of the pioneers, hardened in the period of rugged individualism, absorbed in the creation of material wealth, often looks down contemptuously upon his son's interest in history, literature, or even theoretical physics. He considers such inclinations a sign of decline, particularly if they do not produce adequate material rewards." In other cases such unacceptance of the rival son may, however, result in the father's discontent with the son's lack of interest in intellectual achievements, provided the father himself has attained intellectual goals. The specific attitudes may vary, but the basic mechanism appears to be intolerance of the father for the son, possibly rationalized in a desire of the father to "harden his son for life . . ." or, "I didn't have it easy . . . life is not a bed of roses."

The underlying anxiety can be also transformed into protective and solicitous attitudes. The father will encourage a role of dependency by "I want my children to have it easier." But he becomes disturbed by any sign of emancipation.

Case 3

A successful business man, aged 55, is the son of Russian, Jewish emigrants. The parents had come to a small southern town and were very conscious of their minority role. They worked hard and had little time for the children. The father was a strict disciplinarian; considerable tension existed between the parents. The patient entered the father's business at an early age. He married at the age of 20; he had three sons. He made great demands on them, insisting on high grades in school. After they had finished school, he made his sons junior partners in his business. When one of them showed other interests, the patient called him ungrateful, reminding him of the great sacrifices he, the father, had made in raising him and his brothers. When the two older sons planned to marry, the patient objected to their fiancees, finding fault with them or considering the sons to be too young for marriage. When he realized their determination, he became rather solicitous, presenting them with real estate next to his own home. He helped them finance the building of their homes. After their marriages he continued to demand their frequent visits to his home next door. Finally, the oldest son broke with the patient, leaving the business and moving to the West Coast. The father became increasingly depressed, and this depression culminated in a suicidal attempt.

In summary, the patient suffered severe rejection from both parents during his early childhood and felt particularly threatened by his father. He was unable to handle his relationship to his own sons, controlling them by keeping them in roles of dependency. Marked anxiety and feelings of depression were elicited at middle age when his oldest son established an independent role.

The emotional conflicts do not always reach proportions of clinical magnitude. The anxieties or depressions appear as the late manifestations of unresolved Oedipal conflicts. If such conflicts are resolved, however, the middle-aged man can accept the younger man. And only then will he be able to live and work with him as an equal without needing defenses against potential threats.

Treatment has proved to be difficult in all the writers' cases. The cultural limitations in some cases presented the obstacles to be expected to effective psychotherapy. The treatment of comparatively simple anxiety reactions proved to be rather problematic in middle age, even if cultural limitations were not present. To give the patient insight into only the simplest dynamic mechanisms, intensive psychotherapy had to be carried out over one to four years.

The depressed patients showed considerable resistance to therapy. Electric shock treatments have been considered successful, in other cases, in the various depressive reactions. But in these patients, courses of 12 to 15 ECT's produced only temporary results; the remissions lasted not more than a few weeks. Further ECT did not produce additional benefits.

Case 2 had two courses of 12 ECT's; the second course was given six months after the first. The patient appeared temporarily improved after each course, but he continued with alternating moods of elation and depression without any days of actual comfort. Psychotherapy was started. The treatment goal had to be set in accordance with the cultural background (described in the foregoing). It was aimed to give him an understanding of the interpersonal relations to his father and mother, the continuing authoritative father role assumed by the oldest brother and the patient's relation to his own son. Treatment progressed considerably slower than in other patients of similar intellectual ability and cultural background. The interviews extended over a period of four years averaging two interviews weekly. Gradually the mood changes became less frequent and intense until, finally, the patient reached emotional stability.

Electric convulsive therapy produced a marked personality disorganization in several cases. Memory defects were more marked than usual; the affect became somewhat blunted. Increasing excitement was noticeable. Finally, the patients became disoriented, confused, and at times untidy. Some of them showed auditory hallucinations and had persecutory ideas. When electric shock therapy was discontinued, these symptoms disappeared spontaneously within two to four weeks.*

Summary

The emotional problems of the middle-aged man result either in anxiety or in depressive reactions. His own unresolved Oedipal conflicts make him vulnerable to his role as father. The birth of a child, particularly of the first child, may reactivate his conflicts, resulting in overt anxiety. When the son reaches adolescence the underlying conflicts may again mobilize his anxiety or produce a depressive reaction. The rivalry with his real or symbolic son (younger co-worker, etc.) is of basic dynamic significance. Certain cultural attitudes may reinforce the existing conflicts. Treatment aspects have been discussed.

---

* It may be of interest to note that the authors have never observed similar reactions in women patients.

A TYPE OF POST PARTUM ANXIETY REACTION

Murray DeArmond

The use of the term post partum psychiatric reaction as a diagnostic category does nothing more than place these disturbances in a temporal relationship to the termination of pregnancy. Such a grouping includes a wide range of clinical manifestations. There are frank psychoses and there are milder neuroses. All of these symptom complexes have been considered schizophrenic reactions by some and the post partum period a favorable time for the appearance of the pathological symptoms. Such a conclusion would seem far too casual in light of the broad base of causative factors to be suspected as well as the widely divergent clinical pictures. It is recognized that profound changes occur in the hormone balance during pregnancy and afterward but what effect this may have on nervous functions is yet to be determined. The inherent stability of the personality and its capacity to withstand the experience of pregnancy and delivery as well as the problems of motherhood must be evaluated. There are also environmental stresses and the question of conflict in interpersonal relationships to be considered when an attempt is made to explain the psychiatric reactions of the post partum state. If each case can be critically and impartially studied a more orderly classification can be made and a more specific therapeutic program applied. It is intended to discuss a type of anxiety reaction represented by carefully selected cases from the post partum disturbances. These cases were picked because the presenting clinical pictures were practically identical. The course of the reaction was strikingly similar, none developed any psychotic symptoms and all recovered in a relatively short period of time. In addition there were no tangible causative factors from the physical, physiological, situational or personality standpoint.

Anxiety was the predominant symptom. The anxiety was related to the mother herself. Cases which showed undue anxiety related to the child were not thought fit for the dynamic formulation to be considered. It should be emphasized that only a selected type of anxiety reaction is being evaluated.

Whereas anxiety was the predominant symptom, depression was also evident at times. However, the depression was of secondary importance and seemed to be a resultant rather than a causative force and was never a problem in the therapeutic program.

The onset of the anxiety was early, either appearing in the hospital or shortly after the patient went home. Sometimes there was sudden panic-like fear without precipitating cause. Sometimes there was gradual onset with a sense of uneasiness and apprehension accompanied by a feeling of unreality. There was usually some disturbance in the sleep pattern. There was neither any dissociation nor loss of contact with reality. There was never any loss of control although the patients suffered from a serious threat to their control. These reactions were severely incapacitating.

These patients presented their complaints frankly and with intellectual insight. There were indications of the attempts to deny the existence of the symptoms on a reasonable basis. Comments such as, "It is so silly for me to feel this way" or "I ought to be able to throw these feelings off" were frequently offered. At times it almost appeared that they were discussing another person, except that they could never detach the accompanying affect. The description would be given with an occasional apologetic smile but with the eyes filled with tears.

As mentioned before the anxiety was related to the patient herself and expressed as a lack of confidence in her ability. Thus the concern over the problems presented by the infant was not out of proportion so far as the infant was concerned. The concern was over the patient's capability in meeting these problems. This resulted in a reluctance to be alone. These mothers felt incapable of carrying out the routine household duties as well as performing activities outside the home. As the efforts to surmount the conflict failed, the incapacity was recognized and the anxiety became more acute. Fears of loss of mind were frequently expressed.

The patients in this select group were above average in intellectual status. The family histories were negative for indications that might provide a basis for unstable reactions. The personal histories were free from such tendencies. Some of these women had established themselves in jobs where they showed initiative and independence before marriage. Their marital state was free from conflict. The children were either planned or wanted. These families would be considered average or above in social and economic levels and no undue stress was indicated from these sources.

All had prenatal care, were healthy, had normal pregnancies and uneventful deliveries according to their obstetricians. Some of the anxiety reactions followed delivery of the first baby while in others it ocurred after the second delivery, whereas the first post partum state had been entirely free from such disturbances. The sex of the child did not seem to be a relevant factor.

The following case history is presented in detail to illustrate the symptoms and problems of the entire series since it is typical for all except with minor variations:

A 27 year old mother, a college graduate, met her husband while he was in service during World War II. She was a Red Cross worker at that time. After marriage they established their home in Indianapolis where her husband was employed as a chemist. Their social and economic status is adequately secure. Their first child, a girl, age 3, was born after a normal pregnancy and delivery and the post partum state was normal.

The second child was a boy. There was no anxiety or emotional stress during the second pregnancy and delivery. Shortly after the second delivery, while still in the hospital, the patient became apprehensive and was tormented by fears of losing her mind. She was able to conceal her emotional stress until she returned home. Then she was unable to be alone without extreme tension. She felt unsure of caring for the children. She was unable to drive her car. She could only go out with her husband. Even then the discomfort was so severe that she preferred to suffer with her symptoms at home.

When she was referred for psychiatric evaluation she expressed a fear of insanity, a fear that she would lose control and become violent. Her sleep was generally unsatisfactory, being interrupted and disturbed by disquieting dreams. She expressed the feeling of depression and despair occasioned by her husband's absence from the city, and at the same time deplored her weakness and inability to rise above her dependency.

Since there was no indication of a psychotic tendency, this was accepted as an anxiety reaction and a plan of treatment on an out-patient basis was instituted. It was apparent that she needed support, encouragement and direction to alleviate the sense of failure, the guilt, and the tension which resulted from her ineffective attempts to pull herself together. Arrangements were made for frequent interviews which necessitated her visiting the office. A moderate amount of sedation was given on a regular schedule to reduce her physical tension and improve her sleep. She was encouraged to accept some curtailment of her activities and reduce the time that she would be home alone.

During the office interviews she was allowed to express her feelings freely and put her problems into words. Reassurance was given generously at every appropriate opportunity, but the chief aim of the interviews was to give her a more objective appraisal of herself and correct the introspective distortion which had occurred. As the anxiety began to subside during the course of the interviews other evidences of increased emotional reactions began to come to her attention. She recognized and described new experiences in her desirable responses to her children, her husband, and her friends. There were flashes of happiness which she had never experienced before. Her emotional reactions were quite volatile and mixed and this confused her all the more. She began to realize that the ease with which her emotional responses could be aroused and the new intensity as well as the fluctuation constituted a threat to her sense of control. That her emotional pattern was undergoing a reorganization is supported by this volunteered description of her reaction. She expressed with some concern, "I seem to feel different toward Barby (her daughter). It used to be when she hurt herself I felt as if the hurt had happened to me and I felt the pain myself. Now I don't. Of course, I'm concerned if she is hurt, I'm sorry for her and I take care of her just the same but I feel different. I wonder if I don't love my daughter as much as I used to."

This is only one example out of many which indicates the individual's difficulty in identifying herself and relating herself to her environmental situations. Such opportunities were used to give her a clearer definition of the picture of herself in her role as a mother. She was encouraged to accept the new thrill of fondling her baby and given some explanation of an accompanying anxiety to help her cope with it should it arise. She was also encouraged to extend her emotional participation in the activities which tempted her to experience new heights of happiness. Under this relatively simple therapeutic program the troublesome symptoms began to subside. She became more comfortable and confident. It also seemed apparent that she stabilized herself in a new plane of functioning which was effective and gratifying. This was accomplished in a few months.

The other case histories might be fitted into this protocol with a few minor changes. They were all managed in the same way. All were able to restablize themselves in a period varying from a few weeks to three months.

These post partum conditions can be evaluated promptly and differentiated from the more malignant reactions. Treatment is relatively simple, can be pursued confidently, and the outcome is gratifying.

This type of anxiety reaction is reported for the purpose of discussing the role of the body image in the production of unstable emotional states. Since the concept of body image can be nebulous an attempt will be made to bring it into more tangible form. Body image has very little relationship to that reflection of the body we see in a mirror but rather embraces what we feel ourselves to be. It is more of an emotional attitude making its existence evident by its influence on the behavior pattern. It may be integrated into the intellectual functioning in a harmonious union or its divergence may create a state of conflict, confusion and a sense of unreality.

The body image is a transitional entity and its form is molded by the experiences of the individual personality. It may become arrested at any stage in its development and remain unchanged by subsequent experiences. It also seems to undergo phases of disorganization and reorganization.

With this definition some illustrations may further clarify the concept. The behavior of children shows the presence of a very fluid body image subject to the influence of fantasy. The boy who gallops along on his broomstick shooting Indians from their ponies with his deadly aim feels himself to be the heroic cowboy as pictured by the glamorous tales of the Wild West. Or on another occasion, bedecked with fantastic trappings and a flowing robe he becomes the space man. Of course these are fantasy experiences and leave no lasting residuals, but we can all recall some of our childhood experiences and appreciate the creation of a temporary concept of what we felt ourselves to be.

The temporary fantasy concepts leave no lasting impression on the body image because they are not related to reality situations. The experiences and concepts which are properly related to reality contribute to the enduring body image.

To illustrate the relation of the body image to behavior it may be said that we walk with one body image but drive a car with an altered image to fit the situation. The experienced driver operates a car with a great deal of feel. It is as if the body image incorporates the car. The driver's being then extends from bumper to bumper and fender to fender. When the pilot flies a plane by his feel in the seat we are saying that he feels the plane as a part of him or that his body image extends from wing tip to wing tip and nose to tail enabling him to set the wheels on the ground as if they were his own feet.

Pregnancy is a normal process accompanied by drastic physical changes and profound emotional experiences. It is a process which develops gradually over a period of nine months and is terminated abruptly at delivery. This affords a unique opportunity to speculate on the changes in the body image and the influence of these changes in the production of post partum symptoms. Certainly the woman must incorporate the infant in her body image during the nine months when it is a part of her body—part of her being. The emotional qualities of her state of being are more important than her intellectual concept. That the emotional concept may be disorganized at delivery is based on the separation of the child from her body and supported by the feelings of unreality in which she cannot identify herself. It is this disorganization and lack of identification which appears to produce anxiety.

The presenting symptom of anxiety subsides as reorganization occurs and the personality becomes stablized. It is proposed that the patient is then able to identify herself in her new role of motherhood and her body image conforms to this new reality situation which has already been accepted on an intellectual basis.

Since Schilder and others introduced the concept of body image in organic brain disease it seems feasible to accept it in the interpretation of certain functional disorders. Pregnancy seems to be a particularly appropriate event to study the mother's experience in terms of body image. It is conceivable that the experience may bring about, first very little change in the body image; second, a partial change, and third an adequate reorganization. Which of these conditions prevails appears to have a definite influence on the behavior pattern of the mother. In the first instance the mother acts much as if she never had the baby in that her attitude indicates she cannot identify herself as a mother to the child. It might be said that the infant was never incorporated in her body image.

In the second there is an identification of herself to the child as if it were still a part of her being. Here the infant is incorporated in the body image and remains so even after delivery.

The third instance represents a mature state of motherhood where she accepts the child as a part of her which has been emancipated and this highly emotional relationship is both comforting and satisfying. This is the desirable sequence of events in which the body image first incorporates the infant but at delivery reorganizes with a separation of the child's personality from the body image. The reorganization may occur without symptoms but sometimes it may produce anxiety.

In summary, a particular type of anxiety reaction in the post partum state is presented and discussed in terms of alterations of the body image. This formulation appears to afford a deeper insight into the dynamic mechanisms and to provide greater confidence in management of the symptoms.

THE ADDITION OF CHLORPROMAZINE TO THE TREATMENT PROGRAM FOR EMOTIONAL AND BEHAVIOR DISORDERS IN THE AGING

Benjamin Pollack, M.D.

Not all of the emotional and behavior disorders in the older person are caused by organic degenerative lesions. Many situations which he must face have a direct and pronounced emotional impact because of the increasing limitations of age. Unless there has been a preparation to replace former activities with more suitable outlets, much distress may result. Some of the obvious difficulties arise from an unwillingness to slow down, lack of preparation for retirement, and failure to adjust activities to physical needs. Many aging persons have a tendency to live in the past and to serve others only in accordance with the precepts of their own generations. Others cannot adjust to the reduced income of later years or overlook the need to learn something new. They refuse to face reality until it is too late, and fail to recognize that aging is a gradual process which is characteristic of the entire adult life span.

The older adult should be kept flexible in his thinking and up-to-date regarding modern technologic and social changes. He must have accurate information regarding sources from which help is obtainable. The fantasy of retirement and old age as a period of a "grand loaf" must be erased, for nature always eliminates those who have relinquished their usefulness.

All aging people are concerned with their emotional and financial security. They are often confronted with traditional myths and distortions about the so-called uselessness of the older person. If they are to continue to have a feeling of normality, community ties must be maintained and proper outlets for leisure time must be provided. Like younger persons, they need an outlet for affection and expression of affection. Of course there may be limitations imposed because of physical or other defects, so they cannot engage in their accustomed leisure-time activities and in the same type of responsibilities or creative experiences. Continuous adjustment and substitution are necessary in accordance with the stern and realistic demands of the environment, culture, and society in which they live.

Who is this old person? Is he 35 or 75? He is actually any age at which the degenerative or emotional changes have occurred, and these changes are greatly influenced by the community's concept of an aging person and the difficulty that is found in obtaining and retaining a job, because of artificial standards of age. When a person is faced with physical difficulties or frustrations, his previous personality defects become exaggerated by the added stress and enforced idleness. The common policy of requiring retirement at a stipulated age, such as 65, no longer meets the demands of a country with the vast resources of our own, since it prevents men and women from contributing to the younger generation their accumulated wisdom and experience. This type of philosophy adds a load of nonproducers which must be carried by the producers of our economy. When people wake up in the morning with a sense of belonging, with planned activities and interests, they remain in much better physical and mental health. Unrealistic retirement may be an important factor in the premature failure of a worker's physical and mental faculties.

Rationale for Treatment

This preface bears an important relationship to the rationale for treatment of such disturbing emotional conflicts with tranquilizing drugs. All the problems of everyday living are still present in the old person and often are exaggerated by the factors we have discussed. In the situations involving anxiety, fear, and apprehension, these drugs can be of inestimable value.

This anxiety is not only destructive to the morale of the individual but also to that of his family; relieving it will make life much more tolerable in the home.

There are many emotional changes of aging which are not primarily the result of physical changes but are subject to the same laws which govern emotional changes and behavior disorders in youger persons when faced with stress and frustration. Older persons with such disorders can be treated at home by the general practitioner with much benefit and with great relief to the family. Judicious counseling by skilled workers adds immeasurably to the benefits which can be expected from the use of small doses of chlorpromazine.

It is often forgotten that the elderly can suffer from purely functional emotional conditions not directly related to physical changes. However, there are other groups in which the degenerative changes have produced either temporary or permanent organic defects. The attitude of the person to such defect plays a considerable role in the final evolution of their emotional and personality distortions. Obviously a person who is accustomed to an active and energetic life is distressed at the prospect of a chronic, disabling illness. A patient with such an illness may be cared for at home but often this is impossible because of the patient's intense emotional reaction to his disability.

There is a large group of patients whose emotional disorders are linked much more directly with the presence of degenerative diseases, particularly those with brain degeneration caused by cerebral arteriosclerosis or senile changes. There is thus added to their emotional distress other factors which make their care difficult, such as confusion, lack of judgment, difficulty in thinking, and inability to learn, retain experiences, and follow direction. Such illnesses may vary in intensity from time to time or may be characterized by continuous and steady progression. To these milder symptoms there may be added frank psychotic symptoms such as hallucinations, delusions, and accusations against relatives and friends.

This creates an extremely distressing situation for members of the family and the constant supervision and observation necessary deprives them of their everyday routine, environment, and equanimity. Many grown children will sacrifice themselves and their children for long periods because they feel that they must repay their parent for the loving-kindness shown to them in their own formative years.

The presence of great restlessness and a tendency to wander adds to the already intolerable burden. The reversal of the sleep pattern imposes a still greater strain. Older people of this type frequently eat an inadequate diet because of emotional distress, to which may be added confusion, lack of interest, and perhaps suspicion concerning their food. This frequently complicates a physical balance which has already broken down.

Such devoted families become frantic because they can no longer care for their aged parent. With much feeling of guilt, they often make arrangements to send the aged parent to a nursing home, home for the aged, or a state hospital. As is well known, these institutions have become overcrowded with the tremendous demand that is placed upon them by the community. Many of these patients are difficult to care for because they suffer from chronic degenerative physical disorders, accompanied by much emotional distress, associated with irritability, suspicion, dissatisfaction, hopelessness, and resentment. There may be definite mental changes such as confusion and disorientation, which may be progressive or have periodic fluctuations in clarity. Some of these changes may be caused by feeding difficulties, lack of proper vitamins, and deficiency of protein intake.

However, with newer therapeutic treatment and stress upon rehabilitation, older concepts must be changed from hopelessness to optimism. Such persons should no longer be admitted to institutions with the thought that they are to remain there for life. The ultimate goal must be physical and mental restoration. The initiation of active rehabilitative measures may make them more comfortable and result in discharge of a considerable number. The ultimate goal must be physical and mental restoration.

It has been demonstrated frequently that when elderly persons engage actively in creative, recreational, and other activities, their physical and emotional states improve much more rapidly or symptoms advance much more slowly than when they are treated only for a specific physical disorder.

Today we are learning to look not at the sick but at the well, not at the idle but the busy, not at the unloved but the loved, not at the hopeless but at those who are instilled with a feeling of faith. No longer do such individuals enter homes for the aged or state hospitals with the thought of sitting and waiting for death.

Clinical Study—Materials and Methods

What can be done in this field is exemplified by the program of the Rochester Jewish Home and Infirmary, a progessive institution with more than 200 patients. Active rehabilitative measures, consisting of occupational therapy, recreational therapy, and a volunteer program bringing contact with the outside world, have been used for some time. Half of these patients suffer from chronic physical disorders which require bed care. Many of the ambulatory patients have emotional disturbances which make their care difficult because of cantankerous, irascible, and suspicious attitudes. Clubs whose membership included both in- and outpatients were established, but there still remained a large number of patients who could not cooperate because of confusion, excitement, restless behavior, and feelings of hostility.

In October 1954, chlorpromazine was added to the rehabilitation program, in order to make these people more amenable to other treatment measures. Over 100 patients from the infirmary and other wards were treated with chlorpromazine, and to date 33 are still under treatment. The drug was administered initially to those who were depressed, apprehensive, fearful, aggressive, noisy, or resistive. In addition to this group there were many patients suffering from physical disorders in whom anxiety states or hostile attitudes had developed because of the chronicity of physical ailments. Others were suffering from much pain, associated with terminal carcinoma.

Results

The use of chlorpromazine produced a rapid and pronounced change in the atmosphere of the Home. The patients began to eat and sleep better, were calm, agreeable, and sociable and, with associated rehabilitative measures, began to take an interest in their environment and in life itself. Many lost their confusion, possibly because of decreased activity and increased appetite, with a more varied and adequate intake of food. Complaints of pain decreased. The effect upon the other residents of the Home was noticeable, with obvious decease in the disturbing noises and behavior previously characteristic of the wards.

With increasing cooperation of such patients, it was possible for employees to take part in other activities for the betterment of the patients. There was also an improvement in their morale, since they worked under less tension and in a more agreeable environment. The attitude of the personnel changed from that of routine custodial care to one of interest and personal concern, with emphasis upon the everyday activities of the patients and attempts to get them well. Under this change it was possible to send to occupational and recreational therapy many patients who had been unable to partake in the full facilities of the Home because of their confused or belligerent attitudes.

These patients also became more accepting of family relationship and greeted their families with anticipation instead of resentment. This resulted in a discharge of patient to their homes or permitted them to go home on short visits. The morale of the family also improved, as they had fewer feelings of guilt for having sent their relative to an institution.

Still another result which was noted was a pronounced decrease in the use of analgesics and sedatives, such as barbituates and paraldehyde, despite the fact that the dosage of chlorpromazine was often very small, averaging 30 to 200 mg. per day. The drain upon employees' time was also decreased in that a great many of the patients became tidy in their habits and no longer wet or soiled. The night shift also had more time to attend to the physical needs of other patients, since the majority of those receiving chlorpromazine were now able to sleep through the night.

One of the great problems of state hospitals today is the overwhelming number of admissions of the aged for mental illness. At present, this number comprises 40 to 60 per cent of all admissions. Many patients are difficult to care for because of confusion, excitement, suspicions, hallucinations, and resistive and poorly cooperative behavior. At the Rochester State Hospital, over 200 patients of this type were treated with chlorpromazine in the past two years, out of a total group of over 1,500 treated patients suffering with mental illnesses from other causes. Older patients were selected because of difficult behavior and emotional reactions, and this is the only type of patient who was treated with chlorpromazine. The improvement in behavior shown by many of this group was again unexpected, as well as the improvement in mental conditions shown in some cases.

Complications and Side Effects

The treatment of the elderly patient with chlorpromazine is not without some degree of danger. As is well known, administration may be followed by hypotensive reactions which are much more pronounced when the medication is given parenterally and less so when given orally. These reactions occur less frequently than was first anticipated and appear chiefly in persons with an unstable vascular system, often associated with hypertension which varies from day to day. Since it is seen most often as an orthostatic reaction, it is wise to have the patient lie down for an hour or two for the first two or three days of treatment. If this reaction is to take place, very often it does so in the first few days of treatment and then, like other complications, will disappear following an interval of treatment. The patient can be up and about without this precaution after it has been noted that the hypotensive phenomenon is no longer present. Infrequently premature thrombi or emboli may develop if this precaution is not observed.

Jaundice occurs in 0.5 to 5 per cent of treated patients. Why there should be such a variation is difficult to understand, but this has been demonstrated in our series. The frequency varies not only in the different periods of the year but also in similar seasons and similar settings. It produces few symptoms, although there have been some complaints of general malaise, chilliness, pruritus, and gastrointestinal distress. Although the general practitioner views this jaundice with alarm, it is our feeling that the jaundice is self-limited and requires little treatment. There have been no complications from jaundice in our series. It appears to be caused by the body's attempt to restore its balance. The temporary reaction consists of a swelling of the bile canaliculi chiefly through the invasion of lymphocytes, causing biliary obstruction. Chlorpromazine, if continued, probably does not aggravate this condition, but it is our practice to discontinue its use. We have treated such patients again at a later date, and, except in two patients, there has been no recurrence of jaundice.

Dermatitis in the form of maculopapular eruptions, particularly on the exposed parts of the body, occurred in 4 per cent of our patients. Nurses giving intramuscular injections often develop a contact dermatitis and should wear gloves when giving chlorpromazine.

Hypotensive changes may be noted in complaints of headache, dizziness, or occasionally of fainting. Fainting is uncommon, but in patients with an unstable cardiovascular system it is well to give the initial dose with the patient lying recumbent, particularly if the medication is given intramuscularly and less so when it is given orally. Some elderly patients show a tendency to persistent drowsiness, which may be overcome by the judicious use of dexedrine, 5 mg. once or twice a day, either in single tablets or in the form of spansules. At times, patients may complain of blurred vision, tremor, or unsteadiness. Reflexes are not as prompt at first, so that outpatients under treatment should be warned against driving cars or working with electrical machinery. Most of these symptoms disappear within a week or two when the body has established a new balance.

Other patients may complain of dryness of the mouth, stuffiness in the nose, and occasionally of gastritis and constipation. The last complication must be guarded against, particularly in older patients. From time to time there may be tachycardia. Cardiovascular collapse is rare, but has been noted particularly when the initial dosage was high and was administered suddenly without preliminary testing with smaller doses. If no complication occurs the first time, then symptoms associated with the heart or vascular system do not usually appear. Improvement in appetite is the rule, so that patients begin to eat well and gain weight.

Parkinsonism is unusual, except in cases in which dosages are high, usually 800 mg. or more. Such high dosage should never be used in elderly people. In a few rare instances parkinsonism has occurred, however, with relatively small doses of 200 to 300 mg. per day. It is well to regulate the dosage according to the needs of the patient. Sleep can be promoted by giving 10 to 25 mg. chlorpromazine about an hour before the expected time of retirement.

It is wise to begin chlorpromazine therapy by using small 10-mg. doses three times a day. It is often surprising that small doses in the elderly person may be quite effective, but if these are not, then dosage may be increased to a maximum of 100 to 200 mg. per day, given in three to four doses with the last at bedtime to promote sleep. After a period of treatment, it may be necessary to give only one dose of 25 to 50 mg. at night which may be adequate in itself and persist for the entire day.

Discussion

Many pronounced changes have occurred in the behavior patterns of such disturbed patients, particularly in those who are suffering from a psychosis caused by arteriosclerosis, and to some degree also in those with senile psychosis. Unexpectedly, a number of such patients improved not only in behavior, but in mental capacity, so that they lost their delusions, hallucinations, and even their confusion. In many patients, however, confusion and disorientation persisted with great improvement in behavior. Thus they were less of a problem from the standpoint of supervision, feeding, sleeping, and cleanliness. Chlorpromazine improves the appetite, so that following adequate intake of food and decreased restlessness and excitement, these patients gained in weight and improved physically. The changes which occurred in behavior and psychoses in this group of patients are shown in the accompanying table.

	Behavior	Psychosis
Recovered	4%	0%
Greatly improved	33%	9%
Much improved	37%	21%
Improved	5%	25%
Unimproved	21%	45%

This table includes only patients who were admitted to state hospitals because of frankly psychotic symptoms which made it impossible to care for them elsewhere. It can be noted that 74 per cent of carefully selected patients demonstrated a noticeable improvement in behavior. Coincident with this, and also because of increased rest and better sleep and diet, mental symptoms improved in 30 per cent of patients. In a few patients, improvement was of such degree that they could be returned to and cared for at home. In some, mental symptoms seemed to disappear entirely, but this number was very small.

It must be remembered that when such patients are released to their homes they must be continued on small maintenance doses of the drug. This same type of therapy can be given to the aged person in his own home or in a nursing home.

This field has opened up a wide avenue of treatment for the general practitioner, who is often faced with urgent demands by family members for some type of effective therapy to control the restlessness and emotional turmoil of an elderly relative. This is a field of great usefulness and one which is now being explored and developed more thoroughly.

It must also be emphasized that chlorpromazine therapy should at all times be under the guidance of a physician. When indicated, superficial and supporting psychotherapy, counseling, and guidance must be provided to enhance the effectiveness of the medication. By means of chlorpromazine, the patient who is faced with supposedly intolerable emotional distress is made much more tranquil and anxious to accept guidance and help.

Conclusions

This paper is a brief report indicating various factors which may produce emotional changes in the elderly patients. In this way the rationale for treatment of such situations with tranquilizing drugs and the use of counseling and environmental manipulation becomes apparent. When rehabilitative measures are instituted in addition to the use of chlorpromazine, much greater and permanent results can be obtained. The need for continuous supervision by a physician is emphasized.

With proper therapeutic measures, it can be anticipated that old persons who have required care in a nursing home, in a state hospital, or home for the aged primarily because of emotional and behavior disorders, may improve to such a degree as to make possible their return to care in their own homes. Chlorpromazine is not a cure-all, but can help reduce the emotional and behavior problems of older patients and make life for their families much more pleasant. It must be emphasized that to obtain effective result there must be a careful selection of patients for treatment.

AN OUTLINE OF THE PROCESS OF RECOVERY FROM SEVERE TRAUMA

Harley C. Shands, M.D.

This discussion is an attempt to draw together into a single formulation many separate parts of an experience gleaned during two years of interviewing patients suffering from severe malignant illness of one sort or another. We were impressed at the time, and have continued with increasing interest to be impressed, with the manner in which, after the imposition of intolerable stresses, the resultant strains point up the basic similarity of human patterns in personality disintegration and in the restitution which follows. Further, we may by analogy make certain inferences about early personality development.

In the field of research into human developmental patterns the direct experimental imposition of stress of a degree sufficient to impose strain upon the resources of the individual is impossible: Either the stress is inadequate to present any major adaptive problem to the individual, or else the conditions of the experiment are apt to exceed the limits of the taboos upon experimenting with human beings. However, the transactions taking place between a patient and his physician in the course of the treatment of a malignant illness present an opportunity for study of reactions of strain which is a reasonable facsimile of an experimental situation. In early cases the informational stress is maximal when the patient discovers the nature of the lesion, and during this period, when the patient remains in good health otherwise, much may be learned of the manner in which informational stresses are managed; on the other hand, with the increasing severity in the lesion and the growing disability of the patient, much may be learned about the somatopsychic problem, i.e., about the manner in which the increasingly morbid process affects the state of mind of the patient and his relation to himself and his environment.

Lest it seem that this program is entirely devoid of any quality of human kindness, it may be noted in passing that one of the most reassuring and gratifying parts of the experience of this period of interviewing was the discovery that the interest displayed in the patients by the interviewer was for the most part welcomed by the patients; many of them spontaneously expressed feelings of gratitude at being able to talk to someone. Indeed, it is entirely probable that in a project such as this, some degree of self-interest on the part of the patient is an indispensable motivational element; particularly in advanced states of disability patients are quite unable to display the altruism involved in giving of information without hope of reward. In accepting the report of the patient's experience the interviewer functions as an important tension-relieving device for the patient. One patient remarked that she had become entirely unable to have any feelings that her family understood anything of the distress through which she was passing, and the surgical staff had no time to listen, so that she was greatly relieved by the attention of the psychiatric interviewer.

The process of restitution, beginning with the imposition of the trauma, may be formulated as a single process which demonstrates from beginning to end an increasing ability on the part of the patient to discriminate in his experience, to differentiate those things which belong together from those which should be separated. In general, it appears that the process is, rather, one in which a whole becomes gradually more and more analyzable into parts than it does one in which new parts are added one by one to construct a whole; by analogy, we may say that it appears to us that a human being characteristically is first aware of the forest and gradually aware of the trees which make it up, with an eventual full awareness both of the individual parts and of the whole.

The formulation which we desire to present in the course of this paper is one which rests upon, and attempts to point out a number of relations among, the work of a number of investigators. The general concept of personality formation and the dynamics of the processes in mentation were formulated in the most influential and striking way by Freud; Goldstein has been concerned with the consequences of brain injury, and especially with certain aspects of the problems of abstraction and concreteness; Melanie Klein has been most instructive in her presentation of the early stages of the organization of the ego, particularly in her formulation of the paranoid position, the depressive position, and the manic defense.

This presentation is necessarily an approximation of a hypothetical solution broad enough to cover the whole process of restitution. It is an effort to describe an abstract, idealized process closely modeled upon the contributions of the investigators we mentioned, and there was no single patient in whom all of the manifestations to be discussed were observed.

The process of recovery can be described in three phases, each of which may be divided into two steps. The first phase is that of the immediate response; the second, that of "total defense," and the third, that of a reintegration of the self. In the first phase, with its steps of chaos and of depersonalization, the patient describes feelings of nonexistence; in the second, the patient defends himself by the exclusion of the unbearable information in stages of projection and of denial, and in the third, in states of depressive anxiety and of novel ego identifications, he describes the loss of his old idea of himself and the construction of a new version which includes the painful information.

A. First Phase

First Step: Chaos.—In those patients who were suddenly apprised of the nature of their lesion, there was a remarkable stereotypy of immediate response: Almost every patient said he experience was like being struck a heavy blow over the head. Other descriptions included being "stiffened out," paralyzed, made speechless. In all of the patients without other complications, this phase of the response was a very dramatic, but transient, one.

Second Step: Depersonalization.—The immediately succeeding period was characterized as being one of numbness, "going through the motions," feeling as though in a fog. The patients felt remote and alienated from themselves, although able to act in a rote mechanical way. The symptoms are indistinguishable from symptoms of depersonalization encountered elsewhere.

In a case complicated by extensive operation, the two steps could be distinguished, but here the first lasted for several days, during which time the patient lay almost completely inert, responding only to very strong stimuli. When she began again to respond, she described a very marked inhibition in all emotional processes during this period, followed by a feeling of being "all in pieces," of being afraid to look at the region of her wound for fear that she would find "nothing" there.

B. Second Phase

First Step: Projection.—In patients affected by this particular traumatic situation the examples of undiscriminating defense that we have seen have been primarily projection and denial. It appears that such a symptom as amnesia, seen so frequently in other traumatic neuroses, might also be classified under this heading, but we have not observed it in this group. Both these mechanisms appear to be attempts to deal with the dangerous information by separating it from the self; the attempt is more mature than the preceding one of fragmentation because of the maintenance of a functioning organization which is possible with either projection or denial.

We have been impressed in this series by indications of the more primitive nature of the mechanism of projection, both from the standpoint of the character structure of those patients using this defense rather than another, and by the greater frequency of manifestation of projective mechanisms in the terminal period of the illness.

The defensive use of the mechanism of projection and its sudden collapse on several occasions could be clearly seen in a woman who tended to develop sudden very strong dependent relationships to doctors. When she was relieved by x-rays of a cervical carcinoma, she announced aggressively to everyone what a wonderful man her doctor was because he had cured her cancer; when the cancer recurred, she became very depressed and changed doctors. A second physician promised not to leave her, but after an operation he went to a medical meeting and she became depressed. When seen in an interview for this series, she first reacted with intense gratitude, grasped the therapist's hand, and said no one had listened to her before; but upon the next day's visit, she was very hostile and withdrawn—she said, "Go away, I don't want to see you again; you stirred me all up and made me feel so unhappy yesterday."

While this problem is of immense importance from a theoretical standpoint, it is of equal importance from a practical point of view in the management of patients with cancer, since these patients are on the whole prone to react thus. As a rule, the severer the state of illness, the more likely is the patient to respond by projecting the evil inside onto the external world; but where his world is the hospital, this projecting, leading as it does to a rather paranoid response to the therapeutic personnel, is extremely costly in all ways. Patients report many instances of panic in relation to doctors and nurses; these panic reactions are commoner the sicker the patient, the less sensitive the therapeutic personnel, and, interestingly enough the more the instance in question takes place in the middle of the night.

A patient in the advanced stages of metastatic illness told us that the nurse was crazy. Another woman reported a very severe panic when awakened in the night by the delirious rambling of a neighboring patient—she wondered what terrible things doctors were doing to her: this woman had severe anxiety when the service changed, since she was afraid of strange doctors; on another occasion she reported that a nurse in giving her a back rub had dug her fingers all the way down to the bone, a feeling which terrified her.

Second Step: Denial.—The second of these undiscriminating defenses, that of denial, is of less importance from a psychotherapeutic standpoint for two reasons: In the first place, it is a defense which does not, as in the case of projection, lead onward in a vicious circle to greater and greater distress—the patient dismisses the problem by denying its existence and the process tends to come to a stop until further events occur; in the second place, for some patients a stabilized position of denial in the face of a hopeless lesion is as good a situation as can readily be attained. Where the defense of denial carries with it the most malignant possibilities is in the early stages of the illness, in which the relationship between denial of the existence of a lesion and delay in seeking treatment is of very considerable practical importance.

C. Third Phase

First Step: Grieving.—The third phase, again, may be divided into two steps, an earlier one of the expression of feelings of grief, and a subsequent one of a readaptation by means of the assumption of new ego identifications, in which the painful information may be included in some manner. Although the identifications which serve as "vehicles" for behavior vary greatly in degree of maturity, they all have in common the quality of including, rather than (as in the former two stages) excluding, the problem. Where the situation has to be precariously stabilized by the exclusion of information, the patient is constantly on the alert to keep the painful topic out of mind and consequently suffers from a considerable restriction of interest in the world in general; here, on the other hand, the potentialities of adaptation remain considerably more varied.

The expression of a feeling of grief with crying is a regular part of the process by means of which the prior adaptive identifications are abandoned and the new ones taken on. One patient described a violent reaction of depersonalization followed by a flood of tears (while visting a neighbor) and a subsequent assumption of the idea that she had a year to live, an idea based on the history of another neighbor with a lesion similar to the patient's.

The mourning period is an essential step in reorientation in relation to the changed situation. To us, it appears that the grieving is a response to the loss of a whole system of assumptions and expectations upon which human beings build a view of the world. In some manner the weeping reaction displayed by the patient above serves to help "dissolve" the old system in such a way that it can be replaced by a new. Where the grieving is blocked for any reason, the patient has to adopt some precarious defensive sort of adaptation rather than attempting, after clearing the site, to make a new construction with the materials at hand.

We believe, further, from our experience with these patients, that the grieving reaction is possible only with a personality structure of a sufficient maturity and that it is greatly facilitated by the presence of a sympathetic listener. This listener supplies in the situation a predictable and nonthreatening human being who serves as a leader; the patient, in a human context because of his relationship to this supporting figure, can allow himself to experience and discharge tension in a disorganized way with some confidence in the prospect of being led back to safety with the help of the other person.

Second Step: Identification.—Since the emphasis in this brief communication is upon outlining the course of the recuperative process, we have not attempted to discuss at length the ways in which the ego identifications may themselves assume pathological significance. We may point out in passing that where the identification assumed by the patient is one the model for which is a relative or friend who has died of cancer, the hopelessness engendered by the assumed identity is a serious bar to treatment. Several patients mentioned that as soon as they knew they had malignant lesions, they thought there was no use doing anything about it, since "my father" or "the woman across the street" or "my sister" had had cancer and died of it.

Of the identifications which may be observed, there are as many separate possibilities as there are important figures in the life history of the individual, but, for purposes of description, we may separate out a few of what appear to be common types of identification which make it possible for the patient with cancer to construct for himself a life with some possibility of gratification. Three sorts which we have seen adopted with some success from this standpoint have been the assumption of the role of the good child, that of the physician, and that of the good parent, in an increasing scale of maturity. It, of course, goes without saying that to describe the process in any such fashion as this gives an entirely too structured and static impression of the kaleidoscope of events seen in dealing with a patient.

The first category, that of the good child, is well illustrated by a young woman with Hodgkin's disease. In spite of a great deal of difficulty with her family, it could easily be seen that she wanted very much to be good and to be approved of by them. In the early days of her illness, when the family first discovered the malignant nature of the lesion, the patient abruptly exchanged roles in her relationship to a younger sister: The direction of the relationship had been symbolized by gifts of clothes from patient to sister, but upon reception of the news, the patient took to her bed and the sister brought her a negligee. The patient was told she had only a few months to live, and she and the family planned about this prognostication; when she lived on and on beyond the prediction, she became depressed and felt that she was a disappointment to them. In a series of interviews planned to help her to modify some of her attitudes, she demonstrated after some initial resistance a great enjoyment of the status of patient; so wholehearted was this reaction that she brought in all the other members of her family to the psychiatric clinic and she herself abandoned all other doctors. It was something of a problem to persuade her to be faithful to her appointments in the medical and tumor clinics.

In the second of the types of constructive identification mentioned above, that of identification with the doctor, there were two very prominent examples in this series. One of these was a woman who had survived a very long time after an operation for an ovarian cancer with metastases. In the interim she had devoted herself to reading about cancer and allied diseases and said there was little with which she was unfamiliar. She spoke in interviews several times of the unhappy fate of the poor doctors who had to get up early and work hard while she could take it easy in bed. The other patient had previously exhibited an adaptation on this basis in her profession of dental assistant, when she felt pleased if allowed to perform minor procedures under the supervision of the employer. In the hospital, she felt best when she was able to take care of the other patients; in several instances she accomplished a good deal with patients on the ward by interviewing them in a manner similar to that in which she herself had been interviewed.

In the third of these categories we have observed several instances of a really creative adaptation to the illness in patients who had solved for themselves the problem of dying. These patients had managed to accept the inevitable with cheerfulness and to direct their attention toward helping other patients and their own children to get through the difficult time. These patients had an inner security of such a nature that they did not need to borrow artificial status, as did the former patients. It was striking to note how much of a benign influence was exerted by one woman in the breast tumor clinic as she simply sat on the benches and talked freely to anyone who wished to speak to her. She said that she had decided since she was going to die she wanted people to remember her as a good person, and she presented this picture in a very effective manner.

Comment

The three phases which we have described above may be seen to be variations of a general statement a patient makes about his relationship to the threat: (1) "This is not me" (2) "This alien thing is no part of myself," and (3) "I have the wrong idea of myself and shall have to change it to get along." In terms of Freudian theory, the first phase is that of helplessness, or primary anxiety, and of the immediately succeeding response; the chaotic reaction appears to us indistinguishable from what Goldstein calls the "catastrophic reaction." The first step of the second phase corresponds to the "paranoid position" described by Mrs. Klein, with the denial representing, it seems to us, a version of the "manic defense"; the patient presents what Goldstein refers to as a "concrete attitude," in that he relates the information to some specific entity and then operates upon that entity as though it were the lesion. In the first step of the third phase we are reminded of Mrs. Klein's "depressive position"; the process involved is the internalization of the traumatic information, with the consequent destruction of the old idea of the self and the necessity of a reconstruction, a process of the formation of a new basic abstraction.

It is manifestly impossible to discuss in an exhaustive way the implications of the findings presented in this sketchy way. For the purpose of pointing up the suggestions we are interested in, we may confine ourselves to the second and third stages, representing, it appears to us, the processes of restitution which fall into what is described in classic psychoanalytic terms as ego functioning.

The first of the four phases, that of projection, is of immense interest from several standpoints; it represents a developmental epoch in which the facts are interpreted by the patient in a solidified, concrete representation of a type which demonstrates the poor definition of the "ego boundary." The threat to the integrity of the concept of the self is met by the assumption that the dreaded fragment of the ego is a foreign or alien object introduced from outside and therefore in no way the responsibility of the individual himself. Especially to a cultural group with strong puritan leanings, this device is of great value in assuring the individual of his own blamelessness, and, moreover, it provides an explanation which satisfies to some extent the need for a satisfactory explanation of a puzzling situation.

This solution to the problem is a notably poor one, however, as repeated efforts must be made to ensure the separation of the alien portion which follows the individual as surely as his shadow. The foreign portion has been described under the general term of "bad internal object"; this term in itself is an abstraction which covers an immense variety of concrete manifestations at all levels of human functioning. Such a "bad internal object" is the "devil," of which the sick and the evil were thought to be possessed in primitive times; and, in community terms, the witches of Salem, who were executed in an effort to purge the community of evil thoughts and deeds.

In these patients of ours, the shifting referent of the bad internal object could be seen in a wide variety of manifestations; we were particularly interested in one salient observation, that of the identical process but inverse manifestation in patients with cancer and with cancerphobia. In cancer patients, as exemplified above, the individual sought in many instances to formulate the situation by transferring his concern from the somatic lesion in his body to the image of a distressing close relative, child, spouse, or parent in most cases, whereas the patient with cancerphobia maintained an uneasy relation to some relative by transferring his concern to an imagined lesion inside. The essentially abstract nature of the concept of the self is nowhere better illustrated than in this connection, since for the purposes of this mechanism of defense the image of the malignant relative is equivalent to the image of the malignant process.

To illustrate even further in an effort to clarify this difficult conception, we may cite some further material. One of these patients described the last illness of her father, in which he was suffering from a cerebral lesion which was characterized by convulsions and by a total inability to communicate with the family. The patient was horrified by her fantasies of his experience behind the immobile mask; she became unable to go into his room without a severe anxiety attack and after several days became totally aphonic. When he died, she was relieved of the aphonia and was able to care for the body without any great distress. She endeavored, if our interpretation is correct, on the one hand, to isolate herself from the uncontrollable alien person her father became in his nonhuman state, and, on the other, participated in his illness by her vicarious loss of voice.

Another patient, a severe borderline neurotic woman with an operation habit, attempted time after time to relieve herself of her internal object by means of surgical removals of various organs. She was fat, but she denied any responsibility for her obesity by saying she was not hungry, she merely was following the demands of an implacable stomach; she told of ideas of having something black and horrid inside her, like a tapeworm. After years of work with the problem, she remembered terrifying attacks of rage against her father, in which she wished to tear him limb from limb, when she felt that in urinating he purposely left the door open to taunt her with his possession of an organ she had been denied. Another woman with a similar problem described fantasies of "black brains" in her head and wondered if it might be the best treatment to open her skull and scoop out the diseased areas. Both these women dealt with black things inside to avoid the intolerable effort of understanding themselves as persons capable of harboring murderous impulses against a parent.

The stage of simple denial is of less interest from a theoretical point of view because of the immensely reduced color in the material, as well as because of the reduced complications suffered by these patients, due to the relatively stable adaptive situation which is possible with a bland denial of the presence of the lesion. We suspect that the relatively emotionless denials of these patients are attenuated versions of the florid denials vividly seen in the "manic defense," in which the patient so flagrantly states his ideas of his own importance and happiness. We have not seen in our series, but have heard reported by surgeons with a wide experience, cases in which the patient in a terminal phase displayed great hopefulness, which we suspect is similar to the spes phthisica which used to be observed in terminal cases of tuberculosis.

The depressive position is of the utmost importance in the restitution of the ego because of the necessity of "vacating" a previous state of adjustment before it can be filled by a successive state. One of the most impressive aspects of this state is the severity of the anxiety which accompanies the emptiness. It appears to us that it is the intolerable character of this depressive anxiety which makes the patient think of suicide as a quick and certain method of terminating the suffering. (A very large proportion of patients have reported that at the moment of learning of the diagnosis, or in anticipation of learning it, suicide appeared to be a useful solution.) It may be noted here that a great paradox occurs, in that it is the inclusion within the idea of the self of the alien, foreign, intolerable object which leads to the sensation of emptiness; we believe it possible to resolve the paradox by noting that the emptiness is observably an inability to act or to plan action: The emptiness is one of purpose. The individual becomes aware of himself as including entirely new and alien potentialities, and so immense is this inclusion that none of his previous patterns of action can be carried out without an initial period of hesitation and checking on possibilities.

Finally, in the new adaptation made possible by a novel ego identification, the patient fills in the emptiness in his action pattern repertory by some sort of view of himself which includes the new, initially traumatic, information and begins to go about his business again in some manner. As we have noted above, it is usually easily evident afterward from whence the new action pattern has been derived, although it is frequently difficult or impossible to predict in advance which of the many models available to him the patient will select as the appropriate one for him, and it is equally difficult to say in advance whether the new ego identification will offer a method of gratifying the human needs of the individual. This reconstruction of an ego, or of a self-concept, or of a useful repertory of behavior patterns, to put it in a variety of ways, is an enormous achievement in abstract thinking and planning.

REASSURANCE

Paul Chodoff, M.D.

"The patient should be reassured." How often is this advice given by psychiatrists to each other, to nonpsychiatric doctors who want to know how to cope with the nonorganic problems which make up such a formidable percentage of their practices, to social workers, ministers, and many other nonmedical dealers in human difficulties. It is advice which often results in a glow of accomplishment on the part of the adviser and a feeling on the part of the recipient that he has been told something of value which he wishes to put into effect. It is the intent of this paper to investigate the effects of this "reassurance" on the sick individual on whom it is practiced, to attempt to define what is meant by the term and how it works, and to assay the extent of therapeutic benefit derived from its use. I was motivated to study the problem of reassurance by observing how loosely and ambiguously the term has been used, by becoming aware of how often what is meant to be reassuring has a very different effect on the patient, and by noting the multiple, sometimes unexpected, ways in which beneficial effects are actually brought about when they do occur.

Reassurance is defined by the dictionary as the restoration of confidence. For psychiatric purposes it may be considered as a maneuver, usually verbal, designed to bring about the more or less immediate alleviation or relief of mental perturbation and the reinstatement of at least comparative euphoria. It is of course true that the relief of anxiety and the production of a feeling of well-being is part of the ultimate goal of any well-managed psychotherapeutic program. But it is not in the sense of a hoped-for end result of treatment that reassurance is used here, but rather as a deliberate technic which attempts to bring about such a result quickly and summarily, with a minimum of participation on the part of the patient and without regard for other therapeutic goals. This is done in various ways: by telling the patient not to worry or that he has nothing to worry about, by giving a seemingly rational, usually superficial, explanation of apparently incomprehensible difficulties, by minimizing the problem, and by universalizing it—the "you're not the only one" approach.

When statements of this sort cause the patient to feel better, there arises the question of why this happens. It seems clear that the actual content of the reassurance is insufficient to explain the comfort-producing result. Patients are not often fools, and it is demonstrably false that any neurotic person has nothing to worry about. Telling him to stop worrying adds nothing to his knowledge and must be a reiteration of something he has told himself uncounted times. When ignorance of facts about his body or about the material outside world is responsible for anxiety, explanation can be salutary and has a legitimate function. Too often explanation and information are useless, because what the patient is worrying about consciously bears only a symbolic relationship to its unconscious roots. Anyone who has ever tried to explain to a paranoid or phobic patient that his delusional belief or fixed fear is not based on present external reality will realize the futility of such an exercise. Minimizing or pooh-poohing the problem falls in the same category as telling the patient he has nothing to worry about, while the information that one's troubles are not unique would seem to provide a very tenuous basis for happiness.

Yet experience has shown that this type of reassuring discussion is sometimes, at least temporarily, effective. If we cannot accept what is said as the operative factor, we must look elsewhere for an explanation of this. All of the methods mentioned above carry as a common assumption that the person doing the reassuring is wise and powerful and that the patient is to relin quish his troubles to this omnipotent figure with the tacit assumption that something will be done about them. It seems then that it may not be the verbal content of the reassurance itself which is effective but that the effect is brought about by something in the role taken by the reassurer and in the constellation of factors which constitute the interpersonal situation between him and the person reassured. In such a situation, the reassurer is doing something positive and definite, cutting peremptorily through the tangled skein of doubts and ambivalences which confuse the patient and render him incapable of dealing effectively with his problems. The doctor or therapist may become to the patient the firm, decisive parent he wished for, or the harsh, authoritarian father he consciously rebels against but for whose uncompromising certainties he may unconsciously long. Vis à vis such a figure the patient is relegated to a trusting, childlike posture which can be very comforting and which enables him for a period to be less disturbed by his anxieties. The unconscious assumption made by the patient is that a promise has been made to him that his questions will be answered, his problems solved, his wishes gratified. The hidden promissory note here is that he will accept the omnipotent role of the reassurer and his own inferior status. This kind of relationship, applied particularly to the German people under the Nazi dictatorship, has been described by Erich Fromm in "Escape from Freedom"; and it seems likely when someone feels better after being reassured that this tendency, so widespread in our troubled times, to abdicate responsibility to whoever professes to have the answers, is being called into play.

When this kind of reassurance is beneficial, the comforting effect is often transient. It is clinically observable that in most cases it is simply ineffective. In addition, there are certainly many instances in which reassurance backfires and becomes a precipitant of increased anxiety. It may be that the reason for this is implicit in the authoritarian relationship described above, which carries within itself the seeds of its own destruction. Put in the most general terms, the cause of the failure is ignorance on the part of the reassurer of the dynamic personality factors involved, both in himself and in the patient. As mentioned, when the patient puts himself in the hands of the reassurer as a powerful authoritarian figure, he has made certain unconscious assumptions and he has a bill to present in the form of demands, which stem from the time when he was in fact an infant dependent for his gratifications on the parental figures in his environment. It may be that he has acquiesced in accepting the omnipotent role of the other in the hope that his own infantile need to be omnipotent can now be gratified. The wishes pressing through the defense barriers breached by the seductions of the authoritarian reassurer may be of various kinds, depending on the individual's psychopathology, either sexual or hostile. In any event, these wishes cannot be gratified, and the inevitable crashing of his aroused hopes will be felt as a cruel rejection, or as a confirmation of the patient's secret fear that he is worthless and unlovable, or as another betrayal at the hands of the capricious and enigmatic figures who surround him. Thus, even when temporarily seemingly helpful to the patient, its ultimate failure places the "reassurance" in the category of yet another of the succession of disappointments which have first established and then reinforced his neurosis.

In addition to the inevitable inability to assuage the patient's stimulated infantile demands, certain personality characteristics and needs of the person employing authoritarian reassurance may interfere with the relationship and thus with beneficial results. The use of such methods may be a defensive reaction of the reassurer who keeps his own pervasive unconscious doubts and ambivalences out of awareness by assuring someone else that the world is simple and that answers of a black or white character are easily arrived at. In doing this, he may be really reassuring himself more than he is the patient, especially if he is unconsciously frightened by the fears which the patient is expressing. Such reassurance may also serve as a vehicle for discharging unconscious hostility, since there can very easily be something denigrating and contemptuous in the omnipotent stance of someone who so lightly implies his ability to take over the problems of another as if they were really not very important and as if the person concerned with them must be weak and inconsequential. Another concomitant of such an attitude may be a rather considerable grandiosity with its attendant impatience and poor judgment. It is of course by no means inevitable that everyone employing authoritarian reassurance is motivated by unconscious doubt, hostility and grandiosity, but to the extent that unresolved conflicts of this kind are responsible for the choice of reassurance as a method of treatment any therapeutic usefulness to the patient will certainly be seriously impaired.

An example of how unconscious hostility can disguise itself as "benevolent" reassurance is illustrated in the case of a profoundly devious and manipulative woman with a psychogenic colitis who after two years of psychotherapy suggested that her hours be cut down. The therapist, who was finding himself increasingly irritated and frustrated by the patient, agreed to this with the "reassuring" comment that in view of recent symptomatic improvement, actually slight, he felt that she would be able to handle her problems adequately even with the decreased help. The patient interpreted this as a rejection, and at an emotional level she was quite right, since the therapist had used what was actually a testing maneuver on her part as an opportunity to express resentment resulting from his failure to understand her.

Another patient, an obsessive-compulsive woman, developed almost incapacitating headaches which were felt at first to be organic. Later she was seen by a psychiatrist who, as subsequently described by her, "patted me on the back, told me I had nothing to worry about and that a woman with a husband and children should be happy." The patient quite consciously felt his attitude as patronizing and contemptuous and was further confirmed in her deep belief in her own essential worthlessness. Her headaches, which were in large part occurring because of her inability to be aware of or express anger, became worse under the influence of the repressed resentment resulting from this treatment.

Simple reassurance fails also because, without knowing a good deal about the patient, one cannot know just what a given statement will mean to him. Without a thorough knowledge of the previous life experiences of the patient, any statement made with the intention of being reassuring can be nothing more than "a shot in the dark" and may be so at variance with the facts of what has happened to him and what he knows about himself as to be ineffective or even malevolent. If this is true in regard to the conscious remembered experience of the patient, attempts at reassurance are even blinder stabs if account is not taken of the transference relationship between the patient and doctor. What parental role the reassurer represents is of a great deal more moment to the patient than the content of what is said to him. If he is experienced as the firm, confident father whose positive and definite qualities were a refuge against the insidious exploitations of a doubt-ridden infantile mother, the effect of a therapist's reassurances will be quite different than if he stands for a bellicose, fanatical parent who could brook no opposition. In the former case the patient will be at least temporarily reassured, while in the latter his anxieties will be increased, but in any case it is only when the history is known and a solid transference basis established that a therapist can rationally elect to make a reassuring statement with some confidence in the effect it will have.

An actively disturbed woman, whose symptoms included inability to make a decision, feelings of unreality and depersonalization, and depression, was most alarmed by the development of compulsive ideas that she might strike her child with a knife. She fled to another city where she was induced to consult a nonpsychiatric doctor in the hope that something physical might be found to account for her symptoms. Physical examination proving negative, the doctor spoke to her for a few minutes and ascertained that her obsessive perfectionistic attempts to care for her baby left her very little time for herself and interfered with her sleeping. He thereupon told her in a peremptory manner that because the baby was a burden to her she had feelings of resentment which she buried in something called her unconscious, from which they emerged as lethal impulses. To the patient the doctor sounded very much like her impatient, capricious father who had proved completely unreliable during her childhood. She had had drummed into her, particularly by her mother, that any kind of hostile feelings meant loss of control, which in turn was close to insanity. What she got from the interview with the doctor was that she had been told she was losing her mind by an impatient person who wanted to get rid of her and her unwelcome demands for help. She reacted by an increase in intensity of symptoms and an abortive suicidal attempt. The doctor in the case was not only unaware of the rejecting paternal role he represented for the patient, but in his ignorance of the facts of her history he could not know that his pseudoanalytic explanation, intended as reassuring, would be heard by her as a threatening accusation.

In contrast to the type of handling described above, knowledge of the background and of the transference position may facilitate the deliberate use of reassurance for a definite purpose. An example is the case of a woman who, while in analysis, developed an exacerbation of a previously mild phobia of driving in automobiles just before a trip which was of considerable importance to her. In the hour in which this was brought up she reviewed with her therapist the traumatic events, previously touched upon, which had precipitated the phobia. At the end of the hour the therapist, who was aware that at the time he represented to her a benevolent, idealized father figure, mentioned the difference between conditions at the present and as they had previously been, and suggested that perhaps it wasn't necessary for her to fear driving anymore. This had such a sufficiently reassuring effect that the patient was able to make the trip in relative comfort, even though later on the kind of dependent relationship which made the remark successful had to be attacked analytically.

The case reported above illustrates the possibly deleterious effects of the employment of reassurance in psychotherapy even when the maneuver has been effective in bringing about symptomatic relief. Tendencies to dependency are always fostered by this technic, especially in patients with important personality components of masochism or with passive, submissive identifications. If any attempt at lasting or definitive psychotherapy is to be made, this dependency will have to be analyzed, and the therapist may find that for each occasion he has used reassurance there will be a subsequent struggle with the hostility which is so inextricably intertwined with dependent attitudes.

Another danger inherent in the attempt to assuage anxieties by the use of reassurance lies in the fact that by so doing one forfeits the opportunity of finding out what deeper fears may be behind the patient's superficial worries. By being told that what he complains of is nothing to worry about, the patient may possibly be made to feel better, but he certainly will have his curiosity stifled and will have authoritarian sanction to drop the subject, discussion of which, on a plane of interest and acceptance, might have led back to the roots of the conflict which produced the symptom. Cohen has given a hypothetical instance of such an occurrence when he describes how a patient after tremendous nervous alarums and excursions finally manages to blurt out to his doctor that he thinks something is wrong with him because he eats his dandruff. The startled doctor quickly replies that there is nothing wrong with this, that some of his best friends are addicted to this practice. The patient is reassured at the time, but since the dandruff eating is actually only a psychic straw man covering up problems which are not in his awareness, no permanent benefit is brought about and the chance to inaugurate the investigative process has been lost. If the situation is one in which the doctor has no interest in helping the patient examine his problems and their origins it will be of little moment to him that discussion is cut off and dependency increased by his attempts at reassurance, but in such an instance the possibility of effective help will be so remote and so much a matter of accident that saying nothing at all will be the wiser course. This will at least do no harm, will not add another blow to the patient's fragile self-esteem, and will not discourage him from seeking help elsewhere, whereas well-intentioned attempts to magically exorcise complicated problems in human living by the use of reassurance may have these unfortunate effects.

Reassurance is a valid psychotherapeutic technic. Like any other potent method, it has its dangers and limitations. Because it is apparently so easy to use, there is the risk of its being employed uncritically, as it were, in an interpersonal vacuum, without a proper regard for the harm it can do both by its intrinsic limitations and by its effect in shutting off further exploration of the problems involved. Of special importance is the need for the person doing the reassuring to be aware, to the best of his ability, of his own feelings and motivations and of the nature of the relationship between the patient and himself.

A RATIONALE FOR PSYCHOTHERAPY IN ANXIETY, OBSESSION AND DEPRESSION

George Winokur, M.D.

With the growing popularization of psychiatry and the influx of well-trained, serious workers in the field of psychotherapy, it has become increasingly obvious that a change of outlook in basic cause-effect relationship is not only in order but necessary for the promotion of an art into a science that can be used effectively by all those treating mentally ill persons. As the number of intensively studied cases increased, doubts were expressed in psychiatric publications as to whether ideas propounded earlier were not to a greater or lesser extent incorrect. Many schools of psychiatric thought have arisen, but a fusion of workable propositions has been prevented by the presence of obsessively hostile feelings on the part of the workers in one school toward any other line of thought. The purpose of this paper is to assist in the unification of many of the concepts that appear to have validity, and to fill in some of the gaps with ideas which might contribute to a better understanding of clinical material. In response to a question which may arise, namely whether this paper purports to propose a new way of handling patients psychotherapeutically, the answer is definitely in the negative. It attempts, in the form of a theory, to suggest ideas of what is transacted in a therapeutic relationship, ideas which further observation and discussion might either convert into general laws or relegate to obscurity.

Perhaps primary among the thoughts brought up for revaluation is the question of the efficacy of insight. Its labile nature might lead one to assume it to be of little if any value in patients' varying personalities and conditions. However, to call it completely without use in a therapeutic relationship would undoubtedly be wrong for it does form a link between the patient and doctor and provides a setting for long-term, unverbalized, emotional re-education. Conditions such as schizophrenia, by their very manifestations, often prevent communication on any consensually valid level and, therefore, do not lend themselves to a therapy in a setting in which the aforesaid corrective emotional experiences might occur. In other words, *ability to communicate new material* and not the new material itself may be the important factor, and without this ability the setting for a long-term emotional change may not be possible.

At this point a clarification of the *production of symptoms* is in order, so as to show best the relation between the genesis of symptoms and the application of treatment. The symptom that is most dramatic and best known on an experimental basis is anxiety; and here it is rather obvious that the psychiatrist is dealing with a large number of "anxieties" rather than with a single entity. One type is the reaction to frustration well exemplified by the work of Gantt and Maier. Its nucleus is the difficult differentiation or the unsolvable situation; in addition to anxiety, this particular type of experimental milieu seems to cause compulsive behavior, the organism being seemingly unable to cope with an overwhelming amount of frustration. While this is the explanation of one type of symptom formation, other anxieties might well be produced by placing the organism in a situation which it has in the past perceived as threatening or as particularly gratifying. This, in its totality, has all the aspects of a learning sequence and it, too, has been discussed by Maier. However, further elucidation of one part of this type of experience seems to be necessary for more complete understanding of the problem of anxiety. Most of the time, this feeling is associated with relationships best described as interpersonal. A person's conscience, ideals, and essential value systems are the result of contacts with various authoritarian people. The individual adopts these patterns of response because it is economical and valuable to do so—as far as his feelings of pain and pleasure are concerned. Because of biological needs, occasionally, and because of human interaction, more often, the person finds it difficult to fulfill the requirements of the value system adopted, by a painful process of learning, from parental refusal to conform to the actions of the child. The fear of losing the ideal, and the attack on the system superego caused by a situation formed exclusively by interpersonal relations, are based essentially on a fear of desertion by early authoritative people and tantamount and equal to anxiety. In outline this is:

$$\left.\begin{array}{l}\text{Value system produced by fear of desertion by parents}\end{array}\right\} = \text{Conscience or Ideal } vs \left\{\begin{array}{l}\text{(a) Interpersonal relationship which threatens value system.} \\ \text{(b) Biological needs}\end{array}\right.$$
$$\longrightarrow \text{Anxiety}$$

In other words, the person is threatened with loss of emotional support from the important past person if the value system is not upheld. Actually, there are elements of frustration in this too, because the individual is placed in a situation where it may be almost impossible to fulfill the requirements of the value system. If there is complete defeat of the value system, with no hope of recovery, a depression results.

Depression = Complete defeat of ideals or conscience.

Anxiety = 1/strength of value system (in battle with the value system antagonist).

Complete defeat, however, produces depression and an alleviation of anxiety. This substitutive relationship between anxiety and depression has recently been observed on a physiological level by Leo Alexander. Here obsessions and compulsions play a different part than in the frustration-provoked anxiety. These mechanisms are called into play because, in the past, they have provided satisfaction in the interpersonal relationship between child and parent. They have no symbolic significance but are selected as a result of the qualities of the environment which are perceived in their totality; they may have no actual bearing on the gestalt which produces anxiety.

What then is the possible explanation for the efficacy inherent in psychotherapy? Of probable value in this type of treatment is the fact that the corrective emotional experience may extinguish previous conditional responses. This is to say that the neurotic symptom is a remnant of a situation in the patient's past that either threatened his life or culminated in something quite pleasurable for him. The same situation at a later date, while it does not have the same life-or-death significance to the person, may produce similar types of reaction. This process may be completely unconscious; and the work of the Freudian free association may be the reactivation of the old and unused pathways which, however, may or may not eventuate in psychic painfulness on their admission into the bulk of conscious thoughts.

Whereas it is obvious that ideas and feelings that are not available to awareness on advancing to this state may produce a painful response, it is equally true that suppressed or conscious ideas and feelings may also produce a potent emotional response; for this reason we should not believe that the striving for consciousness of these factors is the only or even the most important producer of anxiety. Nor can it be stated with assurance that these "out-of-awareness" components can form anxiety until they are completely conscious, that repressed feelings can produce anxiety by merely striving for consciousness. This type of assumption, an excellent example of teleological reasoning, must of course have no place in a tight system of psychopathology. Perhaps this would explain why insight produces no change in the symptoms and is, indeed, of no value except to the therapist inasmuch as it helps him to formulate his own role in therapy. If the idea is accepted that improvement is due to a corrective emotional experience which is synonymous with re-education connected with extinguishing and reconditioning of experiences, it is important to clarify the role of the therapist. Here the concept of transference attains primary significance; because of certain aspects in the psychiatrist's make-up, a mass of previously formed conditioned reflexes in regard to important past people come into play and the transference situation develops. This may be "immediate transference," a distortion due to certain obvious physical attributes, character traits, and inherent positional qualities of the physician, or "delayed transference"—a phenomenon due to more subtle emotional aspects of the therapeutic situation. An immediate transference could shorten the treatment and, perhaps, be the stronger and more lasting of the two types. The delayed transference would be a more labile process which would have a less dependable effect on the patient.

The transference situation makes the patient conditioned to the therapist as he had been toward the person in the past from whom the transference is made. *The past person has undoubtedly been important; but if the patient's current problem is not in the realm of this past person's influence then the extant therapeutic situation is probably not one which will benefit the patient.* In other words, if the total situation produced in therapy is not sufficiently similar in its aspect to the one which originally produced the neurosis, a deconditioning process probably will not take place. The realm of the past person's influence can often be somewhat extended by continuity and clarification on the part of the psychiatrist. However, if, playing the role of the past person, the therapist finds himself beyond the problem which had originally concerned the past person, little improvement can be accomplished.

An example of the above can be seen whenever the therapist represents an authoritative figure. In such case, with the aid of a strong transference, a substitution of a new set of standards can occur and the patient's basic attitudes can change considerably. The change might be in the form of a real situation (the doctor actually threatening the patient with some disaster), or it might depend on a previous, stronger-versus-weaker-figure situation. Similar mechanisms might operate in other areas.

The preceding paragraphs may offer some explanation for thus far unsatisfactorily explained events, events which hitherto were accepted uncritically. Further clarification may depend on more intensive concentration on principles rather than on single psychological situations.

THE STATES OF BEING AND AWARENESS IN NEUROSIS AND THEIR REDIRECTION IN THERAPY

Bernard Zuger, M.D.

In psychotherapy today the major emphasis is placed on content. In general, the objective would seem to be for the patient to attain awareness of attitudes, differently acquired according to the various schools, which no longer serve his best interests. Free association and the therapist-patient relationship are tools with which to achieve this objective and are subordinate to it.

Alongside this development there have been currents in psychotherapy with little emphasis on content or in which content has been employed differently. These are less easy to classify but in a rough way may be divided into two kinds. In one the aim is to direct the patient's awareness to body tenseness or muscle patterning. The procedures followed may not be imbedded in any elaborate theoretical framework, though the relief that follows is said to be psychological as well as physical. Among the technics employing this approach may be mentioned those advocated by Jacobson, F. Matthias Alexander and perhaps Reich. In the second kind, content, with none of its importance reduced, is nevertheless used for attaining something thought to be more crucial. Rank early replaced content with the therapist-patient relationship as the dynamic force in therapy. He also recognized neurosis primarily to be a problem of the development of consciousness. Moving also in the same general direction have been some of the teachings and practices of Eastern philosophy, according to such students of the subject as Watts, as well as, more recently, the application of gestalt theory to psychotherapy as attempted by Perls, Hefferline and Goodman.

This paper deals with some theoretical and practical formulations for psychotherapy which resemble those of the last mentioned authors. More specifically, it is the objective of this paper to explore the possibility that in neurosis:

1. There has been an impairment in the reciprocal relationship between what we shall call for the moment the larger unconscious whole of the personality and its smaller conscious part, and a tendency to shift to the latter aspect as a basis of operation. The purpose of therapy would then be to repair this impairment and reverse this shift.

2. Free association and the therapist-patient relationship are means of reversing this shift, but are themselves intrinsic parts of the process of therapy.

It is also thought that the present formulations add to the understanding of some concepts often used in psychotherapy, such as alienation, faith, spontaneity, growth and some others.

This paper is divided into four parts. Part 1 deals with the theoretical aspects; part 2 with their possible clinical significance; part 3 with the goals of psychotherapy in the light of these formulations; and part 4 with some technical points. Pathogenesis is not considered, though a beginning formulation has already been attempted elsewhere.

1. Theoretical Aspects

It is important first to recognize the difference between being, on the one hand, and consciousness or awareness (used interchangeably) on the other. (There are difficulties in the use of all of these words but it is thought that their meaning will become clearer through the context rather than by entangling definition.) Being, as such, excludes awareness; that which is in awareness is an extrusion of being, separated out of it, and, as it were, appearing on its surface or periphery. For the moment that something is in awareness it is alien to being. To put it differently, the being does the awareness and cannot be aware of itself at the same time. The following may illustrate the point: as long as the stomach is part of the individual's normal functioning or being, it is not in awareness. If it malfunctions and gives pain, it becomes the object of the rest of the individual's awareness. Furthermore, the being is the reservoir, the whole of the person, and that part of which it is aware is its product and that of the environment, and disappears within it as other awarenesses succeed it. Being is like the ocean and awareness its outgoing and incoming waves.*

The relationship between being and awareness needs to be considered further. Being is more or less constant while awareness is a continually changing phenomenon resulting from the impingement on being of the continually changing internal and external environments. Awareness is essentially, each time, a different phase of the organism in action—that is, how and what the eye sees, or the stomach feels or the "mind" thinks will be according to the nature of the whole person. At the same time the organism in turn is affected by the changing awareness, probably concurrently as awareness emerges and as it disappears into unconsciousness each time. This effect of awareness on being may perhaps be ever so little at certain times and be much greater at other times, depending on the nature of the interaction, but being cannot remain unaffected. In gestalt terms the process may be best described as the interaction between ground and figure, with ground itself changing to produce changing figure.**

---

* This is not different from William James's stream of consciousness concept except that the experiencer of the stream and its phasic content are especially dealt with here.

** Physiologically this is suggestively similar to Adrian's conclusion ". . . that the mass effect of cell aggregates play an important part in determining the patterns of activity which can be formed in the central nervous system." ". . . in the cerebral cortex there are no through routes, and here the incoming signals lose their identity as soon as they have left the receiving areas. They are dispersed among the crowd of active units which form the bulk of the brain, and the larger the bulk the more complex will be their effects in the various cell groups which have come to beat in unison." Adran, E. D., The Control of Nerve-Cell Activity, in Physiological Mechanisms in Animal Behavior, Cambridge University Press, p. 90, 1950.

In this interchange between ground and figure it is predicated that no other energies (or "will") need be mobilized. The dynamism is the product of the inherent excitability of protoplasm and the energies of the environment.

Several principal assumptions may now be made as to the functioning of the healthy individual in terms of being and awareness.

1. The healthy individual is more or less identified with being. In a sense then he is whole and consistent. His major functioning is therefore unconscious, about which more will be said later. He is organic. He need no more direct his intellectual functioning with one part of himself than he need direct such other functionings of his as breathing or heart-beating. The more he surrenders to himself, the more he surrenders to his functioning and the more he becomes his functioning. The more he becomes the functioning the more effortless it is.*

2. Awareness connects being with the "here and now." The here and now is meant not only to include time and place but also the organism's experience up to that point with what confronts it in the here and now, and what is relevant to the here and now, including consequences, values, goals, etc. The organism can be totally in the here and now only to the extent that it is unconscious of itself, viz., that it is in a state of being unrestricted by set awareness. The release of the organism from any part control within it (which is consciousness) makes it possible for it to be completely influenced by that which impinges on it in the present, and to produce a figure which is most relevant and appropriate for the organism in that environment.

3. As long as the individual remains identified with being, decision for action is a function of being and not of awareness, and up to the point of execution, unconscious. (Action itself

* Predicating the healthy individual as identifying with being obviates the difficult psychological (and philosophical) problem, How much of myself am I? Such a question is based on the premise of the identification of "I" with consciousness.

is included in awareness.) Decision is here regarded as a neuromuscular reaction and occurs only as the result of a total reorientation of being. Two examples may clarify this point. An individual is awakened by the alarm clock. He knows he has to get up but he is still sleepy and tired. Thoughts of the importance of getting up in time pass through his mind—catching the train, making his appointments, etc. He feels his tiredness. Other thoughts, apparently irrelevant to his getting up, also come up. Suddenly, that is, not preceded by any conscious decision to do so, he gets out of bed. The second example: A 37-year-old man has not been able to drive a car for some 18 years although he has had a driver's license for as many years. After six months of therapy during which time many of his problems were taken up as well as his inability to drive but without uncovering any specific reason for it, he buys a car and drives it. He knows no better now why he couldn't drive before nor why he can now.

Knowing the appropriate action doesn't necessarily lead to execution. People often ask themselves after the fact why they had not taken certain obviously indicated steps of which they were fully aware. On the other hand action taken from awareness may seem appropriate one day and totally inappropriate the next. It is a common experience among individuals with neurosis to decide carefully on a course of action and to regret it the moment after it is executed.

The difference between acting from awareness and from being may come out in certain physiological functioning, like defecation or parturition. Although aware of them as developing ends, these acts will be impeded if the individual deliberately tries to expedite them instead of allowing inner bodily changes to occur by themselves for their execution. Similarly, individuals intensely aware of everything they do may find it difficult to carry out the simplest acts, e.g., a college graduate who couldn't give the correct change out of a five-dollar bill; a Phi Beta Kappa graduate who got confused doing the simplest household chore.

4. In the individual who is identified with being there is free interplay between being and awareness. The release of the organism from any restrictive internal controls allows being's reaction to the environment, awareness, to be complete; in turn, the resolution of awareness back into being can be complete. Awareness may then modify being and play its part in decision and new awareness. There is thus change in continuity which is growth. This is to be differentiated from reflex response, which is best elicited when the rest of the organism is distracted, or from "thinking out," which is making available for participation only certain parts of the organism by some other "supervising" part and according to some predetermined pattern or "logic". In either case there results a part that has reacted and a part that has not reacted. There is thus division and accumulation of tension, which are absent when all of being has participated fully in determining the emerging awareness.

These two ways of functioning may also be seen in terms of Lewin's field forces. Awareness would be the resultant of the forces operating on the organism from within and without, as against an accumulation of potential which would of necessity build up in the organism its opposite or ambivalent force.

5. The concept of the healthy individual as one who remains with being while permitting free interplay between being and awareness may be expressed in another way. One may say that what the individual is really doing, at any one time, is polarizing his unconscious functioning in accordance with the here and now, and, over any stretch of time, making his conscious unconscious.

What is crucial then for healthy functioning is the individual's complete release of himself to himself, allowing himself to become whatever the internal and external forces determine. Whatever comes up from within or from without is purely phenomenological and exerts an influence on being by what it evokes, per se, without any intervention on the part of any subdivision of the organism. Because the individual is thus totally involved, no one part of him determines the outcome. The outcome is in fact unpredictable. It is in this way he learns what faith really is, the logic of the organism that is he and its deep preference for the healthy. Just as he doesn't have to have his breathing or walking predictable, so too the interplay of being with awareness will occur according to its own most valid logic.

2. Clinical Significance

A neurosis may be looked at as a disturbance in the being-awareness relationship. On the one hand, there is no longer more or less full identification of the personality with being; on the other hand, there is increasing identification with awareness. This state of affairs has many manifestations.

The individual cannot trust himself to a new outcome according to the newness of each moment of his living. He must therefore have fixed ways from which to operate, and generally constricts his field of operation. The fixed ways are the fixed attitudes of the individual and the nature of the predominant ones give the coloring to his "character structure" (e.g., the typologies of Freud, Fromm, Horney.) Within these attitudes the content itself may be quite rich, emotional and give an appearance of being spontaneous. But it is essentially predetermined, and lived like an actor's part, instead of being each time a new creation according to the forces at play within and upon the individual at any one time. Usually the content itself is also constricted.

There is a general adherence to the past or a failure to move on to the new. The patient justifies this by what happened in the past. In therapy it may often come up in the patient's reverting to one or two incidents as crucial. In some patients the words themselves may be repetitious from one session to the next. In these and other ways the individual is indicating his sense of being static and of necessity tied to the past.

Equally important is the fact that the individual doesn't

grow, no matter how varied or potentially rich his experiencing may have been. The individual has never really let his experiencing affect him; it was accumulated, as it were, and no matter how extensive or abundant, has remained essentially outside the personality and has not changed it. Clinically this is seen in the general immaturity which characterizes all neurotics side by side with physical aging and sophistication in this or that aspect. Subjectively the neurotic feels younger than his contemporaries. There is also indecision and inconsistency because his full experiencing has not and does not play its part in each act of his living. It is perhaps in this way that alienation is to be understood, that each act of his living is not a new outcome each time of all that he is, but either only a part of what he is, or to a large extent a result of fixed attitudes. The emotional range in any act of an individual's living would then depend on how much of himself is involved anew in it, each time he lives it.*

As a result of his experiencing being an accumulation and not a continual becoming and changing, the individual is subject to increasing strain. He must keep himself circumscribed and guard himself from fully letting go toward further experiencing. The neurotic individual has difficulty in initiating action, though once begun, he may do quite well in it. (This is to be differentiated from what occurs at the extreme end of the being-awareness equation, when the individual operates even more from awareness, in which case he may initiate easily but carry out very superficially.) He may resent other people's relative freedom of action for one reason or another, e.g., their being "pushy," "inconsiderate," "selfish," etc. He may attempt to control others.

He must hold on and have access to his experience very much like a school boy must hold on to information he crammed in the night before an examination in place of

---

* The more the individual gives up control and the more he is involved in what he does, the more the "I" of the person is the involvement and the less the alienation.

digesting and metabolizing it in the course of the year. He feels uneasy. He must keep himself together lest he fall apart, ". . . almost as if I'm holding my breath and afraid to let go," according to one patient.

He must consciously match appropriateness of reaction to new experience. This too makes him fearful of entering upon a new experience. This may be especially marked in the case of the neurotic adolescent, faced with new situations and people. He tends to avoid them because he is afraid he wouldn't know what to say or do, that he will make a fool of himself or that people will laugh at him. This may be present regardless of the amount of actual social experience such an adolescent may have had.

There is a general hyperawareness of oneself in relation to others. This the neurotic individual experiences as "self-consciousness" and he often expresses the wish to be rid of it. With other determinants (e.g., self-hate), it may be externalized to one's functioning (feeling inept, clumsy), or to one's appearance, overemphasizing slight bodily differences (e.g., of nose, ear, scarring due to acne) to momentous proportions. (Its projection to others and inanimate objects, and events may possibly be a factor in the production of ideas of reference.)

It is these and similar operations that may be responsible for much of the anxiety from which the neurotic individual is suffering. (The general fear of "letting go" may be imbedded in different context—fear of growing up, giving up one's dependency, shattering one's idealized image of oneself, etc.) Theoretically he may cope with this increasing anxiety by further organizing himself, which will give him some consistency and a kind of controlled "automaticity." (This would be in line with a general compulsive need for organization seen in many neurotic individuals. They cannot leave things open, undecided, but must have an answer and close every gestalt, no matter how forced.) But the very further attempt at organizing means a shift to further identification with awareness. The individual seems to act only from mind. Psychotic individual often give expression to feelings which it is tempting to use as descriptions of what may be going on in such instances. One individual said that he felt dead all over but alive only in his head and afraid that it would spill over. Another thought the thumping of a washing machine was his heart beating.

At the further end of the being-awareness equation may possibly be included cases of phobias and obsessions. It is almost as if the organism to protect itself must substitute some form of control against mind and immediate action, for to such an individual mind and thought are more and more reality and action. The phobia or the obsessive act would then be a symbol of limits and control.

This formulation also allows some understanding of certain schizophrenic symptoms though it is not meant to imply that it "explains" the process. Acting from awareness and no longer from their total organic being, they bring up their alienated organic being as hypochondriasis. (Similarly with the schizophrenic's understanding of dreams.) It may also explain part functioning (e.g., impulsiveness, verbigeration) of the deteriorated schizophrenic, since he no longer operates from being or total functioning. The further organizing of awareness into a kind of artificial "being" with which subsequently to metabolize experience including his own past experience would resemble the state of affairs seen in the paranoid states.

3. Goals

From the above formulation of neurosis it follows that the goal of therapy is to make it possible for the individual to identify with being. This has several corollaries.

It has the objective of helping the patient gradually give in to his functioning and release the parts under control to the whole of himself. He can thus more and more became his functioning.

As part functioning takes a subordinate place in a field of other forces, its compulsive nature is diluted. Fixed attitudes and obsessive formations are modified as decision and action is determined each time anew by the totality of forces at play.

Apart from the specific content of these forces they acquire two general characteristics. One is their being shifted to the present. As the individual give in to himself, being is polarized about the present by the awarenesses that succeed each other and this includes the individual's life experience. The individual learns to become available to himself in the present. That is the real meaning of the here and now. It is a biological phenomenon, in that the individual can release himself to the present and allow the forces acting inside of him and outside of him to form an entirely new outcome which, as already indicated, he cannot completely predict. The unpredictable element of the outcome is a crucial characteristic of the here and now.

The second general characteristic of the forces constituting his functioning is their operation before another person. Heretofore his relations to people were such as to keep him alert and watchful. He could not therefore let go of himself completely for any outcome that the immediate present and immediate configuration exclusively would determine. In the patient-therapist relationship he can. With a gradually growing feeling of being safe, he can let go with his fears, irrationalities, hostilities, etc., and again experience identification with being. This would not be possible without the presence of another person, nor if that person were any other than the therapist.

It is important to note at this point that what is crucial at first is not the analyzing of the fears or irrationalities but rather their full emergence so that they will become part of the configuration forming in the present. Interpretations which do not primarily forward the patient's releasing control over himself might not serve this purpose.

As in the case of faith and the here and now, creativeness and spontaneity are biological phenomena. By the individual's identification with being and its total interaction with awareness he is constantly becoming something new. Thus, however slightly each time, the individual is both creating and is the product of his creativeness. Similarly with spontaneity, the releasing himself to inner and outer forces, without a part of himself held in reserve to keep him tied to the old configuration, makes it possible for him to come up with the unpremeditated.

The presence of the therapist and his inclusion in the configuration is an important aspect contributing toward the patient's maturing. The neurotic individual has up to this point in his life mostly reacted to people (e.g., Horney's "toward," "away," and "against" formulations), but he has never really fully allowed himself just to be with people, nor allowed them to play their respective parts in his life. This is seen in how little, and for how short a time, other people really have a positive influence on the individual with neurosis in spite of apparent closeness to him. As the individual allows himself to be himself, he can allow others to be themselves, and to include them as they really are in his configuration.

The individual's staying with being, as awareness merges with it, gives a biological basis for psychological growth. Growth is then not merely accumulation in mind but a total change. Putting it differently, the *long-term* objective of therapy is not to make the unconscious conscious, but the reverse, the conscious unconscious.

4. Technical Points

Some technical aspects of free association and the patient-therapist relationship, useful toward achieving the goal of therapy outlined in this paper, may now be discussed.

The usual ways of encouraging free association need not be gone into in this discussion, nor the difficulties often encountered. The objective of free association is ordinarily considered to be the uncovering of material for one reason or another not then available to the patient. The objective according to the theory described in this paper also includes complete surrender to oneself, to one's functioning (staying with being) through whatever comes up in awareness, before whatever person the patient may make of the therapist. Free association therefore becomes a much more comprehensive process. It includes not only verbal free association but also bodily feelings and functions, verbalizable or not. When the therapy situation otherwise permits it, an attempt is made to indicate to the patient that at times it may be less important for him to verbalize a feeling than for him to fully feel the feeling. In this connection it may be helpful to use a term like "amorphous" to indicate to the patient that the therapist recognizes that there may be bodily feelings that may not "say themeslves" and counsel him to stay with them. An attempt is also made to get across to the patient to let the words come up from the feelings, and not to work hard at fishing for words, that is to allow an inner need to arise for speaking to the person before him, like waiting for hunger to arise as against the taking of food because it is lunchtime (though that could be one awareness in being for eating). Thus a fetish is not made of verbalization as such. It is important for the patient to know how much inner manipulation is going on in respect to verbalization, which he will often confirm when attention is called to it. Other manipulations may be quite apparent, such as kneading his brow to "think things out," or straining his eyes, or tensing muscles of arms, hands and jaw and those used in posture.

Often such phrases as, "What shapes itself out in you," "What forms or creates itself in you," may help; or "Feel it more," "Focus on it," "Let it spread out more," "Let it take you over," may get the idea across. Patients may get panicky and say they don't understand what is expected of them or that they can't do it. One patient said, "I've never really dared to let myself go like that."

Interpretations are generally geared to the same end, namely to indicate to the patient that what he is doing "makes sense," and encouraging him to give in more and more to his functioning. (The "rational" nature of his productions may best be communicated to him via content or psychodynamics.) Hostility, accusations, embarrassing feelings, sexual reactions to the therapist, in whatever other ways they may be dealt with, are also considered from the point of view of fears of the patient's giving up control over himself. Their coming into the flow of the patient's awareness and his staying with being is the primary objective.

As he gives himself over to the functioning that is he, including all that he thinks, sees, hears, feels, remembers, prefers, hopes, (without intervention or "partisanship" in the outcome) several phenomena may take place. The order in which they will occur is not yet clear, nor which in one patient and which in another. There may be a tightening up of the facial musculature which is not unpleasant and which may spread to involve the whole body. The tightening-up may be followed by a feeling of drowsiness. More often the latter is preceded by a deep sigh or yawn and stretching. Sometimes this sigh or yawn is preceded by almost palpable anxiety which the sigh or yawn does not necessarily relieve.

More localized bodily states are common. Some patients may become aware of headaches which they were not aware of before the session; others may lose the headaches they came in with. Similarly with tenseness across the eyes, "bands" across the chest, tenseness over the abdomen. Some may sneeze and drain from the nose. One patient felt relieved from what had been a continuous "sinus" condition and could breathe easily through both nostrils during the hour, though the condition returned subsequently.

Other patients may begin to feel drowsy and actually go off into sleep, feeling greatly relaxed upon waking. A drowsy-sleepy phase will sooner or later appear in most patients.

These phenomena occur without conscious psychological insights accompanying them. It is of course known that they may occur in response to psychological insights.

The bringing to awareness of conflict and the patient's seeing and feeling the incompatible elements remains important.

But its management is also aimed at furthering the patient's realization that no solution is possible by thinking and figuring out, adding up advantages and disadvantages. Only by letting conflict take him over, so that the resultant decision may come from his larger self, is there in a sense a "solution."

An obstacle invariably encountered to the patient's identifying with being is a fear of what would happen if he should let himself go outside the therapy situation. It is here that an explanation of the general principle of field forces determining action in a particular situation is helpful. Giving concrete examples, the patient may be told that the more he gives himself over to the here and now of a situation, each particular situation will bring up its own forces in awareness for appropriate decision in being. Action would therefore not be from impulse or be simply reflex, but would have its own determining forces in the particular present which would take their place with the larger, continually enduring purposes of the individual's being.

Summary

Neurosis is discussed from the aspect of the identification of the individual with awareness and mind instead of "being" and unconscious functioning. Much of the symptomatology seen in neurosis can be based on such a premise. The objective of therapy is seen then not only as one of dealing with the content of the patient's productions but also as one of helping him to shift his functioning back to being.

THE PLACE OF SEDATIVES IN THE TREATMENT OF PSYCHONEUROTICS

Robert Arnot, M.D.

As psychiatrists we find our desks littered with advertisements and samples of new sedatives with which to treat the psychoneurotics. The purpose of this paper is to determine what is good, current practice as to the use of sedatives. When are they indicated? Which drugs are believed by their users to be of most benefit?

In an attempt to answer these question 3 methods were used: A review was made of the recent books on psychiatric treatment; correspondence was carried on with psychiatrists known to be interested in the problem; and a summary was made on the principles and methods of the writer's own practice.

Before the observations are reported, we shall consider the nature of the psychoneuroses and the type and function of the sedatives. From clinical observation a psychoneurosis may be considered as a psychophysiologic disturbance. The condition is one both psychologically and physiologically of tension and unrest. Traditionally anxiety is considered the basic factor, but actually tension and depression may be of equal or even more fundamental importance. Either may precede or follow the anxiety. In most cases the 3 factors coexist in varying proportions.

To these physiological disturbances are related the psychological expression of thoughts of inferiority, of guilt, apprehension about responsibility, indecision, and excessive concern with what others think. Psychological problems can lead to physiological disturbances and vice versa. Psychophysiologic tension state is really more descriptive of what we see and what the patient experiences than is the term psychoneurotic.

We shall not review in detail the nature of the psychological and physiological disturbances which are well discussed by Hoch. Gellhorn has worked for many years on the nature of the physiological disturbance and believes that there is an "increased excitability of the central nervous system in the psychoneuroses."

In current practice the barbiturates are the drugs most commonly used as sedatives to reduce this hyperexcitability. According to Goodman and Gilman, all the barbiturates have a similar depressing action on the entire cerebrospinal axis, with the cortex and reticular activating system being the most easily affected. These drugs act to elevate the threshold of neurons by stabilizing the cell membrane and prolonging the time for recovery from excitation.

In summary, the sedatives, and particularly the barbiturates, act on the psychoneurotics to reduce the increased excitability of the central nervous system, which, speaking clinically, means that the tension and anxiety are reduced.

Psychoneurotics with Acute Anxiety

In everyday practice with psychoneurotics there are times when sedatives are indicated and times when they are not. The largest portion of the cases that come to a psychiatrist doing a "general practice" can be diagnosed as psychoneurosis, mixed type, with tension, anxiety, and depression. Obsessive-compulsive elements are also present in most cases. Hysterical elements are more rare. If the psychoneurotic has passed into a phase where the diagnosis of acute anxiety state is made, sedatives are, in my opinion, definitely and promptly indicated.

We are all familiar with the patient who is riding on the commuter train or who is shopping in the department store and suddenly becomes "panicked." Her heart is pounding. She is terrified that she is about to faint or die. If a careful history is taken, we find that the illness did not "come out of the blue" as the patient may at first state. Prior to the onset of the attack, she has become increasingly tense and fatigued. Definite evidence of depression such as loss of weight, failing appetite, and difficulty in sleeping will often be reported before the attack. The history discloses that she was always plagued by "feelings of inferiority" and that she has been a very "conscientious," "perfectionistic" person. She has tried too hard to get along with all people, even those whom she does not like. Resentments have piled up. Below is a typical case.

A 38-year-old, single assistant professor of zoology was hurrying to teach a class, for which she was afraid she would be late, when suddenly she became "terribly afraid and felt I had to run." She parked her car as quickly as she could and hastened to the home of a friend where she described the "tension that I was getting." This extremely hard-working perfectionistic teacher had gone to her department head 6 months before to ask for the trained assistants whom she knew she needed for her popular course. When she was refused "because of the budget," she said nothing. "I got constriction in my throat" and walked out. "That has been the ruination of me. I'll have peace at any cost." For many years she had worked to 2:00 or 3:00 A.M and gotten up again by 6:30. But she began to feel more tired than she ever had in her life. At night she would "cry a great deal. . . . And I'm not the kind that cries." Two days before the attack her physician told her that she had a "first-class physical exhaustion." On the morning of the attack she had had to leave the room when she heard some club women arguing about a children's project that was most important to her. "It was the loud-voiced meeting which set into motion the whole chain of events."

No evidence could be found that "repressed" sexual forces were about to "break through." The patient in her tenseness was afraid that something "crazy" would happen. She might shout in public. She might suddenly use a knife or a darning needle to hurt someone. The problem was chiefly one of handling anger.

She was placed on Serpasil 0.25 mg. t.i.d. by her medical doctor. "I'm sure that it has quieted me. I feel very sure of that," she said on her first visit to my office. But she did not really lose the tension until she was placed on barbital 0.6 gm. at 8:00 P.M. and Dexamyl 5 mg. at breakfast, lunch, and 4:00 P.M., essentially as advocated by Myerson. Although Dexamyl increases anxiety in some patients, more often it decreases it by alleviating the depression. Further, the evening barbital hangs over into the next day to counteract some of the Dexamyl excitation.

Psychotherapy consisted of ventilation, explanation, and reassurance. The patient was filled with resentments, but these were not "unconscious." She had in the beginning failed to associate her new symptoms with these other feelings which were definitely known, although not fully acceptable to her. A knowledge of the nature of her illness was most helpful in quieting the fear.

The barbital was discontinued after 4 weeks, as was the Dexamyl, except for an occasional dose when the patient noted some depression. Chloral hydrate 0.5 gm. was used for those few nights when she had difficulty falling or staying asleep.

Sargant and Slater's preference of a drug for this latter situation and actually for the whole acute anxiety state is sodium amytal:

This is the drug *par excellence* for the minor emergency. It is useful both as a sedative (gr. 1 to 2) and as a hypnotic (gr. 3 to 6). In the latter capacity it is the drug of choice for the patient who has difficulty in getting to sleep; and it may also be taken in the middle of the night by the patient who wakes up after sleeping well for a few hours and cannot sleep again.

Sargant and Slater also use amytal for those patients who, having once suffered an acute anxiety attack or actual frightening experience, are afraid of specific situations such as travelling by train.

The neurotic who is compelled to avoid particular situations because of his fear of fear can guard himself by taking gr. 1 to 2 of amytal about an hour before the situation has to be faced. The very fact that he knows that he has the relief available may save him hours of misery and persuade him to tackle his particular phobia afresh. This effect was particularly noticeable in treating neurotic patients during the period of heavy air raids on London.

They believe that by using sodium amytal to suppress the autonomic responses these patients can be "deconditioned" to unpleasant situations. They also use the sodium amytal to help an overworked patient, such as the zoology teacher, to return to work when she may get panicky just thinking about the responsibility. Gradually they reduce the dosage until finally the patient is just carrying a few capsules for emergencies.

There is not, however, uniformity of opinion among psychiatrists about the use of sedatives in the manner described by Sargant and Slater. Von Salzen writes:

I use very little in the way of sedation in my office practice. Dexamyl spansules, Eskabarb spansules and Seconal make up the major part of my prescriptions. I have been using Thorazine and Serpasil, but I have found them slender reeds. I place greatest reliance upon a full hour of psychotherapy which seems to reduce the need for sedatives.

When asked, "Do you let patients have Seconal to meet anxiety situations?" he replied; "No—merely to *encourage sleep*. I tell them there are no miracle drugs—that the control of anxiety lies within their own capacity to find and face their conflicts."

Although Fleming uses sedatives, he does not like barbiturates. He writes:

For the past couple of years I have used Benadryl (diphenyl hydramine) (dosage 25 mg. p.r.n. or 25 mg. t.i.d., a.c. and 50 mg. h.s.) far more than any other drug for daytime and nighttime sedation. I rarely use a little chloral hydrate; *never* use barbiturates or paraldyhyde. I am finding Thorazine helpful and use more and more of it; am trying Serpasil but have not decided about it yet.

We conclude this section on the use of sedatives in acute anxiety states with a paragraph from a letter by Whitehorn.

In regard to one aspect of the use of sedatives, my clinical impression is very clear, that is, one should use enough to get a demonstrable effect, and avoid token doses. These are very likely to become the focus of a power-struggle or demands for "kindness," *i.e.*, favoritism, to the neglect and detriment of more important and constructive startegy.

The admonition to use a large enough dose to be effective is also made by Ross and by Sargant and Slater.

Psychoneurotics with Chronic Anxiety

In the cases diagnosed psychoneurosis, chronic anxiety, the problem is similar to that in acute anxiety, with some important differences. Again the clinical picture is one of tension-anxiety-depression, which in these days of initials might be called the TAD syndrome. Terms such as neurasthenia, cardiac neurosis, and hypochondriasis also apply to some of these patients. They are the same perfectionistic, overconscientious people who get the acute anxiety attacks. In fact, often they have had an acute anxiety attack that has been allowed to become chronic. In other cases the tension has slowly risen to the point where they have demanded help from their physican and then from the psychiatrist, as illustrated in the case below:

A 27-year-old mother of 3 children, who had had an acute anxiety attack in a restaurant at a time of extreme fatigue 3 years previously, says of herself, "I feel tense and nervous. . . . I'm very much afraid to be alone. I always had a fear of loneliness. I feel rather dizzy and weak." In the morning she is often so tense that she vomits before breakfast. Her appetite is poor when she is nauseated. She has recently lost 10 pounds as the condition has become worse.

She complains of headaches that have been present for most of the 3 years. "My headaches are not just a physical pain. It's a feeling of tension." She is referring particularly to the muscles in the suboccipital, posterior-cervical region.

She cannot go shopping alone beause she feels frightened of being with people. This feeling is even more pronounced in church. "It's not the church; it's the people. I feel smothered as though I couldn't get out if I had to—as though I were going to faint. I sit there and clench my fists and my jaw, and I tap my feet continuously. I read furiously, trying to find some outlet." Although she has forced herself to continue to go to church for the 3 years, there has been no improvement.

She says she has "periods of great depression, unhappiness. I cry a great deal for no apparent reason; just feel so miserable and helpless. I think I've had this emotional instability a long time. It's just these past 3 years that its manifested itself this way. Ever since I was a child, I've been reticent and afraid to express my opinion or talk freely to people until I know them quite well. Everyone thought I was just bashful. Facing an audience was always an ordeal."

The patient is an unusually attractive, olive-skinned woman who is married to a teacher, her high school beau. She considers the marriage very successful, although in the first 6 months she could not "enter freely into the marital act," because she was too tense. No significant frictions with her husband or with her in-laws could be discovered. But she does have real apprehension about her own father, who was a chronic alcoholic, and from whom the mother obtained a divorce when the patient was 9.

Ventilation, explanation, reassurance, and barbital 0.6 gm. at 8:00 P.M. promptly quieted her and left her sleepy into the middle of the next day. Her intense fear that she was about to either commit suicide or go insane was allayed. But more definitive treatment, which we shall discuss below, was required before she recovered.

Prior to being seen by the psychiatrist, she had been treated by the general practitioner with phenobarbital ½ gr. t.i.d. At first the medication seemed to help "slightly." "It kept me a little calm; a little drowsy; more relaxed." But then the effect "diminished. It didn't help at all. I began to feel steadily worse."

This is an appropriate point at which to discuss the use of phenobarbital in these chronic anxiety cases, especially those in whom the depressive element is less marked, in whom such phobias as of church, restaurants, elevators, crowds, and trains are the chief features.

Sargant and Slater write of phenobarbital:

It is of value in the treatment of anxiety (and, of course, of epilepsy), but is of little use as a hypnotic. Nevertheless many anxious patients sleep much better when taking regular dosage throughout the day, as they go to bed in a less plagued and worried state. It should be prescribed as a basic sedative, and not *pro re nata*.

Kraines has a different opinion about how to use phenobarbital (also barbital 2½ grains and sodium bromide):

Sedative medication should *not be given routinely* or at regular hours for there are many times when the patient has no need for sedation. Instead, I tell the patient he can take the sedatives when he feels the need, taking them every half hour but never using more than 4 to 6 tablets a day. "Avoid taking medicine," the patient is told, "unless it is absolutely necessary.

This is an appropriate point to bring up the problem of barbiturate poisoning in the psychoneurotics.

Rinkel writes:

The overwhelming majority of patients with anxiety neuroses come to my attention after they have been treated, over a long period by their personal physicians, frequently including one, or two, or more psychiatrists. They have received large amounts of barbiturates, and some of the patients I have seen at my office were in a state of chronic barbiturate poisoning. . . . From this experience alone, it may be obvious that barbiturates do not constitute an adequate treatment for anxiety neuroses because they enhance the anxiety, cause serious disruption of sleep, and decrease the patient's mental acuity.

I do not wish to make the statement that barbiturates should be completely excluded from the treatment of neuroses. In exceptional cases, and particularly if the patient has not been under barbiturate treatment previously, Seconal or Nembutal may bring about most needed sleep, but I have found that to maintain barbiturate treatment for any length of time is most detrimental to the patient.

As Rinkel indicates, the therapy with the chronic anxiety states is more likely to require the withdrawal of barbiturates than the giving of them. The chronic psychoneurotic may demand the sedative; whereas, the acute anxiety patient may be afraid of medication and sometimes will not even get a prescription filled. A simple rule, which is as contrary as the neurotic himself, is: Give the sedative to the patient who does not demand it, and withhold it from the one who does.

Practically, withdrawing the barbiturate may not be difficult because by the time these patients get to the psychiatrist they have found out for themselves that the medicines filling their cabinet have not worked, and they are refreshed to hear the doctor say that sedatives are not the answer.

The patient is told, "What you are really dealing with is an emotional problem—a state of tension. The excessive anxiety that bothers you now is an accompaniment of this tension and of the depression that is also present. You will find that by focusing on the tension instead of on the fear and by gaining understanding you will improve.

"The *first* step is to recognize what is wrong with you. Your trouble is not just imaginary, not just in your mind; it is real. The *second* step is to learn to identify the various psychological factors that set off your emotions and produce your symptoms. You will need to observe your human relations more closely and become aware of what it is that produces the tension and anxiety in you. In the beginning you may say that you are thinking of nothing, but you will find that just the thought of a report that is due tomorrow will cause you to tighten up, as will also the recollection of the resentment you felt today when you were criticized and dared not answer back.

"Having learned what is wrong and what triggers it, you are then in a position to learn the *third* point; namely, how to handle your tensions and anxiety. You will not faint, die, or 'go off the beam.' You will be able to say to yourself that it is just tension, and you will thus interrupt the cycle of tension leading to fear leading to more tension, or fear leading to tension leading to more fear. You will also learn ways to relax your muscles as from Jacobson's *You Must Relax*. *Fourth*, and most important, you will learn to depend on yourself to manage your own life and symptoms. You will stop reaching out for your husband, your doctor, or your sedative. You will act in situations out of strength, because you want to, and not out of fear, because you ought to."

Obviously this is not delivered as a single compact lecture. Rather the points are made, sometimes over several interviews, when the appropriate material makes the point pertinent and likely to be understood.

These psychoneurotic patients in the review of their personal history can learn what faulty attitudes have produced their defective human relations; how they failed to settle issues promptly; and how thereby they let intolerable situations build up. The anxiety-laden, guilt-producing events can be reviewed so that the patient is less sensitive to them. The full effect of the anxiety-producing people in their lives can be brought out.

Undoubtedly these may sound like rather simple ways to approach the psychotherapy of the chronic neurotic, and the acute as well. But they are effective.

Returning to the case of the 27-year-old mother with the chronic anxiety state, actually she was too depressed, too tense, to respond to sedatives and psychotherapy. Electroshock treatment was necessary. A series of 10 treatments was given using sodium pentothal, Anectine, and the Medcraft machine set at 170 volts and 1.0 second. Marked anxiety about having the treatments was not produced. Tension and depression were relieved. She was then better able to handle the reduced anxiety and to begin again to enjoy life. Psychotherapy during the recovery period and later was important.

Many present-day psychiatrists are themselves anxiety-ridden about giving electroshock to patients with anxiety. They believe the treatments aggravate the condition. But as a matter of fact electroshock is the unfailing physical sedative. The patient must go to sleep. The tension goes. The poor results are probably obtained by stopping the treatments between the fourth and the eighth, or by using a machine that does not produce a full discharge, a complete convulsion.

With the Anectine, the doctor's own anxiety about using a machine such as the Medcraft is reduced.

There are, to be sure, some chronic anxiety cases that are made worse by electroshock. Alexander says these may be identified by the anxiety produced when 0.025 mg. of epinephrine is injected intravenously in the Funkenstein test.

The cases that may require electroshock are those in whom depressive element is clear. However, many of these will respond without shock to the routine of psychotherapy plus barbital 0.3 gm. at 8:00 P.M. and Dexamyl 5 mg. at breakfast, lunch, and 4:00 P.M.

Psychoneurotics Who Become Psychotic

Finally, there is another type of psychoneurotic with whom sedatives are urgently needed. Neuroses do lead to psychoses. Although we can assure most of our tension patients that they are not going insane, the old German statement "No psychosis without neurosis" is also true. In much the same manner that the psychoneurotic drives himself into an acute anxiety attack, he can also drive himself into a mental illness. Because of his perfectionism both in his work and in his human relations, he will drive himself too far. He will work day and night, and come into a period of the most extreme fatigue of his lifetime. He will not be able to sleep. Tension and anxiety will mount. Depression may develop. Ideas of reference may appear. If they do, delusions as of persecution and auditory hallucinations may follow. These patients can be helped if the seriousness of the development is recognized by the family physician, when the patients first come with somatic complaints, as they often do. Too often they are treated with reassurance and a mild sedative such as Seconal, Nembutal, or chloral hydrate. This is not enough. Prompt, heavy sedation, as with barbital 0.3 gm. or 0.6 gm. is needed, together with psychotherapy on the current problems in human relations. If this treatment were given in the early stages, many psychoses could be prevented.

Sargant and Slater write about barbital:

The best type of patient for Medinal (soluble barbitone) medication is the man who goes to sleep fairly easily, but tends to wake up in the early hours of the morning, unable to get to sleep again; or the man who sleeps throughout the night, but restlessly and disturbed by dreams and is unrefreshed in the morning. These types of insomnia are particularly frequent in depressives and the lasting effect of medinal suits them very well.

In obsessive-compulsive neuroses and in hysterias, heavy sedation early in acute phases will help. But when these conditions are in a chronic phase, barbiturate sedatives will be of little value and may be quite habit forming.

Summary

Psychoneuroses may be considered as psychophysiologic tension states. Treatment consists of a combination of physical and psychological methods. General principles for use of sedatives are given. Methods for effective, short-term psychotherapy of psychoneurotics are presented.

EVALUATION OF PSYCHOTHERAPY

With a Follow-up Study of 62 Cases of Anxiety Neurosis

Henry H. W. Miles, M. D.,
Edna L. Barrabee, M.S., and
Jacob E. Finesinger, M.D.

Patients ill with psychoneuroses have been treated by a wide variety of procedures, ranging from those designed primarily to effect physiologic changes to those which have been considered purely psychologic. A great need exists for methods of comparison and appraisal of therapeutic results obtained in various types of cases by various types of treatment. Burchard, Michaels, and Kotkov have recently discussed group therapy from this viewpoint in a comprehensive critique. In the present paper we will concern ourselves with individual therapy of the psychoneuroses, only mentioning briefly other forms of treatment.

When one attempts to evaluate the efficacy of psychotherapy it becomes apparent at once that the task is enormously complex. The prognosis in a particular case depends not only upon the treatment but also upon the interrelationship of many variables, imponderables, and unknown factors; complete elucidation may be impossible in the present state of our knowledge. Sciences may be said to develop through three evolutionary stages: first, the theological or mystical; second, the empiric or

---

The authors wish to thank Dr. Stanley Cobb for his suggestions and helpful criticisms during the course of this study. Thanks are due also to Dr. Samuel Waldfogel for valuable assistance in evolving the rating scales and applying statistical procedures and to Dr. Henry Musnick, Mrs. Robert Bigelow and Miss Claire Swift for technical help.

taxonomic; and third, the positive or dynamic. Psychiatry has only recently advanced to the second stage and is still upon the threshold of the third. Precise measurements, accurate predictions, and formulated laws are not yet possible. Nevertheless the problem of testing therapy is of vital importance and one cannot beg the question because there is no full answer. It is desirable to examine critically the methods and technics which are available.

We have reviewed the literature dealing with the results of psychiatric treatment of the psychoneuroses to find out how others have approached the problem in the past. No attempt was made to collect all references concerned with clinical impressions or discussions of the nature of the problem. Follow-up reports of patients at completion of treatment, or after varying intervals, are surprisingly scarce, and are not readily comparable to one another. One is struck by the paucity of carefully planned, objective studies and by the general lack of definition of terms. These points will be discussed in more detail later.

To evaluate the treatment of an illness one should know its etiology, natural history, and untreated or "spontaneous" recovery rate. In regard to the neuroses such information is fragmentary. In certain medical diseases, lobar pneumonia for example, these things are now known fairly accurately so that evaluation of a therapeutic agent can be carried out by comparing patients who have received specific therapy with untreated controls. This method has not been employed in psychiatric research, although it was suggested in 1935 by Cheney and Landis, who outlined a plan for testing the results of psychoanalysis. There are many reasons why such a study would prove technically formidable. The matching of two groups (controls and patients) would be almost impossible. Diagnostic categories are still largely descriptive, and as Masserman and Carmichael have pointed out, "psychiatric syndromes are so protean in their manifestations as to be differently classified by competent observers with only slightly different orientations." Landis observed that there may be disagreement as to the cause of the illness, the dynamic mechanisms operating, and the factors influencing the course of the illness. He then approached the problem from the standpoint of the so-called spontaneous recovery rate. (The word "spontaneous" is used in an inexact sense to mean recovery or remission without planned psychotherapy.) He was impressed by the constancy in the number of psychoneurotic patients in state hospitals who were reported "recovered" or "improved." This figure remained within fairly close limits from year to year and from state to state. Since psychoneurotics are not usually committed to state hospitals unless their illness is severe, and since psychotherapy in such institutions is usually very limited, he concluded that the reported recovery rate could serve as the best available index of a so-called *basic amelioration rate*.

In Table 1 are the statistics quoted by Landis.

TABLE 1
The "Basic Amelioration Rate"

	New York 1925-1934	U.S. 1926-1933	Annual Variability 1926-1933
Number of patients recovered or improved per 100 cases admitted to the hospital	70	68	62-72
Percentage of patients discharged as recovered or improved within 1 year of admission	New York 1914 68	U.S. 1933 66	

The two sets of figures, while not exactly equivalent, are comparable, since 85 per cent of all patients discharged as recovered or improved were hospitalized less than a year. Admittedly the selection of this basic amelioration rate as an index of spontaneous recovery cannot take into account such important variables as type and severity of the neurosis, socio-cultural levels of various groups of patients, or the criteria used in different hospitals for defining improvement. Nor does it take into account what happens to the patient after he leaves the hospital.

Thus we do not believe that Landis' figure can be used as a *general* standard for measuring the effectiveness of psychotherapy in a *particular* group of cases, and would disagree with his statement that "any therapeutic method must show an appreciably greater size than this to be seriously considered."

To test further Landis' conclusions we have tabulated for comparison a series of reports dealing with follow-up studies of psychiatric patients (Table 2). It is obvious that only a crude comparison of these reports is possible. The various authors have rarely described the groups of patients accurately, diagnostic categories are mixed, goals and methods of treatment have not been discussed in detail, and there has been no uniformity of meaning in such terms as "recovered," "much improved" and "slightly improved." A number of writers, however, stressed the difficulties in setting up criteria for evaluation of the patients' status. From some studies one gets the impression that the therapeutic zeal of the writer has caused him to relax his critical judgment.

In an attempt to bring about more uniformity we have modified some of the figures and percentages in Table 2. For example, where a follow-up has been done on a mixed group of psychiatric cases we have included only those cases in which a diagnosis of *psychoneurosis* was made. (In some reports the information has not been detailed enough to permit this, and these have been omitted.) Under the heading *total number of cases* (Column 1) we have included only the cases actually followed-up, omitting those who were not traced or had died. This produces differences from the figures in the original publications. Because of discrepancies in the criteria for evaluation, we rated degree of improvement only in two broad categories: those cases reported "recovered" or "much better" in Column 2, and those cases reported simply as being "better" in Column 3. The authors' criteria were often so vague that the term "better" sometimes means "a lot better" and sometimes "a little better." The figures in Column 4 indicate the total percentage of cases showing improvement; they are the sums of figures in Columns 2 and 3.

Follow-up Studies of Psychiatric Patients
(Part One)

Author and source of material	1. Number of cases	2. Percentage "recovered" or "much improved"	3. Percentage "improved"	4. Total Percentage showing improvement	5. Type of treatment	6. Follow-up interval	7. Remarks
Orbison: Private patients	30	83	10	93	Physical conditioning	Not stated	Criteria for evaluation of results not stated
Coon and Raymond: Stockbridge, 1910-1934	422	69	21.5	90.5	Re-education, inspirational talks, explanation, etc.	1-20 years	Follow-up by questionnaire—only 40% replied; evaluation done by patient
Denker: Equitable Life Assurance Co., 1921-1936	707	—	—	90	Treatment mostly by family doctors. Tonics, sedatives, reassurance, suggestion, etc.	Up to 15 years	Criteria are vague, and "improvement" is not defined
Landis: N.Y. Psychiatric Inst, 1930-1935	119	40	47	87	Psychotherapy in hospital	At completion of treatment	No details regarding criteria for evaluation
Huddleson: Veteran's Bureau, 1922-1923	200	46.5	40	86.5	Brief out-patient psychotherapy; sedation, reassurance, etc.	1 year or more	No details regarding criteria for evaluation
Hamilton, Varney, and Wall: N.Y. Hospital, Westchester Division, 1927-1937	100	66	17	83	State hospital routine	5-15 years	Criteria for "improvement" are not strict or very specific
Yaskin: Private patients	100	41	41	82	Brief psychotherapy; encouragement, suggestion, etc.	Not stated	No details regarding criteria (author reports a 24% "recurrence rate")
Wenger: General OPD, Vienna	50	50	32	82	Brief out-patient psychotherapy	6-30 months	No details regarding criteria for evaluation
Matz: Veteran's Bureau, 1922-1928	775	1	80	81	Hospitalization in Veteran's Facility Hospitals	At completion of treatment	No details as to criteria for evaluation or type of treatment

TABLE 2

Follow-up Studies of Psychiatric Patients—Continued

Author and source of material	1. Number of cases	2. Percentage "recovered" or "much improved"	3. Percentage "improved"	4. Total Percentage showing improvement	5. Type of treatment	6. Follow-up Interval	7. Remarks
Shapiro and Freeman: Geo. Washington University Hospital	30	50	31	81	Metrazol shock	2-11 months	Criteria for evaluation were fairly specifically stated
Bond and Braceland: Pennsylvania Hospital, 1927-1928	35	60	20	80	Mental hospital routine	5 years	Criteria vague; indirect information used mostly, as few patients were actually seen for follow-up
Ross: Cassell Hospital, 1921-1933	1055	51	28	79	Nonpsychoanalytic therapy; persuasion, hypnosis, etc.	1 year	Follow-up by questionnaire; 89% replied
Wilder: Private patients	54	50	28	78	Various types of psychotherapy	1½-6 years	No details regarding criteria for evaluation
Mapother: Maudsley Hospital, 1932-1935 (in-patients)	641	19	58	77	Nonpsychoanalytic therapy in hospital	At completion of treatment	Many cases were selected for their value for teaching purposes
Schilder: Bellevue Hospital OPD	31	29	48	77	Psychoanalytically oriented group therapy	At completion of treatment	No details regarding criteria for evaluation
Curran: St. George's Hospital, 1933-1934	49	37	37	74	Brief out-patient psychotherapy	1-3 years	Follow-up by questionnaire, only 40% replied
Landis: N.Y. State Hospitals, 1917-1934	5700	32	40	72	State Hospital routine	At completion of treatment	No details as to diagnostic breakdown, type of treatment or criteria for evaluation
Bennett and Semrad: U. of Nebraska Hospital	100	—	—	70	Not stated	Not stated	No details as to type of treatment or criteria for evaluation
Harris, H. I.: Boston Dispensary, 1938	272	—	—	68	Group psychotherapy	At completion of treatment	No details regarding criteria for evaluation

Follow-up Studies of Psychiatric Patients—*Concluded*

1. Author and source of material	2. Number of cases	3. Percentage "recovered" or "much improved"	4. Percentage "improved"	5. Total Percentage showing improvement	6. Type of treatment	7. Follow-up interval	Remarks
Hamilton and Wall: N.Y. Hospital Westchester Division, 1927-1937	100	51	17	68	State Hospital routine	4 years or more	No details regarding criteria for evaluation
Neustatter: Maudsley Hospital, 1933	50	—	—	64	Brief out-patient psychotherapy	At completion of treatment	Evaluation based mainly upon symptoms
Masserman and Carmichael: U. of Chicago, Hospital Division	29	—	—	62	Hospital routine plus various types of brief psychotherapy	1 year	An objective study with definite criteria
Hardcastle: Guy's Hospital, 1931	21	14	48	62	Not stated	Up to 2 years	Evaluation based upon a detailed follow-up interview
Harris, A.: Maudsley Hospital, 1924-1926	107	35.5	26	61.5	Brief out-patient psychotherapy	10-12 years	Only 50% of cases could be traced; criteria for evaluation are not specific
Luff and Garrod: Tavistock Clinic, 1928-1931	406	32	29	61	Brief out-patient psychotherapy	3 years	70% of cases were traced. On the whole, a good, careful study
Mapother: Maudsley Hospital, 1932-1935 (out-patients)	1529	10	48	58	Brief out-patient psychotherapy	At completion of treatment	Criteria for evaluation not specifically stated
Carmichael and Masserman: U. of Chicago Clinic, 1935-1937	66	35	20	55	Psychoanalytically oriented out-patient therapy	1-2½ years	Each case interviewed at follow-up; criteria strict; an objective, careful study
Slater: Sutton Emergency Hospital, 1939-1941	239	—	—	53	60% of the cases received no psychotherapy; the rest received little	Not stated	Evaluation based mainly upon symptoms
Jacobson and Wright: Elgin State Hospital	22	—	—	50	State hospital routine plus group psychotherapy	At completion of treatment	No details regarding criteria; the group consisted of severely ill patients
TOTALS	13,039	—	—	73			

The series is arranged in order of total percentage of cases showing improvement and when one studies it several interesting facts are noted. One is struck by the infrequency with which authors have defined their criteria for evaluating results. When the various studies are compared in terms of thoroughness, careful planning, strictness of criteria, and objectivity there is often an inverse correlation between these factors and the percentage of successful results reported. Masserman and Carmichael using strictly defined criteria and depending upon personal interviews with each patient at follow-up, found 62 per cent and 55 per cent improvement in their two studies. Luff and Garrod's appraisal of a much larger series was a careful, well-planned study and showed an improvement rate of 61 per cent. Going to the upper end of the table, one notes the 93 per cent improvement rate reported by Orbison in a small series of cases. In his paper, however, he gave no details concerning selection of cases or method of evaluating improvement. In the large series of Coon and Raymond the follow-up was accomplished by means of a brief questionnaire which provided no space for the patient to describe his condition as unimproved or worse. Three choices only were included in the questionnaire: "well," "much improved," and "improved." One might question such a technic on the grounds that an element of suggestion undoubtedly played a part. Furthermore, response to the questionnaire was only 60 per cent; the status of the missing 40 per cent of the group was not determined.

The marked variations in favorable results shown in Table 2 are not due only to the different sets of standards employed by different authors, but must surely be influenced also by such variables as those already mentioned: (type and severity of neurosis, social, educational and economic levels of groups of patients, etc.). It is interesting that the *mean figure for all cases showing improvement* in Table 2 (13,039 cases) is *73 per cent* which is a close approximation of Landis' basic amelioration rate. Such a general figure therefore becomes meaningless when used in the frame of reference of a specifically selected group of cases treated according to a particular plan.

Other reports concerning psychoneurotic patients have dealt with (1) those treated in medical wards or clinics most of whom had received little or no psychotherapy, and (2) those treated by psychoanalysis. These are shown in Table 3.

Patients treated medically showed somewhat less improvement than the groups which had received psychotherapy. Many of these patients had medical illnesses in addition to psychoneuroses and one might conclude that the poorer results were influenced by that. A medically oriented report not included in Table 3 is that of Wheeler, White, Reed, and Cohen who made a twenty-year follow-up study of 173 patients originally diagnosed as having effort syndrome, "irritable heart," or cardiac neurosis. They examined 60 patients personally and found that of this group 11.7 per cent were well, 35 per cent had symptoms but no disability, 38.3 per cent had symptoms with mild disability, and 15 per cent had symptoms with moderate or severe disability. There is evidence that neurocirculatory asthenia is closely related to anxiety neurosis but we do not agree with these authors that one can lump together categorically anxiety neurosis, effort syndrome, neurasthenia, "irritable heart," and cardiac neurosis, all under a single descriptive term. Another paper of interest is Grant's follow-up of 665 cases of effort syndrome seen in soldiers in World War I. Five years after hospitalization, excluding those dead or with organic diseases, there were 556 cases of whom 16.5 per cent were "well" and 19.2 per cent "improved." Treatment in military hospitals had been confined to graded exercises.

The group of patients reported by Coriat was treated by psychoanalysis, but in many cases the duration of treatment was very brief. The degree of improvement was judged mainly upon disappearance of symptoms and upon a lessening of the conflicts as reflected in dreams. By present-day standards, one might interpret many of these "recoveries" as transference phenomena.

TABLE 3
Studies of Psychiatric Patients
(Part Two)

Author and source of material	1. Number of cases	2. Percentage "recovered" or "much improved"	3. Percentage "improved"	4. Total Percentage showing improvement	5. Type of treatment	6. Follow-up interval	7. Remarks
Friess and Nelson: N.Y. Hospital, 1932-1934	237	12	30	42	Half of the patients had some psychotherapy; but in most instances very little	5 years	The patients in this group were treated in a Medical Clinic; many had medical illnesses as well as neuroses
Comroe: U. of Pennsylvania Hospital	100	—	—	40	Not stated; apparently little or none	Not stated	No statements as to criteria for evaluation; follow-up by questionnaire—only 40% of answers were satisfactory
Coriat: Private patients	66	73	13	86	Psychoanalysis (in most cases very brief)	Not stated	Criteria for evaluation based mainly upon disappearance of symptoms during treatment
Knight: Collected cases from various sources. Cases treated 6 mo. or longer	383	63	29	92	Psychoanalysis	Not stated	It is not definite that cases from different sources were evaluated by similar criteria
All cases — including those terminated in less than 6 mo.	534	45	21	66	Psychoanalysis	Not stated	

In Knight's summary of all other reported cases treated by psychoanalysis one can look at the results in two ways. If *all* cases are considered, including those whose analyses were broken off in less than six months, the percentage of improvement is 66. Excluding the group whose treatment was terminated within six months, the figure rises to 92 per cent. When a psychoanalysis is discontinued prematurely it may be because of the patient's neurotic conflicts (resistance) or because the analyst has decided after a trial period that further treatment will be fruitless; so it would seem that some at least of the terminated cases should properly be called "failures." This point introduces another variable not considered in most of the studies; namely the *selection* of cases to be included in the follow-up series. Mapother, in discussing the unreliability of follow-up statistics, stated that the number of patients who are recovered or improved after psychotherapy is limited largely by one's skill in prognosis. In other words one can select from the great number of patients available in a psychiatric clinic a group of cases which will be very amenable to treatment. Statistics that are based upon such a group will show an extremely high recovery rate.

Oberndorf asked a number of experienced psychoanalysts with which type of case each had achieved the most satisfactory results. The answers varied widely: some analysts believed they had most success in the treatment of anxiety neurosis, others, hysteria, and still others, compulsion neuroses. Thus the prognosis in an individual case may have a specific relationship to the particular interests and skills of the therapist, as well as a general relationship to his experience and training.

It would therefore seem reasonable that the basic prerequisite of an adequate follow-up study should include a sociocultural description of the group as a whole (or of each individual patient) and a statement as to selection of cases. A detailed pretreatment work-up of each case should be done including significant factors in the family and social background, the clinical diagnosis and a comprehensive dynamic formulation of the patient's personality structure and important conflicts. The patient's assets and liabilities should be considered: I.Q., physical limitations, the amount of gratification supplied by the illness, his desire to get well, etc. A tentative plan of treatment should be outlined, and after completion of treatment one should attempt to describe exactly what the therapist did and what were the significant elements in the patient's response to therapy. The emphasis, then, is more upon the prognostic determinants and the actual therapeutic process than upon the percentage of patients who are clinically better. This problem was discussed at the Institute for Psychoanalysis, Chicago, and a scheme for case study was outlined. More recently, the matter received detailed consideration in a symposium at the Boston Psychoanalytic Society and Institute. So far, however, these discussions have not borne fruit in the form of a published study nor has any report in the literature as yet demonstrated that the degree of improvement of patients treated by various psychotherapeutic technics can be correlated with the type of procedure used. It may be that the problem is too complex and too subtle to yield an answer, but we believe that by further definition of various aspects of the problem some progress may be made. The present study was undertaken to find out how adequate (or inadequate) are the data available in the case records of a psychiatric department in a general hospital. We also hoped to learn something about evaluating and quantifying certain factors, with an eye to possible revision of our psychiatric case records. Thus the groundwork might be laid for future investigations of the relationship between psychotherapy and the clinical course of a neurosis.

II. Material and Method

A. *Selection of Cases*

A problem which has not been solved satisfactorily is that of picking a homogeneous group of patients with psychoneuroses. The reasons for this are obvious, yet at the risk of seeming naive we should like to emphasize the point that a psychoneurosis is not a simple "disease" related in a clear fashion to some specific etiologic agent. It is more profitably regarded as an illness of maladaption. Disregarding the as yet unknown importance of inherited and constitutional factors, it is striking how the clinical picture correlates with various life situations and stresses. These correlations may be overt or they may be hidden and revealed only through an understanding of unconscious conflicts and fantasies. We do not, of course, imply that the ultimate cause of the neurosis lies in these correlates.

Since there is no *etiologic* classification of the psychoneuroses, the usual diagnostic categories are delineated upon a descriptive level. The syndrome of anxiety neurosis—or "anxiety state," in the classification approved by the American Psychiatric Association—presents a well-defined clinical picture and is fairly common and for these reasons was chosen as the basis of our study. The diagnosis is based essentially upon a constellation of symptoms which are those of fear, except that the patient seldom knows what he is afraid of. There may be chronic, sustained anxiety, though more characteristically, there are episodic attacks lasting from a few minutes to hours or even days. The principal symptoms are palpitation, respiratory distress, sweating, tremors, chest pain, and usually pronounced feelings of impending disaster and fears of death. Between attacks patients feel relieved but not completely well. In this study, we do not use the term "anxiety" to denote vague feelings of tension or subjective distress, nor do we attempt to recognize unconscious anxiety in the psychoanalytic sense.

Case selection was determined by three criteria: (1) descriptive diagnosis, (2) the fact of having been admitted to the Psychiatric Ward of the Massachusetts General Hospital since January 1, 1935, and (3) a minimum elapsed time of two years between discharge from the hospital and follow-up contact. All records bearing the diagnosis "anxiety neurosis" were checked, and those satisfying the second and third criteria were studied in detail. About 35 per cent of this group were discarded because of complicating factors. (Coexistent psychosomatic disease such as hypertension, asthma, or peptic ulcer; structural disorders of the central nervous system; concomitant surgical or medical disease which could have contributed to the symptoms; grossly abnormal electroencephalogram; or a prominent admixture of other psychoneurotic symptoms such as those of hysteria, obsessive-compulsive neurosis, or hypochondriasis were all disqualifying factors.)

Seventy-six cases of anxiety neurosis fulfilled all requirements, and upon them the present study was based. Detailed research records have been kept routinely on psychiatric in-patients which include the psychiatric history, medical history, mental status examination, Social Service reports, summaries of psychotherapeutic interviews, and a transcript of staff discussion. In some cases, psychometric tests and various projection tests have been done. The record includes complete physical and neurologic examination as well as laboratory studies which ordinarily consist of a hemoglobin determination, total and differential leukocyte count, urinalysis, Hinton test, BMR, and chest X-ray. Since 1942, routine EEG's have been done, and 34 patients (45 per cent) had this procedure. In no case in the series was there evidence of any medical or surgical disease which might have been related etiologically to the clinical symptoms. There were, of course, a few minor conditions such as acne vulgaris, dental caries, poor nutrition, chronic cervicitis, refractive errors, etc.

B. *Description of the Group*

Each record was studied carefully and pertinent information was abstracted. A brief description of the entire group furnishes a frame of reference.

Sex distribution: 43 males and 33 females.*

Age at time of hospitalization: Range was 12-50 years with a mean age of 26.8 years. About three-fourths of the group fell into the 20-35 year age span.

Marital status: 20 males were married and 23 were unmar-

---

* It was interesting and puzzling that the group consisted of more males than females. Usually in our ward one sees far more women than men with psychoneurotic illness and this is supported by Denker's observation that among many thousands of persons insured by a large company the incidence of psychoneurosis was three to four times greater among women than among men.

ried. Of the females, 23 were married and 10 were unmarried. Two of the men were separated from their wives, but there had been no divorces in the group and no patient had lost a spouse through death.

Racial and National backgrounds: All patients in the group were white. Seventy (92 per cent) had been born in North America, but 44 (58 per cent) had one or both foreign-born parents. The commonest national backgrounds were Italian, Irish, Russian, and Lithuanian. Also represented were English, Swedish, Portuguese, Polish, Syrian, and Armenian.

Religion: 53 per cent were Roman Catholic, 34 per cent Protestant, 6.5 per cent Jewish, and the remaining 6.5 per cent unknown or expressed no particular affiliation.

Educational level: Three patients had less than 5 years of schooling, and 3 were college graduates. The mean years of schooling for the entire group was 10.2.

Social and Economic levels: It was difficult to decide in many cases how to evaluate the patient's social status. Using various criteria we estimated that about three-fourths of the group belonged to the so-called lower class (working class) and one-fourth to the middle class. Most of the latter would be designated lower-middle class. Among the male patients the occupations were chiefly distributed among unskilled labor, factory or mill work, and semi-skilled labor. There were only a few "white collar" workers or men with skilled trades. There were no executives or men of professional status in the group. Half of the female patients were housewives, and of the rest most did clerical or factory work. One was a teacher.

Most of the patients had relatively small incomes, but very few had been dependent upon public funds or charitable organizations. Our data on incomes and average earnings were inadequate, however. The above points are mentioned because some evidence suggests that one's social class may be a determinant in one's "life chances"—i.e., likelihood of securing freedom, leisure, deference, etc. The social class may also be related to such things as incidence of disabling chronic illness and even to the frequency of certain types of mental disorders.

C. *Follow-up Method*

Our plan was to interview personally as many as possible of the 76 patients, since studies employing indirect information have been less satisfactory.

In developing criteria for the evaluation of cases at follow-up we attempted to be as precise and objective as possible, at the same time remaining aware of the subtleties of appraising symptoms and personality disturbances. The discussions of Hendrick, Knight, Oberndorf and others proved helpful in formulating our goals.

Each patient was interviewed separately by two of us (H.H.W.M. and E.L.B.), the combined interviews lasting about one and a half hours and covering as thoroughly as possible the following topics:

1. *Symptoms:* The patient was asked first to describe his symptoms in his own words and then for completeness was asked specifically about each of 40 symptoms on a prepared checklist which had been compiled from the most frequently encountered psychologic and somatic complaints. The symptoms on the checklist were items understandable both to the patient and the doctor and each was graded as to severity or intensity: 1+ indicated a mild or occasional symptom, 2+ meant that the symptom in question was moderate in intensity or frequently present and 3+ signified a severe or almost constant symptom. Symptoms present only rarely (for example two or three times a year) were not ordinarily considered noteworthy.

The *number* of symptoms of each patient was thus recorded as well as a rough approximation of their *severity* as shown by the arithmetical sum of the +'s which we termed "weighted symptoms." By this means, the pre-treatment and follow-up symptomatic status of each patient could be compared in a fairly accurate manner.

2. *Social adjustment:* For convenience this was subdivided into four separate areas:

A. *Occupational adjustment:* This was discussed in detail, not only from the standpoint of type of job, amount of work done, and salary; but also with a consideration of the patient's degree of personal satisfaction, his efficiency, and his relationships with co-workers and superiors.

B. *Interpersonal relationships:* Relationships with important figures in the family and social orbit were investigated: whether the patient was more or less ambivalent than at time of hospitalization, and whether in general his relationships were smoother or not.

C. *Marital adjustment:* This was considered separately from sexual adjustment in that it encompassed a wider area. Patients were asked about common interests with the spouse, recreation, management of finances, religious problems, problems connected with rearing the children, in-law problems, etc. An estimate was then made of how well they seemed to adjust to each other's personal idiosyncrasies.

D. *Sexual adjustment:* Sexual adjustment was discussed in terms of heterosexual performance, degree of personal satisfaction and that of the spouse or partner. Specifically inquired about by the interviewer were any difficulties that might have been significant at the time of hospitalization, such as premature ejaculations, frigidity, or masturbation problems.

3. *Insight:* An attempt was made to assess the degree of insight: whether the patient could see a relationship between emotional conflicts or situations and his illness, and how well it enabled him to handle everyday conflicts and reality problems.

4. *Life situations since hospitalization:* Patients were also asked about their medical and surgical illnesses during the period since hospitalization, and a general account of their life experiences was obtained; reactions to loss of family members, increasing responsibilities with additional children, etc. We were interested in whether environmental stresses seemed to have increased or decreased, and how the patient reacted to them.

Admittedly such an interview is somewhat formalized; nevertheless it was believed that by so organizing the topics more material could be obtained in the limited time available than if a less pointed technic were employed. The interviews were conducted with as little activity as possible on the part of the examiners, but of course many specific questions had to be asked.

In an attempt to objectify our appraisal of the different areas of social adjustment of each patient so that the method might be useful to independent observers, we constructed 5-point rating scales which were adapted (and considerably modified) from those of Masserman and Carmichael.

We attempted to formulate (for each area of social adjustment) the expectations demanded of an individual in our particular culture. It was then possible, by means of the information we had obtained, to determine how well the patients fulfilled the various roles which were theirs by reason of their particular places in society. The rating scales were defined empirically to fit the available information, and represented a series of steps going from a very inadequate level of adjustment to an "ideal" level—one which, needless to say, we did not regard as a norm.

Definitions which included several possibilities were used where possible so that appropriate extrapolations could be made in cases which were difficult to categorize. The rating scales thus permitted estimates of a patient's adjustment, both for the "pre-treatment" period and for the "follow-up" period. This introduced a complicating factor, namely a time dimension which was not constant in each case, since the duration of illness was different in every patient, as was the period from discharge to follow-up contact. Therefore, we decided to rate adjustment by a sort of "cross-section" which was arbitrarily defined. The "pretreatment" rating was based upon the patient's adjustment during the year preceding admission to the hospital, unless the duration of the anxiety syndrome had been less than a year, in which case it was based upon his adjustment during the course of the neurosis. In those few cases where the neurosis was of sudden recent onset (duration less than one month) a rating was more difficult to assign. The "follow-up" rating was based upon the patient's adjustment during the year preceding follow-up contact. In some cases seen many years after hospitalization, with definite fluctuations in adjustment associated with environmental stresses, such factors were taken into account. The rating scales were as follows:

*Occupational Adjustment**

1 = unable to work because of the psychoneurosis.
2 = unable to work more than 50 per cent of the time, which might include: long periods of continuous inability to work running into weeks or months, or frequent short absences from work such as days or weeks.
3 = able to work most of the time, with only short periods of inability to work such as occasional days or weeks off.
4 = able to work steadily, but because of the neurotic problems there was definitely impaired efficiency.
5 = able to work steadily and efficiently with no significant neurotic handicap.

Interpersonal Relationships

1 = unable to make and maintain adequate human relationships.
2 = unable to make and maintain more than a few adequate relationships: marked ambivalance towards most of the people in the social orbit, or able to maintain relationships only with perpetuation of neurotic symptoms.
3 = able to make and maintain adequate relationships with most people most of the time, but may have marked ambivalence toward a few specific figures in the social orbit.
4 = able to make and maintain smooth and consistent relationships with only minor conflicts.
5 = no apparent disturbances in interpersonal relationships.

Marital Adjustment

1 = completely unsatisfactory marriage; patient and spouse separated because of *neurotic* conflicts. (Separations because of *realistic* factors were evaluated individually and an appropriate rating given.)
2 = difficulties in many areas of the marriage: finances, common interests, personal habits, friends, in-laws, religion, sexual relations, children, etc.
3 = difficulties in a few areas of the marriage.

* Patients who were not employed, such as housewives or students, were rated according to their efficiency and ability in performing their daily tasks.

4 = marriage mutually satisfactory to patient and spouse except for minor problems, or the marriage was satisfactory in all areas except sexual.

5 = marriage consistently satisfactory and harmonious for patient and spouse.

Sexual Adjustment

1 = unable to tolerate heterosexual genital relations: complete impotence, could not permit intercourse (women); able to utilize only perverse methods of gratification; homosexual relations with marked guilt or anxiety; adults who were restricted to masturbation because of neurotic conflicts.

2 = marked difficulties in heterosexual relations: disgust, anxiety, disturbing fantasies, or symptoms which inhibited genital activity; partial impotence, premature ejaculations most of the time, frigidity which permitted rare or occasional intercourse without pleasure or orgasm; frequent reliance upon perverse activity as an adjunct to genital relationship, disturbing homosexual fantasies or conflicts.

3 = able to perform heterosexually, but without consistent pleasure or potency: some premature ejaculations, partial frigidity; satisfaction restricted in various ways by guilt, fears of pregnancy, fears of infection, etc.

4 = able to derive pleasure and satisfaction from intercourse most of the time, with only minor difficulties or dissatisfaction.

5 = able to enjoy a mature, consistently satisfactory heterosexual adjustment without significant conflicts.

Depth of Insight

1 = did not consciously admit psychogenic factors in the illness.

2 = admitted psychic nature of illness but constructed vague rationalizations such as "nerve strain from overwork," "nervous breakdown," etc.

3 = admitted the relationship of emotional difficulties to the illness, but insight was mainly intellectual and a tendency to blame others for inner conflicts persisted.

4 = realized the significance and personal origin of past emotional conflicts, but rejected insight that would occasion severe narcissistic trauma.

5 = deeper insight into ambivalence and inner conflicts, including those arising from erotic urges and aggressive drives previously repressed.

It will now be seen that for each patient the "pre-treatment" status, as determined by study of the hospital record, and the "follow-up" status, as determined by the interview material could be assessed and compared in terms of *symptoms* and *social adjustment*. It was very difficult to rate symptoms on a scale, so we expressed them as "weighted symptoms" and judged the degree of change in a quantitative and arbitrary manner. Because of the relative constancy of the symptom constellations in anxiety neurosis, this seemed to be a satisfactory procedure.

Criteria for Symptomatic Evaluation

Much improved = retained less than one-fourth of weighted symptoms.
Improved = retained one-fourth to two-thirds of weighted symptoms.
Slightly improved = retained two-thirds to seven-eighths of weighted symptoms.
Unimproved = same number of weighted symptoms, plus or minus one-eighth.
Worse = weighted symptoms exceeded former number by more than one-eighth.

Criteria for Social Evaluation

Much improved = total social adjustment (job, interpersonal relationships, marital and sexual adjustment) had improved by more than one level in the rating scales.
Improved = total social adjustment had improved by one level in the rating scales.
Slightly improved = total social adjustment showed less than one level of improvement.
Unimproved = no change in total social adjustment.
Worse = total social adjustment was less adequate than formerly.

The *over-all evaluation* of each patient was then arrived at by a consideration of symptomatic status and total social adjustment as well as degree of insight and ability to withstand environmental stresses. It was a subjective appraisal based partly upon arithmetical additions of the various ratings but not entirely derived from them. Although less easily defined in explicit terms, such an appraisal was more satisfying to us and seemed to give a more accurate, sensitive, and representative picture of the patient. We were cognizant of and attempted to avoid the type of error which Bandler discussed in warning of the dangers of assigning too much importance to symptoms. As much as the data permitted, we tried to understand changes in a patient's status from the dynamic as well as the descriptive viewpoint.

Criteria for Over-all Evaluation

Apparently recovered = recovery from symptoms (except possibly for one or two minor complaints) and marked improvement in social adjustment, with no return of the neurosis even under severe stress. This implied a complete and stable recovery from the neurosis.

Much improved = recovery from symptoms except for a few minor complaints and marked improvement in social adjustment. Under severe stress a transient exacerbation of the anxiety syndrome might occur.

Improved = definite improvement in symptoms and in one or more areas of social adjustment, although some symptoms persisted and patient's total adjustment was still not as good as it had been before the anxiety syndrome began.

Slightly improved = slight or variable improvement in symptoms and/or social adjustment.

Unimproved = self-explanatory.

Worse = self-explanatory.

III. Results of Follow-Up

Forty-nine patients were interviewed, and 4 who had moved to other parts of the country answered detailed questionnaires. The latter were prepared individually for each case, the questions being framed to cover the major interview topics. In 9 cases we obtained reliable indirect information: personal communications from psychiatrists who had treated the patients subsequently, letters from state hospitals, or interviews with members of the patient's immediate family.

Ten cases were considered "refusals" because they failed to keep appointments even though contacted repeatedly. (One of these reported that he was "cured," 3 said they were "better" and one said she was "about the same," but the information was not detailed enough to be considered adequate. Two more implied that they were getting along satisfactorily, but gave various excuses for not keeping their appointments.) Four cases could not be traced despite all efforts. No deaths were known to have occurred in the series.

Satisfactory follow-up was therefore achieved in 62 cases or 81.5 per cent of the entire group. This fact, plus the trend suggested by the majority of the refusal cases, led us to the conclusion that the follow-up patients constituted a valid sample of the total group.

The over-all evaluations of the 62 cases are shown in Table 4.

TABLE 4
Over-all Evaluation of Patients

Over-all evaluation	No. of cases	Percentage of cases
Apparently recovered	5	8.1
Much improved	9	14.5
Improved	22	35.5
Slightly improved	13	21
Unimproved	12	19.3
Worse	1	1.6
Totals	62	100.0

It was believed that patients in the "Slightly improved" category should not be considered *unequivocally better* and so on this basis 36 cases (58 per cent) were regarded as having a satisfactory outcome and 26 cases (42 per cent) were classed as essentially unchanged after their hospital stay.

Each of the patients interviewed, or to whom a questionnaire had been sent, was asked to give a self-rating of his present state of health as compared to his condition at the time of hospitalization. He was requested to choose, from the following list, the expression which best described him:

1. Cured (completely well)
2. Much better
3. A little better
4. The same as before
5. Worse

The correlation between our over-all evaluations and the patients' self-evaluations can be seen from Table 5.

In constructing Table 5 we arbitrarily grouped our own designations as shown because "much improved" implied at least recovery from symptoms, and thus seemed comparable to what most patients called "cured." Even if we had put the designation "apparently recovered" in one box and combined "much improved" plus "improved" in the second box, the correlation would still have been close. This correlation was interesting in

TABLE 5

CORRELATION BETWEEN OVER-ALL AND SELF-EVALUATION

Over-all evaluation		Patients' self-evaluation					
Designation	No. of Cases	"Cured"	"Much better"	"A little better"	"Same as before"	"Worse"	Totals
"Apparently recovered" plus "much improved"	13	9	4	0	0	0	13
"Improved"	18	0	15	3	0	0	18
"Slightly improved"	13	0	3	7	3	0	13
"Unimproved"	9	0	0	0	6	3	9
"Worse"	0	0	0	0	0	0	0
TOTALS	53	9	22	10	9	3	53

regard to the opinion expressed in the Five-Year Report of the Institute for Psychoanalysis, Chicago, that the physician who treated the patient and the patient himself are the best judges of therapeutic results. From our data, psychiatrist and patient at least show a close *agreement*.

IV. ANALYSIS OF THE DATA

The question arose whether it might be possible, from the available information, to determine some of the interrelated factors associated with improvement or failure to improve. Because of the small number of cases, the various categories were condensed into 3 groups:

Group A = cases *markedly improved* ("apparently recovered" and "much improved" designations). $N = 14$

Group B = cases *definitely better* ("improved" designation). $N = 22$

Group C = cases considered *essentially unchanged*. ("slightly improved," "unimproved," and "worse" designations). $N = 26$

For convenience these groups will be referred to hereafter simply as Groups A, B, and C. In testing group comparisons, where the nature of the data was appropriate, we used statistical methods to indicate whether differences were significant. Fisher's t Statistic or the Chi Square Test were employed and the level of confidence expressed by P in the conventional manner.

Comparisons were first made in terms of facts which could be ascertained accurately and concretely:

A. Length of Follow-up

	Range	Mean	
Group A	2-12.2 years	6.3 years	
Group B	2-11.9	6.8	(Differences are
Group C	2-12.2	6.6	not significant)

B. Sex Distribution

	Males	Females
Group A	9	5
Group B	15	7
Group C	11	15

(Differences are not significant)

C. Age at Onset of Anxiety Syndrome

	Range	Mean
Group A	11-37 years	24.1 years
Group B	12-44	24.0
Group C	10-36	22.2

(Differences are not significant)

D. Duration of Anxiety Syndrome Prior to Hospitalization

	Range	Mean
Group A	4 mo.-22 years	5.7 years
Group B	10 days-22 years	4.7
Group C	1 mo.-34 years	6.6

(Differences are not significant)

E. I.Q. (Bellevue-Wechsler Test)*

	Range	Mean
Group A ($N = 6$)	70-133	105
Group B ($N = 16$)	86-141	108
Group C ($N = 11$)	64-117	91

(Significant difference between Groups B and C; $P = <0.01$)

F. Length of Hospital Stay**

	Range	Mean
Group A ($N = 12$)	13-153 days	49 days
Group B ($N = 21$)	8-296	68
Group C ($N = 20$)	10-91	39

(Differences among the 3 groups are slight: $P = 0.1$ to 0.05)

G. Number of Psychotherapeutic Interviews**

	Range	Mean
Group A	6-90	28
Group B	4-175	33
Group C	5-50	19

($P = 0.1$ to 0.5)

From these data, to which statistical treatment was applicable, it was evident that such factors as age at onset, duration of symptoms prior to hospitalization, or sex of the patient were not

* Done in only 33 cases.
** Excluding 7 patients who left the hospital against advice, and 2 who were admitted for diagnosis only.

significantly related to the outcome at follow-up. Patients with low I.Q.'s were more frequently in the "essentially unchanged" group, and when the correlation between prognosis and I.Q. was calculated by the Point-biserial method a positive value (r equals 0.42) was obtained.

In regard to length of stay in the hospital and number of interviews, the slight differences among Groups A, B and C could perhaps be explained as follows: patients who made the most improvement (Group A) were those who responded most quickly to treatment—were "less sick" than those in Group B who improved more slowly and were kept in the hospital longer for further therapeutic efforts. In Group C were a number of patients whose prognosis had been considered poor by reason of low I.Q., very bad environmental situation, etc., and they usually had been discharged after a brief period of supportive psychotherapy. This lowered the mean figures for the group.

The three groups were next compared as regards various family situations. Data such as these were not measurable with enough precision to warrant statistical comparisons, and only the trends have been noted.

H. Childhood Home Environment*

	Good	Fair	Poor
Group A	38%	54%	8%
Group B	45%	45%	10%
Group C	19%	33%	48%

* This was defined in terms of family relationships rather than social or economic level, since the "emotional climate" in the home appears to be a more significant factor in the development of neurosis. Three categories were defined:
  Good: Parents lived together without major conflicts and patient received adequate affection and love. No major difficulties with siblings.
  Fair: Parents may have had occasional serious conflicts and patient suffered some rejection. One parent may have been lost (death, divorce, desertion, etc.) but if so, patient received good care from the step-parent or older siblings.
  Poor: Continuous conflict between parents, perhaps leading to separation, or patient may have lost one parent and been rejected by the other. Patient may have grown up in an orphanage or an unsatisfactory foster home without love and affection. Patients whose parents were both markedly unstable, neurotic, alcoholic, or psychotic would also be included in this category.

I. Loss of One or Both Parents
(before patient was 8 years old)

	Loss	No Loss
Group A	29%	71%
Group B	24%	76%
Group C	25%	75%

J. Size of Family and Patient's Position in Family

Groups A, B, and C were compared as to number of siblings (including the patient) in each family, and no significant differences were found. For the total group of 62 cases, family size varied from 1-16 with a mean approximating 5. The patients' positions in the family—only child, eldest, second, third, youngest, etc.—were noted and were found to have no significance but fitted very closely the random distribution determined by chance.

K. Emotional Difficulties in Siblings*

	Total Number of Siblings	Siblings with Emotional Difficulties Number	Percent
Group A ($N = 12$)	42	11	26
Group B ($N = 13$)	42	12	28
Group C ($N = 10$)	41	7	17

L. Emotional Difficulties in Parents

(Percentages based upon number of cases where information was complete.) These percentages are shown in Table 6.

M. Ages of Parents at Time of Patient's Birth

	Father's Age Range	Mean	Mother's Age Range	Mean	
Group A	26-49	35	24-45	32	(Differences
Group B	22-45	32	21-39	31	are not
Group C	19-47	33	19-45	31	significant.)

* Because of inadequate information our terms were vague, but included under this heading were: marked emotional instability, definite clinical neurosis, or alcoholism. No patient gave a history of psychosis among the siblings. Only the number of cases where detailed information was available were included, thus the discrepancies in sizes of N.

TABLE 6
EMOTIONAL DIFFICULTIES IN PARENTS OF PATIENTS
(Figures in percentages)

	Psycho-somatic disease	Neurosis	Psychosis*	Alcoholism	Marked "nervousness" or "instability"	No obvious difficulties
Group A						
Fathers ($N = 12$)	0	8	8	8	25	50
Mothers ($N = 12$)	0	0	8	8	17	67
Group B						
Fathers ($N = 14$)	14	0	0	14	7	64
Mothers ($N = 13$)	8	15	15	0	39	23
Group C						
Fathers ($N = 14$)	0	0	7	21	21	50
Mothers ($N = 14$)	0	7	21	0	21	50

* Eight parents were found to have had psychotic episodes. The diagnoses as obtained from the mental hospitals were: involutional depression (1), manic depressive psychosis, depressed (2), schizophrenia (2), "paranoid psychosis" (1) and "psychosis with mental deficiency" (1). The eighth diagnosis was not confirmed, but there was no doubt that there had been a psychotic breakdown.

From the information pertaining to family situations, one sees that the early home environment was usually good or fair in Groups A and B, while in Group C about half the cases came from poor homes. The patients who had suffered a loss of one or both parents early in life were evenly distributed among the three groups and there was no significance attached to the patient's position in the family or number of siblings. The amount of "emotional disturbances" among siblings and parents seemed to be about the same for all three groups, although among the parents of patients in Group C there was a higher incidence of psychosis and alcoholism. The age of the parents (particularly the mother) at the time of patient's birth has been thought to have a possible relationship to certain abnormal conditions. Barry noted that in a series of patients with serious mental disease, advanced maternal age was more frequent than in the general population. No conclusions can be drawn from our small series, but of the patients who could give accurate information, there were 5 out of 43 (11.6 per cent) who were born after their mothers were 40 years old. This is about three times the figure for the normal population.

Further comparisons of the groups were made in terms of early neurotic traits, number of operations and details of the symptomatology.

N. Number of Childhood Neurotic Traits*

	Range	Mean
Group A	0-3	1.3
Group B	0-4	1.6
Group C	0-5	2.2

Since one neurotic trait may have an entirely different meaning from another, one cannot compare them statistically, but the above table was constructed to illustrate a trend. The patients in Group C, had, on the average, more overt neurotic traits in childhood than did those in Groups A and B.

O. Operations Prior to Hospitalization

	Tonsillectomy	Appendectomy*	Other major operations	Other minor operations
Group A	75%	23%	15%	23%
Group B	69%	21%	21%	16%
Group C	62%	16%	17%	12%

* Where primary diagnosis had been appendicitis. Cases in which appendectomy was incidental during a laparotomy for other causes are not included.

There seems to be a widely held belief that psychoneurotic patients are frequently subjected to unnecessary surgical procedures. We compared the groups according to types of operations, and obtained operative and pathologic reports whenever possible.

No patient had had more than two major operations including appendectomy, and in the majority of cases there had been pathologic justification for the surgery. Minor operations were

* This includes the common traits such as eating difficulties, tantrums, marked fears, night terrors or bad dreams, enuresis, thumb sucking, nail-biting, walking or talking in sleep, speech impediments, etc.

not investigated so carefully, and the information was probably less accurate. Some patients were likely to recount many procedures such as tooth extractions, incision of furuncles, etc., while others tended to ignore such incidents. Among the minor operations were included several "dilatation and curettages" which apparently had been done upon good surgical indications.

P. Symptoms at Time of Hospitalization

	Number of symptoms		Weighted symptoms	
	Range	Mean	Range	Mean
Group A ($N = 12$)	9-24	16	14-43	24
Group B ($N = 16$)	13-26	18	18-39	28
Group C ($N = 22$)	13-25	19	14-46	31

In the detailed study of symptoms only the 50 most completely studied cases were used and as shown by the figures above, the group differences as to number and weight of symptoms were not striking. Since individual symptoms are by no means equivalent to one another, statistical comparisons were not carried out.

The three groups showed only minor differences in relative frequency of the common symptoms at time of hospitalization. Group A as compared with Groups B and C showed slightly fewer acute anxiety attacks, less complaints of irritability and fewer disturbing dreams. There was also slightly lower incidence of headache, weakness, effort trouble, "choking," and sighing. On the other hand, in Group A there were more complaints of insomnia and anorexia than in Groups B and C.

The incidence of the 30 most common symptoms in the group of 50 cases, both at time of hospitalization and at follow-up in shown in Fig. 1. It should be noted that the *weight of symptoms* is *not* depicted so that in many instances while a symptom may appear almost as frequently at follow-up, its intensity may be less. The amount of symptomatic improvement was therefore greater than Fig. 1 would suggest.

By definition, Group A showed the most symptomatic im-

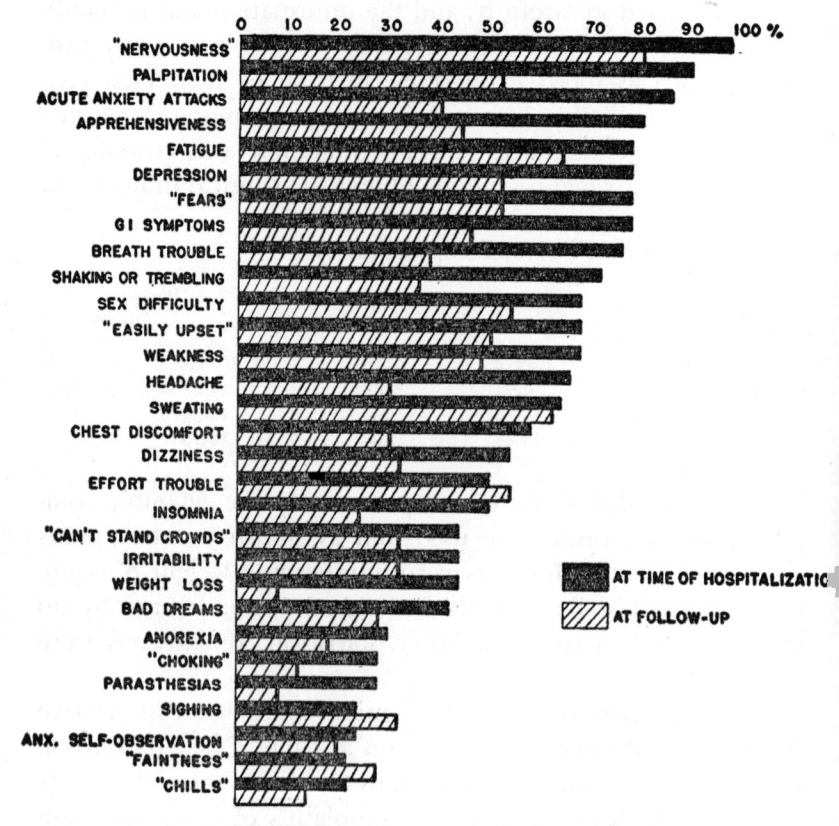

INCIDENCE OF SYMPTOMS IN 50 CASES OF ANXIETY NEUROSIS

FIG. 1.—*Incidence of symptoms in 50 cases of anxiety neurosis.* Many of the symptoms do not require further definition. Of the others: *acute anxiety attacks* = attacks of choking, palpitation, chest discomfort, difficulty in breathing, and fear, coming on abruptly and not usually connected with stimuli obvious to the patient; *fatigue* = feelings of tiredness not related to physical exertion; *"fears"* = specific fears which the patient consciously knows are not realistic; *G.I. symptoms* = such items as nausea, vomiting, diarrhea, and "indigestion"; *breath trouble* = subjective dyspnea or feeling of inability to get enough air; *sex difficulty* = symptoms complained of by the patient (unconscious homosexual conflicts and minor perverse activities are not included); *effort trouble* = difficulty in performing ordinary muscular work; *"can't stand crowds"* = marked uneasiness or anxiety when in a crowd; *"choking"* = a feeling that throat is constricted or blocked, can't get air into larynx; *"chills"* = sensation of being cold and shivery without actual rigor.

provement and Group C little or none. However, at follow-up certain symptoms were found to have disappeared more frequently than others. A comparison of the three groups from this standpoint was interesting. For example, in Group A most of the symptoms associated with *autonomic discharge* had disappeared: no patient at follow-up complained of acute attacks of anxiety or of palpitation, dyspnea, sighing, chest pain, nausea, vomiting, or diarrhea. However, complaints of excessive sweating were only slightly reduced.

Symptoms of a less specific, more *"generalized"* nature, such as apprehensiveness, fears, depression, insomnia, bad dreams, etc., were also markedly improved in Group A; but minor complaints of "nervousness" and "easily upset" persisted in several patients.

Fatigue persisted in a few patients in Group A and was essentially unimproved in Groups B and C. *"Effort trouble"* remained as much a problem at follow-up as at time of hospitalization even in the much improved patients of Group A. *Sexual difficulties* also tended to persist with relatively little change.

The disappearance in Group A of autonomic symptoms probably indicated that the patients' ego defense mechanisms were operating more effectively in handling anxiety, since those symptoms are essentially the somatic component of conscious anxiety. The relationship of anxiety to fatigue is interesting and has been discussed in detail in a monograph by Shands and Finesinger. In 92 per cent of our cases, either acute anxiety attacks or fatigue were among the presenting symptoms, and 80 per cent of these had both complaints. Fatigue was the more persistent symptom; a significant number of patients who at follow-up had lost their anxiety attacks retained fatigue, but none who still had anxiety attacks had lost fatigue. The explanation might be that certain symptoms which tended to persist even in Group A such as "nervousness," fatigue, and sexual difficulties were manifestations of basic personality problems, conflicts which in the dynamic sense were at a "deeper" level than those conflicts associated with the acute episodic manifestations of anxiety. Thus patients could more easily overcome their anxiety symptoms.

The persistence of effort trouble was also of interest. Studies done at this hospital on neurocirculatory asthenia, which certainly closely resembles anxiety neurosis, have stressed the chronicity of the illness and brought forth evidence suggesting physiologic factors which may be constitutionally determined. Individuals with this illness apparently cannot be trained to perform as much muscular work as the "normal" control subject can do.

Q. Social Adjustment

Comparison of Groups A, B, and C in terms of "pre-treatment" and "follow-up" ratings in the various areas of social adjustment is shown in Fig. 2. One must realize, of course, that the various ratings are not actually comparable arithmetically. For example, the patient who is given a 2 rating in marital adjustment is *not* exactly half as well adjusted as an individual who rates a 4. Thus there is a statistical fallacy in the "mean" levels of adjustment which are shown in Fig. 2, but they express graphically the group comparisons and so have been used. The scattergram shows the actual distribution of *before* and *after* ratings in each group and is the more valid representation.

R. Insight

Patients' insight at time of admission to hospital was very slight. The group as a whole had naive ideas about psychiatry and neurotic illness. In most cases patients never suspected that their trouble might be related to emotional difficulties. Some believed that they suffered from a "nervous condition" or a "nervous breakdown" but usually blamed it on a glandular dysfunction or some medical condition which the doctors had been unable to diagnose, or "heart trouble," "leaking valves," etc.

At the time of follow-up, even those patients who were markedly improved had relatively little insight, though the impression gained by our crude rating scale was that Group A showed significantly more insight than did Group C. The characteristics of the group: naivete, frequent lack of introspection,

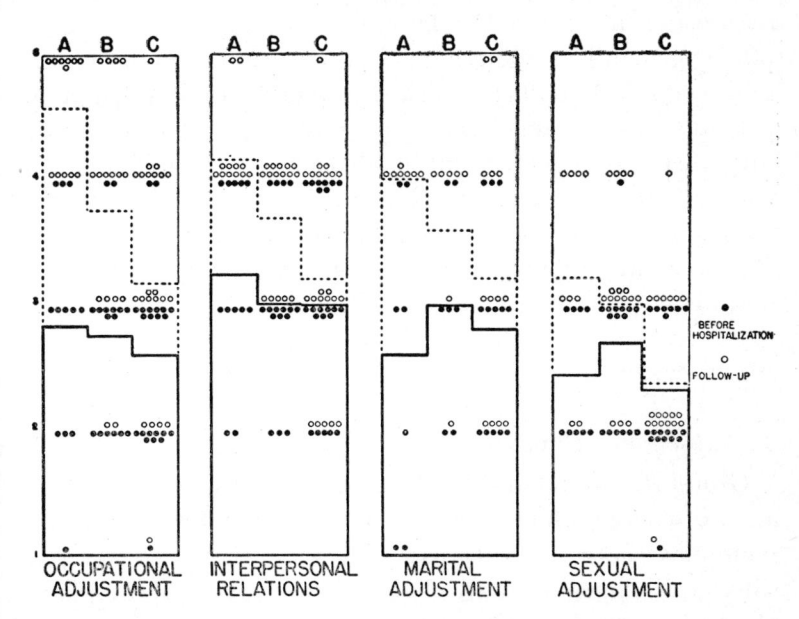

FIG. 2.—This demonstrates the ratings in occupational adjustment, interpersonal relationships, marital and sexual adjustment of the patients in Groups A, B, and C, before hospitalization (black dots) and at follow-up (open circles). The scattergram shows the distribution of ratings in each group and the lines show the "mean levels" of adjustment in each group. (Solid lines for pre-hospitalization and dotted lines for follow-up.)

It can be seen that the pre-hospitalization levels of social adjustment of Groups A, B and C do not differ very much, while at follow-up the greatest amount of improvement has been made in job and marital adjustment.

unawareness of inner thought and fantasies, and the general inarticulateness of many of the patients, may have contributed to this seeming lack of insight. The fact that in successful psychotherapy the patient may "assimilate" interpretations and later not recall much of the therapeutic work or of his conflicts perhaps played a part in a few cases.

S. Clinical Severity of the Neurosis

At the time the case records were studied and abstracted, each patient had been given a rating as to the severity of his neurosis. This rating was the psychiatrist's (H.H.W.M.) *clinical impression,* not arrived at by any specifically defined criteria, but by generally considering symptoms, early neurotic difficulties, severity of conflicts which precipitated anxiety symptoms, patient's capacity for carrying on under the load of neurotic illness, etc. Each patient was graded on a scale of 1+ to 4+, with 1+ representing a mild neurosis and 4+ a severe neurosis. After the follow-up interviews, Groups A, B, and C were compared in terms of this "clinical impression." The trend was, in general, that the cases which showed most improvement were least severe by clinical impression, but no striking correlation existed.

T. Subsequent Illnesses

Group A: No patient developed a medical or surgical illness after discharge which could have accounted for the original symptoms. Four patients had had surgical procedures (tonsillectomy, appendectomy, cholecystectomy, and hernioplasty), all of which on the basis of history or pathologic reports seemed indicated. No patient had a flare-up of anxiety symptoms associated with an illness or operation, and none had a prolonged convalescence.

Group B: Two patients in this group were found to have essential hypertension at follow-up examination seven years and twelve years respectively after hospitalization. Both patients, however, had had transient hypertension with systolic pressure as high as 160-170 mm. Hg and normal diastolic pressure at time of hospitalization.

One patient in the group had been subjected to an unnecessary operation upon a varicocele (present at time of hospitalization) which was not contributory to his symptoms. It was clear that the patient had insisted upon surgery for neurotic reasons.

Four other patients had had operations which were surgically indicated: incision of an infected pilonidal cyst, tonsillectomy, excision of an anal fistula, and resection of a Grade II adenocarcinoma of the rectum. In two instances (pilonidal cyst and anal fistula) there had been delayed recovery apparently neurotically determined rather than on the basis of surgical complications.

Group C: One patient had angrily left the hospital against advice, when in the course of psychotherapy it was pointed out to her that her abdominal pains were not due to appendicitis. She was operated on later at another hospital, and the pathologic report indicated no acute inflammation. She had had several operations subsequently, but the details could not be obtained. Another patient, after discharge, continued to have abdominal pain and had been subjected to two laparotomies, for which there was no clear surgical indication. Six other operations on four patients had been done, all with reasonable indications: 2 "dilatation and curettages," 2 laporatomies, a tonsillectomy, and a submucous resection.

The subsequent illnesses were studied in detail because of statements in the literature to the effect that patients with the diagnosis of psychoneurosis are often found later to have an "organic" illness which was responsible for the "neurotic" symptomatology. We believe that thorough clinical study would minimize such findings.

U. Dynamic Formulations

In those cases where information was sufficiently detailed, we attempted to compare patients in terms of their over-all life adjustments, the types of conflicts most evident and the dynamic mechanisms operating. One point which was apparent at once was that patients in Group A were much more likely to have made adequate adjustments in childhood, with the anxiety symptoms coming on rather acutely as a result of a precipitating situation which seemed to break down the ego defenses. In Groups B and C, more than half of the patients had had various overt neurotic difficulties in childhood and adolescence, eventuating more gradually in the typical clinical picture of anxiety neurosis.

Of the male patients, almost all had the personality generally described as "passive." They had difficulty in expressing aggression, were apt to have been timid at school, avoided rough sports, had perhaps been considered "sissies," and usually brought out many feelings of inferiority. A few were typical "tough guys" in their behavior, but the interviews clearly revealed that this attitude was the result of a compensatory mechanism. Homosexual conflicts were evident in about half the cases, although only 1 patient indulged in overt homosexual practices.

Female patients were less easily categorized into "personality types." Almost half of them had adjusted fairly well until some environmental strain precipitated the anxiety symptoms. The precipitating event was most commonly the increasing load of responsibilities, restrictions, and conflicts associated with a growing family. Fears of further pregnancies, and hostility to the husband and children were often expressed. Many of the female patients had always been shy, timid, fearful, and sensitive. Some were markedly self-sacrificing, with strong masochistic trends. One patient had a definitely masculine orientation, with severe conflicts and difficulties in regard to her heterosexual relationships.

The precipitating factors in anxiety attacks or in the genesis of the anxiety syndrome showed considerable uniformity. In those cases where correlations could be established, the immediate conflicts or situations associated with anxiety were as follows:

1. Conflicts in managing hostile or aggressive impulses; 27 cases
2. Conflicts over disturbing heterosexual fantasies; 4 cases
3. Acute revival of old mutilation fears induced by trauma (2 cases) or combat experiences (1 case); 3 cases
4. Unconscious homosexual conflicts with acute anxiety; 2 cases

While there did seem to be a certain gross homogeneity in the group, the data were inadequate for the construction of detailed dynamic formulations. Usually only the more "superficial" or immediate conflicts were apparent.

V. Changes in Diagnosis (at Follow-up)

Group A: In the descriptive sense in which the diagnosis of anxiety neurosis was made in this study, no patient in this group had a significant neurosis any longer.

Group B: Seven cases in this group would now probably be differently classified: 2 patients showed hypochondriacal tendencies in that they had minor somatic complaints with which they were preoccupied, 1 patient would probably be termed "inadequate personality," and 4 patients, because of changes in symptoms would probably be diagnosed "mixed neurosis," although anxiety was still a prominent feature.

Group C: Six cases would now be differently diagnosed: 3 as "mixed neurosis," 1 as hysteria with anxiety symptoms, 1 as "inadequate personality," and 1 as reactive depression and chronic alcoholism.

In no case was there evidence that a psychotic reaction had developed in the interval between hospitalization and follow-up. Four patients had had state hospital admissions, but letters from these institutions in all cases confirmed the diagnosis of psychoneurosis, severe anxiety neurosis, or mixed neurosis.

W. Subsequent Psychiatric Treatment

Group A: Half of the patients had had further psychotherapy. Of these, 5 had been seen in our psychiatric out-patient clinic for a few interviews (2-5 visits) and 1 patient had been treated for a total of 150 hours by a staff psychiatrist. At the time of follow-up none had had psychotherapy within the past eighteen months.

Group B: Seventy-four per cent of the group had had further treatment, mostly, however, only a few interviews in the out-patient clinic (2-30 visits). One patient had had 2 voluntary admissions to a state hospital which he believed had benefited him much more than his treatment in our ward. Another patient had had 100 hours of psychotherapy with a staff psychiatrist, and was still being treated at the time of follow-up. No others in the group had had treatment within six months of follow-up.

Group C: Seventy-two per cent of the group had received further therapy, including 3 patients who were still in treatment at time of follow-up. Three patients had been admitted to state hospitals, 1 to a private sanatorium, and 1 had been given a series of 9 electroshock treatments.

The above facts complicate one's evaluation of the influence of intramural therapy, but tend to substantiate the impression that among the patients who got better (Groups A and B), those showing the most improvement had the least treatment.

Actually, only 2 patients had had intensive psychotherapy after hospitalization, and in both cases the details of treatment were discussed with the staff psychiatrists concerned and thus we were able to evaluate to some degree the part played by the intramural therapy.

X. Analysis of Intramural Therapy

All patients had been subject to the same general ward regimen. This emphasized participation in group social interaction, occupational therapy, and a regular routine of meals, recreation, and visiting hours. Very little medication was given for somatic complaints, and bedtime sedatives were used only sparingly. Therapeutic interviews of fifty to sixty minutes each were ordinarily carried out four or five times weekly, occasionally less often. A more complete general description of how the Psychiatric Ward functions has been given by Cobb in a report of its first ten years of operation.

In attempting to describe and categorize the psychotherapy used in each individual case, we considered particularly the following:

1. When dynamically significant material was produced in the interviews, was there evidence of strong emotion or lack of emotion?

2. What was the status of the patient-physician relationship: warm, indifferent, ambivalent, hostile, etc.?

3. The amount of experience and training of the therapist.

4. What type or types of psychotherapy were employed? These included ventilation by the patient without interpretations by the therapist, reassurance, explanation of symptoms on a simple physiologic level, situational manipulation to remove the patient from disturbing influences, suggestion (with or without hypnotic drugs), or dynamically oriented insight therapy with limited objectives as described by Finesinger. In many instances a number of technics had been used together, so it was sometimes impossible to know exactly what the therapist had done.

5. The patient's own impression of what had helped him most in the therapeutic process.

The amount of affect displayed in interviews and the patient-physician relationships were about the same for Groups A, B, and C. There was a slight trend in Groups A and B toward more therapists at the resident level or above (two years or more of experience). Of the entire group, 60 per cent had been treated by members of the house staff with one to two years of experience, almost a third by fourth-year medical students under supervision and slightly less than 10 per cent by experienced staff psychiatrists.

When the patients treated by insight therapy were compared to those treated by simple ventilation, reassurance, explanation, or suggestion, it seemed that results were better in the former group. However, in a sense the insight-treated patients were *selected,* since a number of cases had been rejected for insight therapy because of low I.Q., language difficulty, or extremely poor environmental situation. (This might be another factor in the relationship between I.Q. and follow-up results. Patients with good intelligence were more apt to be chosen for intensive psychotherapy with attempts at producing insight, whereas those with obviously low I.Q.'s were likely to have brief supportive measures only. As a general rule if the I.Q. was lower than 90 insight therapy was not attempted; and if one divided the cases on that basis, those with I.Q.'s above 90 averaged 37 hours of therapy, and those with I.Q.'s lower than 90 had a mean of 20 hours.) Discounting the "unsuitable" cases, the group which had insight therapy showed no significant difference from the rest. The numbers were too small, however, to draw any conclusions, and one must also recall the other complicated factors involved.

Patients' statements as to what had helped them most revealed the previously mentioned lack of insight. One woman who had improved remarkably both symptomatically and in her social adjustment was very enthusiastic about her "recovery," but was not able to say how the treatment had helped her. She recognized the fact that her symptoms had been a source of secondary gain and said, "I don't have to have them any more." She was inclined to attribute her improvement to "the doctor's interest and sympathy." It would appear in this instance that the patient-physician relationship was the medium by which therapy was successful, but our information was not adequate to explain how it operated. Another patient who had improved a great deal believed that reassurance had helped her to get better. "I had all those examinations and tests, and I knew there was nothing wrong. That helped."

In attempting to assign values to the numerous interrelated factors, including psychotherapy, it was our impression that the outcome of an individual case in this particular series depended more upon the balance between the patient's assets and liabilities than upon the treatment. Such factors as good intelligence, favorable childhood environment, a reasonably satisfactory life adjustment until severe stress had precipitated the neurosis, all weighed upon the positive side of the balance. Insoluble reality problems, neurotic patterns of behavior extending back into childhood, and inferior intellectual equipment were negative factors.

V. Discussion

In an appropriate context Ruesch states, "It seems that clinical appraisal of the state of recovery is easier than its scientific definition." Many of the studies we have cited bear out this view: certainly the follow-up evaluations were done by clinical appraisal or "intuition" rather than by specifically defined criteria.

In this study we have attempted to make a first approximation of a scientific definition by means of explicit rating scales and criteria. The method is crude and its imperfections are obvious. Criteria are mainly descriptive since they take into account overt behavior and symptoms rather than dynamic mechanisms. This is due in part to the incompleteness of the case material. It is also unavoidable that when one reduces complex areas of human behavior and interaction to discrete categories one may overlook nuances which are important but are not readily classified. It is to be hoped that methodology can be developed eventually to the point where objectivity will be achieved by a conversion of "intuition" into measurable and rational principles. Stanfield points out that, "principles not intuition lend themselves to objectification, revision, pedagogy and broadening practical application."

Our over-all evaluations being done upon a descriptive level with a good deal of emphasis on symptomatic status, it seemed likely that our criteria were similar to those arrived at subjectively by the patients in their self-evaluations. This might explain their close correlation. We then worked out other correlations between over-all evaluation and its constituent elements, expressed in terms of the Contingency Coeffcient (C). Because of the small samples and uncertainty whether the categories being compared were normally distributed, we did not assume that C was equivalent to the product-moment r as it is under certain circumstances, but simply used it as a comparative index for the various correlations.

Over-all evaluation correlated with C

1. Patient's self-evaluation 0.79
2. Symptomatic evaluation 0.72
3. General social adjustment 0.66
   a. Occupational adjustment 0.51
   b. Interpersonal relationships 0.67
   c. Marital adjustment 0.70
   d. Sexual adjustment 0.48

It would appear that symptoms actually counted most significantly in both our evaluations and in the patients', which is understandable in this particular group, since the patients sought help primarily because of their symptoms. In general, psychoanalytically treated patients would show a higher level of intelligence and more sophistication. Such patients might complain less of the somatic manifestations of their neuroses than of difficulties in interpersonal relationships, sexual problems or "character disturbances."

The relatively poorer correlations of occupational adjustment and sexual adjustment with over-all evaluations can be explained. Our follow-up was done at a time when jobs were easily available, whereas at the time of hospitalization of many of the patients working conditions were less favorable. Thus almost all of the patients had better jobs, making the correlation less precise. There was relatively little improvement in sexual adjustment in any of the patients, so again the correlation was lower.

It seemed desirable to investigate the *reproducibility* of our methods because criteria and ratings, if objective, should yield equivalent results in the hands of independent observers. Ten case records were selected, together with the corresponding material obtained at the follow-up interviews, and these 10 cases were classified according to the rating scales by 4 independent observers, as to occupational adjustment, interpersonal relationships, marital adjustments and sexual adjustment. Both "initial" and "follow-up" ratings were done. Considering the total number of individual ratings (77 in all), the 4 observers agreed exactly in 20 per cent, showed a disagreement of 1 point in the scale in 58 per cent, and varied by 2 points in the scale in 22 per cent. There was no disagreement by more than 2 points. These discrepancies partially discounted one another when the observers amalgamated their ratings into an appraisal of the *total social adjustment*. The principal differences were in distinctions among "same," "worse," or "slightly improved." There were fewer differences of opinion between "much improved" and "improved." When the independent ratings were expressed in broad categories corresponding to our Groups A, B, and C, 5 cases were rated exactly the same as our final rating, by all 4 observers; 4 cases showed disagreement by 1 of 4 observers and in 1 case all the observers disagreed with us. If one took a "majority vote" of the 4 independent observers, their opinions would be the same as ours in 9 cases and divergent in 1 case.

In a similar manner, two of us repeated our own appraisals of 15 cases after a lapse of six to eight months to check our consistency. In the individual ratings, one observer (H.H.W.M.) checked his own previous results exactly in 74 per cent of the instances, and showed a discrepancy of 1 point in the scale in 26 per cent. The second observer's (E.L.B.) figures were much the same: 70 per cent checked exactly and 30 per cent showed one degree of variation. In the broad groupings—A, B, or C— there were three changes in the 30 repeated cases. In each of the three instances we gave a higher rating on the second evaluation ("Improved" to "Much Improved"). It would appear then, that there is not enough precision in our ratings, when applied to case records such as described here, to warrant categories based upon finely graded degrees of improvement and for practical purposes three broad groups are sufficient.

It would be interesting for comparison to have several psychiatrists rate the same group of patients at follow-up not on the basis of recorded material and arbitary criteria, but by interviewing them personally and using clinical judgment. This apparently has never been done, although Wilder comments on the results reported from the Berlin Psychoanalytic Institute. The groups followed up by Eitingon and Fenichel overlapped, so that about one-third of the latter's cases had been included in the former's report. Wilder pointed out discrepancies which he believed were due to the fact that the two writers had sometimes differently evaluated the same cases. The degree of inconsistency, however, could not be estimated from the published data.

Meisels followed up a group of psychoneurotic patients at this hospital in 1940, and upon examining her data we found that 15 of our cases had been included in her group. Thus we could check her findings after a further interval of seven to eight years. Her criteria of evaluation were somewhat similar to ours, but not identical, and in 9 of the 15 cases there was very close agreement. In 3 cases discrepancies were clearly explained by environmental and social changes in the intervening years, and in 3 cases differences were due to changes in symptoms which were not readily explained and might be termed "spontaneous."

A critical appraisal of our data in terms of accuracy and reliability reveals the fact that in describing interpersonal relationships, sexual adjustment, basic conflicts, "ego defenses," etc., the material is not only incomplete but is by no means unbiased. An investigation of dynamic factors is unavoidably shaped by the examiner's skill, personality, and theoretical orientation, and it must be remembered that the case material had been recorded by inexperienced examiners. From the psychodynamic standpoint the most significant facts were least accessible, and when obtained were apt to be fragmentary and difficult to evaluate. Factual data concerning age, sex, number of siblings, years of schooling, etc., were reliable but were of course relatively unimportant.

In the analysis and interpretation of the data there were apparent contradictions. In Group C there was a high incidence of poor home environment as compared with Groups A and B, yet there seemed to be little difference in percentage of parents with emotional difficulties, and no difference in incidence of emotional problems in siblings. This probably indicates that our criteria for evaluating such factors (and our anamnestic information) are inadequate to detect any but gross differences.

In the present study it is obvious that what we have analyzed as "'factors" associated with successful or unsuccessful outcome are not discrete factors at all, but are inter-related representations of the constitutional and environmental setting in which the neurosis developed. The early home environment, number of childhood neurotic traits, emotional difficulties in the parents are all inextricably bound up with one another and one is uncertain what to label "cause" and what "effect." That our findings were on the whole consistent with dynamic theory, and contributed nothing not already known was not unexpected. Undoubtedly a better study would have resulted had the records been more complete, as would have been the case if the project were planned in advance as suggested by the Chicago group.

In further considering the general problem it seems to us that the first methodologic step is the accumulation of accurate and detailed information dealing with the entire clinical picture and psychotherapeutic situation. The human memory is such a selective and unreliable recording instrument that complete, permanent recording is desirable. The gathering of material and its painstaking analysis is tedious and regarded by many as unrewarding. Nevertheless there are very few workers who make crucial discoveries by a process of serendipity and even fewer who can penetrate to the heart of a problem by inductive genius. The great majority must pursue a groping, pedestrian course.

Much thought must also be given to problems of defining and quantitating significant social and familial data and of categorizing dynamic factors in a way that will ultimately permit statistical treatment. Methods may then eventuate by which one individual's prognostic assets and liabilities can be compared with another's. The role played by psychotherapeutic efforts would then be easier to evaluate.

The approach to the problem, we believe, must be carried out by psychoanalytic technics since these offer the most sensitive and illuminating method of investigation at present available. That the problem is receiving more and more consideration can be seen from recent group discussions. Particularly has Kubie detailed his suggestions for methodologic advances. One of the drawbacks to such a projected study is the truly prodigious expenditure of time and effort required. It is not unlikely that a major reason why no one as yet has made a full-scale attack on the problem is because of doubts that the results could justify the amount of labor involved.

VI. Summary

1. The problem of evaluation of treatment of the psychoneuroses was discussed, with a review and criticism of previous reports. These have not been comparable to one another, largely due to lack of sufficiently detailed clinical data and precisely defined criteria.

2. A follow-up study was carried out upon 62 patients with anxiety neurosis, two to twelve years after intramural psychotherapy.

3. When evaluated by explicit criteria, 23 per cent of the group were found to be markedly improved, 35 per cent were definitely better, and 42 per cent were considered essentially unchanged. There was a close correlation between our evaluations and the patients' own self-evaluations.

4. In no case was previously unrecognized medical or surgical disease later found to be associated with the sypmtoms and no case had later become psychotic.

5. Analysis of the available anamnestic material suggested that a number of elements were related to the course of the illness. Among these were the patient's intelligence, his early

home situation, early neurotic traits, severity of the clinical symptoms, and capacity for achieving insight. Almost the whole group had been treated by relatively inexperienced therapists but a slightly higher percentage of patients in the improved categories had been treated by the more experienced psychiatrists.

6. The scope of the study was limited by the type and amount of information available in the case records, but our findings were consistent with dynamic theoretical concepts. It is believed that further progress in solving the problem awaits more detailed investigations and methodologic advances in the analysis of data.

THE CARBON DIOXIDE TREATMENT

A Review

L. J. Meduna, M.D.

The carbon dioxide treatment, even though we usually do not think of drugs as having a gaseous form, is a pharmacological treatment. During ancient times, and even during the Middle Ages, any drug had to be given in decoction, or in digeratum, or as tea, all of them liquids. Later, probably in the Renaissance, solid forms of medication—such form as powders, tablets, and pills—were accepted by the lay public as drugs or medicine. Still later, the parenteral administration of medicine through injections came into vogue. Finally, the administration of gases to induce anesthesia was accepted. In the evolution of medication, the next logical development, I think, will be the acceptance of carbon dioxide, and other gases still to be discovered, as legitimate medicaments for treatment for suitable pathologic conditions.

History

I came upon the use of carbon dioxide in a somewhat roundabout way. As I have mentioned in my monograph, in Budapest in 1934 I heard a garbled report of the work of Loevenhart, Lorenz, and Waters.

At that time I knew no English; and so, being unable to read the original reports, I had to follow the rumors that I gathered. According to these rumors, Loevenhart, Lorenz, and Waters had used oxygen in catatonic conditions by injecting it into the cerebellar cysterna. I carried out a series of experiments in which I similarly injected oxygen, but from these I saw no results. Later, in 1937, an English psychiatrist, a Dr. Cook, informed me that the American authors were using carbon dioxide, which they were administering by having patients inhale it. In 1937 and 1938, I administered carbon dioxide to catatonics and other schizophrenic patients, with results identical with those which Loevenhart, Lorenz, and Waters had obtained: some patients seemed to benefit from the carbon dioxide anesthesia; but their improvement lasted, at most, one-half hour, after which time their catatonic conditions reappeared. This, my early experimentation with carbon dioxide, I discontinued.

In 1942 and 1943, we at the Illinois Neuropsychiatric Institute carried out experiments, first on animals, by injecting cyanide intravenously. The convulsive phenomena following the injection led us to believe that cyanide might be utilized as a variant in the convulsive treatment of schizophrenia. Accordingly, we carried out cyanide-injection experiments on, I believe, about 40 schizophrenic patients, each of whom received a fairly long series of cyanide injections and each of whom responded with an appropriate motor discharge. *None of these patients, however, recovered* from their illness as a result of these convulsions, although an expected percentage of the same patients later recovered with electrically induced convulsions. This fact led us to study cyanide convulsions in greater detail. As it developed, cyanide convulsions are not *grand mal* convulsions, since they are not caused by cortical stimulation and followed by downward discharge from the brain cortex. These convulsions are release phenomena because of the fact that the cyanide inactivates cortical integration and inhibition upon the deeper motor centers; thus the normally suppressed or controlled low-motor-center function appears as motor phenomenon of the body.

During my observations of cyanide convulsions, I developed, tentatively, a theory by which I at first tried to explain why convulsions produced by metrazol, picrotoxin, electricity, etc., have curative effects upon psychotic conditions and why inhibition of higher cortical centers does not have similar curative effects. Basic to this theory were my assumptions that psychotic processes are due to biochemical disturbances in the cortex of the brain, which disturbances are self-sustaining; and that psychoneuroses are disturbances of lower structures of the brain, which disturbances upset or distort the emotional values of the concepts formed in the brain cortex. If, in accordance with the latter assumption, cyanide would effect the lower structures of the brain, then, I further assumed, a profound alteration of the psychopathological sypmtoms in neurotics might be achieved.

Cyanide, being a powerful and dangerous drug, did not seem suitable for mass experiments. I had to look, therefore, for some other agent which would produce physiological effects similar to those produced by cyanide. Fortunately, at that time I remembered the work of Loevenhart, Lorenz, and Waters; and, to my joy, I found that these authors had experimented with cyanide at about the time when they were working with carbon dioxide inhalations. Thus, by way of a long detour, I was able to continue Loevenhart, Lorenz, and Waters' work by assuming psychoneuroses as a proper indication for this treatment.

Method

In developing my method, I made initial mistakes: to my first few patients I gave 100 per cent carbon dioxide to inhale. The results were formidable: massive motor discharges, decerebrate fits on the objective level, and horrifying dream experiences on the subjective level. None of these patients ever permitted a second experiment. One of them, in fact, still in a half-daze, jumped off the treatment table and began to run out of the laboratory at such speed that only at the door were we able to catch him and hold him by force until he had calmed down enough to be permitted to leave the building. After a few of these crude experiments, I made the opposite mistake. I administered 5 per cent to 10 per cent carbon dioxide to a number of patients who were willing to take it; but from the inhalations by these patients I saw no results. After many a trial and error, I arrived at two concentrations of carbon dioxide that I found suitable for the treatment. One was a mixture of 20 per cent carbon dioxide and 80 per cent oxygen; the other, 30 per cent carbon dioxide and 70 per cent oxygen. I could not go any higher with the concentration of the carbon dioxide for the simple reason that no greater concentration than that, mixed with oxygen, can be put under the high pressure necessary, into the tanks. If it were tried, a certain amount of carbon dioxide would freeze out from the mixture in the form of dry ice, and the gas mixture would still be one of 30 per cent carbon dioxide and 70 per cent oxygen.

The use of 20 per cent carbon dioxide I discarded early; from then on I used the mixture of 30 per cent carbon dioxide and 70 per cent oxygen. This mixture has the great advantage of producing anesthesia without a long transitional phase from full consciousness to narcosis. Furthermore, the mixture can be obtained commercially without difficulty in almost any country. And, finally, this mixture necessitates the use of only one tank and a few gadgets.

The most important of these gadgets is the reducing valve. In this treatment, no reducing valve that limits the flow of gas to 20 or 30 liters per minute can be used. The best kind of reducing valve is that which has a manometer that shows the pressure of the gas inside the tank and one valve that permits the flow of gas into a rubber tube. This tube is connected with a 10-liter breathing bag, which is connected with the mask. The valve ought to be so constructed as to permit the flow of any amount of gas, depending upon how far the valve is opened. The mask must have an automatic spring valve, or other type of exhaling valve, which opens when the patient exhales and closes when he inhales, thus preventing his rebreathing into the bag.

When the two mixtures—20 per cent carbon dioxide with 80 per cent oxygen and 30 per cent carbon dioxide with 70 per cent oxygen—had proved to be suitable for treating psychoneurotics, my greatest problem was to minimize any autosuggestion in the procedure—a goal which can to some degree be approached but can never be reached. I told the patients not to expect anything from this treatment because I did not know whether it would work. Furthermore, I depreciated any improvement or change in their conditions which they reported, telling them firmly that these changes had been due only to autosuggestion and that during the further experimentation they would evanesce.

Before the first treatment, I found, some explanation must be given to the patient; but the shorter the explanation, the less was his anxiety regarding the procedure. While the treatment was in the experimental phase, I omitted any allusion to its possible efficacy; but I assured the patient that it was utterly harmless. I told him that the gas would produce a special kind of anesthesia, during which he would sleep; that he would be unable to talk and therefore would reveal no secrets; that he might have a dream during the treatment; and that, although the dream would have no particular significance, he should tell it to me after the treatment was over.

Before giving the treatment, I had the patient remove his shoes, loosen his collar and necktie, and lie down upon a treatment table. After I had opened the valve and when the gas was flowing freely, I put the mask on the face of the patient.

For didactic purposes, we may differentiate three phases of a single treatment: the introductory phase, the anesthesia phase, and the transitional phase. The introductory phase may last from 1 to 20 or 24 respirations. The length of this phase I determined by asking the patient, after the treatment, the last count he had heard. (While the patient had been taking the gas, I had counted the number of respirations loudly. He usually did not remember more than 8 to 12 counts.) During this phase, the respiratory rate is increased slightly, and the respiratory volume apparently is increased considerably. Flushing of the face and, occasionally, slight perspiration appear.

The phase of anesthesia is charactedized by various motor and sensory phenomena. The motor phenomena develop fairly rapidly; there is a little difficulty, therefore, in relating the appearance of these manifestations to the amount of gas inhaled. From about the tenth to the thirtieth respirations, indications of psychomotor excitement are often discernible. Occasionally these indications resemble a struggle to escape discomfort caused by the gas; most often the movements of the patient reveal the nature or the tone of mood accompanying his dreamlike experiences.

During the first 10 to 30 respirations, the lower extremities are often flexed at the hip, and the knee joints are slightly abducted. There are also a slight flexor hypertonus in the upper extremities and, frequently, carpal spasm in both hands. During the interim of 30 to 50 respirations, adversive seizures may occur. These consist of conjugate deviation of the eyes and torsion of the whole body in the same direction, usually with flexion of the legs and extension of the arms on the side toward which the eyes have turned. During these adversive seizures, the pupils react to light. Following or preceding these adversive seizures, rhythmic movements of the legs, resembling those in bicycling, may occur. Commonly, there is simultaneously an alternating change in the tonus of the contralateral upper arms, which movements, together with those of the legs, resemble the movements in quadripedal locomotion. During this phase—i.e., the phase of anesthesia—the pupils are usually dilated, and the reaction to light remains prompt.

Simultaneously with these phenomena, the behavior of the deep and superficial reflexes changes. After 20 to 60 inhalations, appropriate stimuli may provoke forced gasping and biting. After 30 to 40 inhalations, the plantar reflexes become less active; and after 50 to 60 inhalations, these reflexes disappear. At this time, Babinski reflex can be elicited. If the inhalation is continued beyond this phase, a decerebrate fit will ensue; but this fit, I assumed, is beyond the therapeutical range. The patient's recovery from the anesthesia usually occurs promptly—within one or two minutes. After the first treatment, usually the patient is confused; he does not recognize the doctor or the treatment room. But tactful handling with reassuring words help greatly; and the patient, usually with a smile, soon signifies that he has recovered his consciousness and recognizes the doctor.

The sensory experiences of the patients during the administration of carbon dioxide are intriguing. I usually call these phenomena dreams, although they do not fit into the category of dreams, hallucinations, or delusions. These sensory experiences may consist of only the three groups of form-constants described by Klüver. The first of these constants Klüver had designated as grating, lattice, fretwork, filigree, honeycomb, or chessboard design. A form-constant related to these is the cobweb figure, which my patients saw as cobwebs, spokes of a giant wheel, converging lines, and streets of huge dimensions. His second form-constant Klüver designated by such terms as tunnel, funnel, cone, and vessel. During the carbon dioxide anesthesia, the patients may feel motionless, and the revolving tunnel engulfs them. The third form-constant of Klüver is the spiral. This form is frequently reported by the CO_2 patients; they have approached a spiral, or a spiral has approached them, or they have felt that they are in the axis of a huge spiral.

A fourth constant of these sensory experiences I have described and named *dynamic-constant*. This constant has been described by my patients specifically. They have seen dots *falling* down in a constant rain or geometric figures sometimes *approaching* them, some of these figures moving on a horizontal plane, others *undulating,* and still others *gyrating* from the center toward the periphery.

Whether these visual and dynamic phenomena correspond to a stimulation of the visual cortex or to the stimulation of some other part of the brain, I cannot say. Some psychosensory experiences of a higher order seem to point to the stimulation, or to the independent function, of the temporal lobes. One of these psychosensory experiences of a higher order is a frequently reported *déjà vu,* which is recognized as a temporal lobe symptom.

Another of these psychosensory experiences is the phenomenon that has been described by Klüver and called by him *presque vu*. This phenomenon is characterized by an event or a visual image pointing in a certain direction, the suggested end of which is not quite reached. Or this phenomenon lacks the proper completion; it does not call forth a "closure" experience. A form, a movement, a pattern, etc, is almost complete; but, since it is never completed, a characteristic *presque vu* experience arises. The *presque vu* sensation may be adjectival to a problem—a problem spiritual, philosophical, or mathematical. To the *presque vu* sensation may be attributed a "special" or "cosmic" importance, as if the sensation were of esoteric importance, individual or cosmic—as if it had a function of divination. The *presque vu* sensation may be carried by any of the constants or may present itself in purity.

Another sensory phenomenon that commonly accompanies the CO_2 treatment is that which I have described under the name of *experience revenant*. This phenomenon may appear several hours or several days after the treatment. It comprises one of two kinds of experience: a sudden remembrance of a sensory phenomenon experienced during the actual CO_2 therapy, or just a feeling that the patient is taking the CO_2 treatment.

Besides the visual type of sensory symptoms, the patient may experience auditory, somaesthetic, or rarely olfactory sensations. Any one of these sensations may develop into a complex dream. In such a dream, one patient saw eccentric rings of blue and yellow suspended from the center. These began to undulate, forming a funnel. The yellow rings appeared and began to wave; and the whole scene turned into a seascape of deep blue with an ultramarine sky and a vibrating yellow light. Another patient saw a circle of light which grew immense and then became a wheel. The patient was the hub; the spokes were made of figures, which represented some planning for which he was responsible. Sometimes in the center of the visual field distant small objects appear and begin going faster and faster, *growing* as they move outward. Sometimes, also, patients have reported micropsias, or a feeling of being small.

When the visual sensations develop into dreams, they often possess strong catathymic components. These dreams are strange, even weird, in a way that sets them apart; they are like some epileptic auras or ecstatic experiences. One normal experimental subject has thus described a dream experience: "I had an impression of being in complete understanding and harmony with God. Seemed like an abrupt awakening of truths I should have known but somehow didn't before. Failures and successes faded into insignificance and I was possessed with an all-consuming Love—so strong and intense and beautiful—everything was right—always had been right. Only human's thoughts, errors, and miscomprehension of the plan distorted facts and made the misery and unhappiness that is part of our lives. In my dream, the latter part of it, my thoughts seemed to disconnect from the divine harmony and I had to struggle to keep from turning the entire experience into a nightmare."

All these sensory phenomena—dreams, hallucinations, *presque vu*,—rest, I am convinced, on some underlying physiologic function of some brain structures, which function operates independently of what, in psychiatry, we call personality. Furthermore, any one of these phenomena, I am convinced, can be secondarily invaded and modified by the psychologic problems and other troubles of the individual.

As to the number of treatments necessary to be administered to a patient—necessary, i.e., for a cure—it is difficult to give instructions. I administer, usually, three treatments a week, one every other day. I prepare the patient not to expect any sign of improvement at the beginning. If, however, after some 20 treatments, he has not reported any improvement, I terminate this procedure and recommend another. The number of treatments that I have administered in successful cases has varied from about 15 to about 200.

Modifications of the Original Method

The great difficulty that one encounters in the treatment of anxiety cases with CO_2 is due to the fact that CO_2, since it affects the medulla and produces hyperventilation, may, in the beginning, increase the patient's anxiety. To remove this difficulty, I modified the CO_2 treatment by using nitrous oxide to introduce anesthesia. The apparatus that I set up for doing so is as follows. A tank of 100 per cent nitrous oxide and another tank of 30 per cent carbon dioxide and 70 per cent oxygen are connected by a single tube, which leads to a breathing bag. In this combination, I do not mix the two gases; but, after first opening the nitrous oxide, I apply the mask to the patient's face and let him inhale this gas for 20 to 60 seconds. Under no circumstances should the nitrous oxide be given longer than 60 seconds because it is a more dangerous gas than CO_2 and because during its administration an anoxemic state of the brain develops. During the administration of the nitrous oxide, I talk to the patient, asking him such questions as: "Are your legs numb?" "Is your face numb?" "Do you still hear me?" During this questioning, I do not lift the mask from the patient's face; his voice is audible through it.

When the patient is unable to answer verbally, I consider the anesthesia deep enough to switch over to the administration of CO_2. And so, without removing the mask from the patient's face, I close the nitrous oxide valve and turn on the CO_2. From then on, counting the respirations of CO_2, I give the required number, usually 20 to 30. Since I introduced this modification of the treatment, I have hardly ever begun the treatment of a patient with a straight administration of the CO_2 mixture; but, for the first 10 or 20 treatments, I have used the nitrous oxide modification. After about 14 to 20 of these treatments, the patient's anxiety has so decreased that I try the administration of the CO_2 mixture without the nitrous oxide introduction. If the patient objects to this straight administration of the CO_2, I do not insist upon using it; many times I have used the nitrous oxide-carbon dioxide combination from the beginning until the termination of the treatment.

My nitrous oxide combination with the carbon dioxide treatment was not, however, the first published modification of my original technique. My original method of administering the carbon dioxide treatment has undergone many other changes, changes initiated by eager research men who have wanted to improve the original method and thus achieve a greater number of recoveries. These modifications I shall designate, for the time being, by the names of those who first introduced them into the treatment.

The first of these modifications to have been published is that of P. Wilcox, who has modified the original therapy by combining carbon dioxide treatment with psychotherapy. His technique, which he has termed "psychopenetration," consists of administering 5 to 10 respirations of carbon dioxide and then asking the patient certain key questions to test the accessibility of the latter's unconscious conflicts.

The modification next published is that which has been worked out by W. Liddell Milligan of Portsmouth, England, and, I believe independently of him, by W. Sargent of London. Milligan has written:

It occurred to me that more use might be made of the "subcortical excitatory state" described by Meduna, and that it should not be necessary for the patient to lose consciousness. The following modified technique was therefore worked out. The patient receives treatment in bed in a quiet room and the procedure is briefly explained. It is emphasized that consciousness will not be lost and that after inhaling the gas he is to "let himself go" and do and say exactly what he wants. It is useful to spend some time in insuring that the patient knows what is required of him. A Boyle anesthetic apparatus is used and the patient is first allowed to inhale pure oxygen, the mask being held a few inches above the face and gradually lowered into position. . . . After a few respirations, carbon dioxide is gradually introduced until 10 to 15% is given. After 20 respirations the amount of carbon dioxide is increased to 30%, and then almost immediately lowered to the former level. The inhalation is terminated rapidly after 25 to 40 respirations. . . . As soon as the mask is removed the nursing staff retires, but should be within call lest any subsequent violence ensues. Some patients abreact immediately, but others recount former incidents for as long as half an hour before any true release of emotion takes place. It is necessary for the psychiatrist to devote at least an hour to each patient and to be content to await results. It is only rarely necessary to encourage the flow of material. When, however, abreaction occurs, it is helpful to increase the drama and attain the emotional atmosphere.

J. D. Moriaty of California has combined the classical carbon dioxide therapy with psychotherapeutic technique. Moriarty's finding:

Carbon dioxide therapy facilitates treatment by brief analytical methods through which the experienced therapist may usually uncover rather quickly the infantile trends that generally constitute the core of a neurosis. . . . Development of the transference situation is hastened by carbon dioxide therapy, and both positive and negative phases more easily worked through. Sometimes a patient who is unaware of his hostile feelings for the therapist is greatly surprised when these rise suddenly to the surface, as he emerges from the carbon dioxide coma, yet as he regains full consciousness 30 or 40 seconds later he retains sufficient memory of these negative feelings to be able to discuss them with much more therapeutic gain than at first. Occasionally the patient becomes flooded with a rush of hitherto buried feelings that disturb him considerably. At such times the therapist may find it advisable to give him another treatment in short order to dissipate this particular reaction. As skill in the technique develops it becomes possible to achieve therapeutic gains of the fundamental nature that equal or surpass those of the painfully slow and protracted psychoanalytical technique of traditional procedures.

A. A. LaVerne has worked out another modification of the carbon dioxide treatment, one which he has described under the name of "rapid coma technique." In this technique, LaVerne mixes a gas of 70 per cent carbon dioxide and 30 per cent oxygen in a 10-liter breathing bag and administers to the patient a single deep maximal inhalation. He has reported:

When the patient gives a signal that he cannot inhale any more gas, the mask is quickly removed. At that time the patient is still fully conscious. He then rapidly enters a carbon dioxide coma, or sub-coma, or hypnagogic state, during which he almost invariably visualizes a geometric, colorful pattern with or without formed symbols. Within a matter of 8 seconds he is fully awake and recalls every detail of the treatment. In the meantime, he demonstrates autonomic and motor body reactions consisting of skin changes, perspiration and flushing, mottling, motor activity and vocalizes without the usual severe exhaustion that follows the multiple breath technique of prolonged carbon dioxide.

LaVerne usually gives three treatments a week, treatments in which he administers 1 to 10 single-breath inhalations and allows between these inhalations intervals of at least three minutes. "Psychotherapy," he says, "may be utilized between treatments if the physician so desires." If, after three or four weeks, this schedule has not produced clinical improvement in the patient, LaVerne, considering that intensive treatment is then required, gives the patient up to 20 single-breath treatments daily for a period of two weeks.

LaVerne has developed a variation of his single-breath technique by using repeated inhalations of high concentrations of carbon dioxide. In this technique, he induces anesthesia by giving nitrous oxide to the patient; after anesthesia has been reached, he administers from 4 to 12 respirations of a 90 per cent to 95 per cent carbon dioxide–10 per cent to 5 per cent oxygen mixture. His best therapeutic results, he claims, he obtains with 6 to 9 breaths of this mixture. "The criterion for the optimum number of breaths is the production of physiological level of coma, with mild twitchings or mild clonic movements of face and body, lasting approximately 10 to 15 seconds. The therapist should avoid production of a deep generalized convulsive level unless the most superficial levels of coma have been ineffective after a preliminary trial of 5 to 10 treatments."

A. I. Jackman was the first to utilize the CO_2 treatment to produce therapeutic convulsions. In his technique, which he calls "carbon dioxide convulsive treatment," he utilizes carbon dioxide inhalation to a point of convulsive reactions in depressed patients who have not reacted quickly to the original carbon dioxide-inhalation therapy. He uses my original method and my nitrous oxide combination but modifies these by continuing with the carbon dioxide inhalation to the point at which the patient develops what could be described as a decerebrate fit.

W. E. Wilkinson also utilizes the CO_2 treatment to produce therapeutic convulsions.

We have used convulsive CO_2 therapy on patients who previously would have been given convulsive electroshock therapy. This group has included patients with schizophrenia, obsessive-compulsive neurosis and those with the manic and agitated depressed phases of manic depressive psychosis. These patients have shown tremendous variations in their convulsive threshold and in the intensity and duration of the convulsions. Following the CO_2 induced convulsions, the patients go through the several stages of the awakening reaction not unlike patients recovering from electric convulsive therapy. Patients who have been treated by this method usually have shown temporary relief of symptoms immediately after the treatment, but in most of them the improvement has not lasted for as long as 24 hours. A few patients have been completely relieved of their symptoms, but all of these were treated in 1952 and we do not know how permanent the relief will be.

W. M. C. Harrowes of Scotland and Z. Selinger of Canada, having reached the same conclusion independently, have achieved beneficial results by giving only 5 to 10 respirations of the 30 per cent carbon dioxide–70 per cent oxygen mixture and thus not producing any anesthesia. The administration of this limited number of respirations they repeat five to ten times during one treatment. The time between the repeated administrations of the gas they use for psychotherapy. Their modification of my original technique they call the "fractional method of carbon dioxide therapy." This method, apparently, can be used only in selected cases.

INDICATIONS

As is well known, it is extremely difficult to construct any adequate classification for the psychoneuroses. Our present-day classifications are more or less descriptive. In my "Alterations of Neurotic Pattern by Use of CO_2 Inhalation," I have listed stuttering, spastic colitis, anxiety neuroses, a feeling of inferiority, irritability, neurotic fatigue, alcoholism, homosexuality, and other character neuroses that are amenable to the carbon dioxide treatment. At the time of the publication of this article, I had not had any success with obsessive-compulsive neuroses and psychoses.

LaVerne claims that with high concentrations of CO_2—concentrations up to 95 per cent—he has achieved results in some cases of schizophrenia; but as to the efficacy of LaVerne's method in psychoses, no useful statistics are available.

Douglas MacRae has introduced the CO_2 treatment into obstetrics, where he uses it both during the pregnancy, in order to treat anxiety about delivery, and during labor, as an analgesic. He claims that "during pregnancy the CO_2 treatments were helpful in controlling the vomiting of pregnancy, insomnia, or unusual nervousness."

G. A. Silver, who has used the CO_2 treatment on a fairly large group of psychoneurotics, has succeeded in curing a woman of 40 "hysterically blind for eight years, who received a pension on the basis of her blindness." Silver has found, furthermore, that while psychoneurotic depressions respond favorably to CO_2 treatment, "it seems valid to make a distinction from the manic-depressive patients, which do not seem to be favorably affected by the CO_2-O_2 treatment."

Leonard J. Liest has found CO_2 therapy to be useful in the treatment of psychotic patients after remission has been produced by the use of shock therapies.

Temple Fay claims good results with inhalations of 20 per cent CO_2-80 per cent O_2 in patients suffering from "true types of rigidity" (parkinsonism and athetosis). Confirmation of his claims is lacking.

A. A. LaVerne claims excellent results in chronic alcoholism if he initiates the course of CO_2 therapy for the alcoholic in a hospital for at least 50 treatments. After giving these 50 treatments, he discharges the patient and puts him on a once-a-week maintenance schedule.

Anna May Smith, who has treated stutterers with the carbon dioxide therapy, has found that 21 of her 33 patients were improved—that 11 showed 100 per cent improvement; 3, 75 per cent; 2, 50 per cent; and 5, 25 per cent.

Jackman reports success with CO_2 treatment in patients with allergy, such as hayfever and asthma.

Contraindications

Contraindications for the CO_2 treatment are few; and these have been arteriosclerosis, hypertension of high degree, diseases of the heart muscle, coronary disease or attacks, and advanced emphysema. Psychiatric contraindications were first published by Simms *et al*, who have stated that "pre-psychotic states were found to be precipitated into open psychoses as a result of these treatments."

Inasmuch as we do not have any test or method that would determine the degree either of a neurosis or of its improvement or cure, for the purposes of this presentation I shall omit the word "cure" from my statistics and designate the results in terms of "improved" and "not improved" groups (Table I).

That these statistics are somewhat misleading is apparent to everybody who has an understanding of statistical principles and has been working with psychoneurotic patients. These figures give an erroneous impression because of the fact that the degree of improvement for the time being cannot be measured; therefore, patients slightly improved, improved, greatly improved, and cured are grouped as "improved" patients. These statistics, furthermore, are incomplete because

TABLE 1

	Improved	Not Improved	Total
Meduna	208	112	320
Kindwall	45	55	100
MacRae	31		31
Milligan	40		40
Pellage	7	3	10
Silver	39	11	50
Weaver et al.	8	5	13
Jackman and Schorr	8	2	10
Moriarty	62	12	74
Silver	174	76	250
LaVerne and Herman	35	15	50
A. M. Smith	21	12	33
Simms et al.	38	34	72
	716	337	1,053

many authors mentioned in their reports "large" numbers of patients whom they had treated, but referred in their statistics to only small numbers; and because other authors merely published that they had treated 30 or 40 patients with excellent results and presented three or four representative case histories, without giving statistical analyses of their whole groups. These statistics, however, cannot fail to convey to the unprejudiced reader the impression that the treatment is effective in different forms of neuroses. Of 1,053 published cases in which the CO_2 treatment has been used, 716 patients (68 per cent) have improved, and only 337 (32 per cent) have remained unimproved. This 68 per cent—a figure arrived at from computing the results of 13 authors who have treated over 1,000 cases—is interestingly identical with the over-all improvement that I published in my monograph, *Carbon Dioxide Therapy:* "Of the 100 patients, 58 were males and 42 were females. Thirty-six of the 58 male patients—that is, 62 per cent—and 32 of the 42 female patients —that is, 76 per cent—have improved from the CO_2 treatment. The over-all improvement is, therefore, that of 68 out of 100, or 68 per cent of all the cases treated."

Total Failures

A few authors have reported total failure in their use of the CO_2 treatment. The reasons would be interesting—if I were able to trace them—for the total failures of some authors as compared with the excellent results achieved by others. Determination of the reasons for these failures is possible, however, in only a few cases. One of these cases is that of Jackson A. Smith, who treated 33 patients with anxiety, hysteria, and depression. Of this group, Dr. Smith has reported, "4 patients responded promptly and sustained their improvement. Eight patients showed slight and usually temporary improvement over a period of 6 to 8 weeks. . . . Twenty-one of the 33 patients received no appreciable help from this method of treatment and in this series the procedure was considered to be of limited value."

The failure of the CO_2 method in Dr. Smith's hands is due to the fact that he apparently did not apply this treatment in a technically correct way. "Six of the patients," he says, "regularly lost consciousness as judged by their failure to recall the last few numbered inhalations." All the authors who have worked out a modification of the CO_2 treatment have agreed that loss of consciousness—that is to say, anesthesia—is an absolutely necessary factor in producing results with the treatment. Doctor Smith's failure to produce anesthesia in about 80 per cent of the cases which he treated explains his meager results and does not controvert the effectiveness of the CO_2 therapy.

The reader must be reminded that Harrowes and Selinger have been using the fractional method of CO_2 therapy, a method that does not produce coma, *in selected cases only;* and that they have been combining this method with psychotherapy.

Hargrove, Bennett, and Steele, who treated 50 patients with anxiety, obtained 17 improvements; but 33 patients did not improve at all. In contrast, they have reported, of 50 patients with anxiety whom they treated by psychotherapy only, 14 recovered,

26 improved, and only 10 showed no change. Their final conclusion is that more patients improved from psychotherapy alone than from a combination of CO_2 and psychotherapy. The shortcoming of these authors' work was that in anxiety patients they used straight CO_2 instead of the nitrous oxide-carbon dioxide combination. Thus, in many cases they increased the patient's anxiety and, furthermore, produced abreactions of such magnitude that the psychotherapist could not appropriately deal with them. By using the nitrous oxide-CO_2 combination and by giving lesser amounts of CO_2, they could have produced abreactions of smaller magnitude, which could have been easily handled by the psychotherapist or by the patients themselves.

Arthurs *et al.* treated 14 stutterers with a combination of nitrous oxide and CO_2. None of these patients recovered from stuttering, nor did their speech improve. With the lack of description of the procedure of these authors, it is impossible to conjecture the cause of their absolute lack of success.

Mode of Action of the CO_2 Therapy

The effectiveness of the CO_2 therapy may be explained by (1) the doctor-patient relationship, (2) autosuggestion and other psychological processes, or (3) physiological effects of the gas upon the whole organism. I cannot help feeling that any explanation that attributes the effectiveness of this therapy to an improved doctor-patient relation or to transference, autosuggestion, abreaction, and other so-called "psychological" processes is no explanation whatsoever, but only a simple description of how the doctor thinks of his work and himself. And his mode of thinking is conditioned by the frame of references which he has obtained through his previous education. Moreover, even if any of the so-called "psychological" explanations that I have designated are partly or wholly acceptable, the physiological basis of the "psychological" explanation should be given in terms of the brain tissue and its function. I do not want to minimize the so-called psychological effects of any treatment situation; but we ought to know that beyond or beneath any psychological function there is the function of the brain, and that unless we can explain our work in terms germane and applicable to the tissue of the brain and to its function, although we may have described a process, we have not explained it at all.

It was known for some time that CO_2 raises the threshold of stimulation of the excised nerve cell, increases its membrane potential, and, finally, increases the ability of the nerve to conduct trains of impulses. It was known, also, that CO_2 delays the appearance of fatigue of the stimulated nerve. Because of recent researches, we now know more of the action of CO_2. Seifritz has found that CO_2 changes the state of protoplasm from sol to gel; that if the concentration of the CO_2 is too high, or if the exposure to it is too long, the sol-to-gel conversion becomes irreversible. Dusser de Barenne, McCulloch, and Nimms have found that the increased acidity of the brain tissue caused by CO_2 is associated with low electric activity and a decreased excitability of the cortex. McLellan and Elliott have found that CO_2 destroys acetylcholine by lowering the pH in the brain. All these effects revealed by recent researches amount to a decreased activity, or a resting state, of the nervous system saturated by CO_2.

From recent researches we have learned of other effects of the action of CO_2 upon the nervous system. Bain and Klein have ascertained that CO_2 enables the brain more clearly to balance energy demands with oxidative processes. K. E. Schaffer has found that if experimental animals are exposed to CO_2, hypersecretion of epinephrine occurs, and that this hypersecretion of epinephrine is followed by hyposecretion, the latter due to a diminished synthesis. Schaffer has found, too, that as an effect of the CO_2 there is a hyper- and a subsequent hypo-phase in the adrenal cortex and in the basophilic cells of the pituitary gland, and that the thyroid gland becomes somewhat inactivated. Pollock, Stein, and Gyarfas have found that CO_2 inhalation produces low-amplitude, fast cortical activity; and that the response of the thalamus to CO_2 is much less than that of the cortex, as is the hypothalamic response, which shows lower-than-cortical amplitudes and slower frequencies.

The data that I have just cited indicate the following trend: (1) increased cerebral inhibition that is repeated in the cortex of the brain at every treatment; (2) decreased excitability of the cortex that is reproduced by every treatment; (3) an effect of the CO_2 upon the carbohydrate metabolism of the brain, enabling it more clearly to balance energy demands with the oxidative process; (4) a changed balance in the activity of the pituitary, adrenal, and thyroid glands. If this biochemical trend is pertinent to the fact of psychoneurosis, it follows that psychoneurotic's brain structure is hyperirritable; and either that the psychoneurotic's brain does not balance energy demands with oxidative processes properly, or that there is a disturbance in the distribution of this process. Finally, we may assume that there is some disturbance in the interaction of at least three important glands—the pituitary, the adrenal and the thyroid glands. These disturbances that appear on the perceptual level to the patient and to the doctor as disturbances of the mind or as psychosomatic symptoms are rectified by the action of CO_2.

On the phenomenological or clinical level, three modes of improvement resulting from the CO_2 treatment are discernible in the patients. Observations of these different modes will lead many a research man to believe that the improvements move exclusively on the psychological level and thus forget that no "psychological" way of improvement is possible unless it is based on cortical, neuronal, or glandular changes.

The first and most frequent clinical mode of improvement during CO_2 treatment is manifested by simple diminution and disappearance of the psychoneurotic symptoms. The patients who experience this mode of improvement show decreased emotionality and decreased sensitivity to internal and external stimuli. These changes are apparent in a decrease in and, later, a disappearance of exaggerated reactions, in improved psychological economy, and, sometimes, in considerable changes in physiological activities. Reduction of frigidity in women, normalization of sexual activity in men, improvement in the texture of skin, nails, and hair, increase in the size of the female breast, disappearance of menstrual cramps, and normalization of the menstrual cycle are common changes in the improved cases.

The second mode of improvement during CO_2 treatment occurs through what appears as abreaction. There are three varieties of abreaction. One is the known realistic abreaction, during which the patient relives a previous experience and discharges, or acts out, pent-up emotions. This variety of abreaction occurs in full consciousness and is recoverable by the patient. A second variety of abreaction, and one which I have observed frequently, I call allegoric abreaction. In this, the patient discharges realistic emotions; but these are connected not with a recovered memory but rather with a symbolic dream. This variety of abreaction is recoverable by the patient, but its real meaning remains hidden unless it is explained to him. A third variety of abreaction is utterly unconscious, inasmuch as it occurs when the patient is in the anesthesia phase of the CO_2 treatment. This variety of abreaction is manifested by the patients having, upon awakening, but a vague memory of some unpleasant experience.

The third mode of improvement during CO_2 treatment is the rarest but the most fascinating one. This mode of improvement I call "spontaneous analysis of the patient and reintegration to a more normal personality pattern." The patient who experiences this mode of improvement may not show any considerable emotional discharge and may or may not have either a symbolic dream, or a vague recollection of some past experience during his dream. Later in the day, however, or a few days after the treatment, he recollects forgotten or repressed childhood memories and other pathogenic experiences and discovers the causal relation of these memories and these other pathogenic experiences to his actual symptoms. As the treatment proceeds, he recovers more and more of his material, and the pathologic symptoms correspondingly decrease or disappear.

It would be an error on the part of the therapist to force any one of the above modes of improvement upon every one of his patients. It seems that some inherent quality of the brain is the factor that will determine the mode of improvement to be followed by the individual patient. If the therapist notices that a patient is inclined, for instance, to produce realistic or allegoric abreaction, he had better switch over to Milligan's and Sargent's abreactive technique, which I have described; on the other hand, there is no use in forcing abreactions upon a patient whose brain has chosen the modality of improvement which I have described as "simple diminution and disappearance of the symptoms." The patient should not be expected to adopt and to adjust himself to any particular method of administration of the CO_2 treatment chosen or preferred by the therapist. Contrariwise, in order to adjust the technique to the need of the patient, the therapist should use the CO_2 treatment and its modifications as flexibly as he is capable of doing.

Strange as the pharmacological method of the CO_2 treatment may seem, I feel that it has not come to us unheralded. May I remind the reader of one of the last works of Sigmund Freud, *Outline of Psychoanalysis,* first published, in German, in 1940. In this little book, Freud, speaking of the failures of psychoanalytical technique, states: "It is true that we do not always succeed in winning but at least we can usually see why it is that we have not won. Those who have been following our discussion only out of therapeutical interest will perhaps turn away in contempt after this admission. But we are here concerned with therapy only insofar as it works by psychological methods; and for the time being we have no other. *The future may teach us how to exercise a direct influence, by means of particular chemical substances, upon the amounts of energy and their distribution in the apparatus of the mind. It may be that there are other undreamed of possibilities of therapy.*"

The first of these "undreamed of possibilities of therapy," possibilities of influencing "the amounts of energy and their distribution in the apparatus of the mind" by administration of carbon dioxide, I offer to those psychiatrists who have the vision and the courage to follow a still-unbeaten path.

THE MODE OF ACTION OF CARBON DIOXIDE TREATMENT IN HUMAN NEUROSES

L. J. Meduna, M.D.

The CO_2 treatment of neurotic conditions consists of repeated inhalations of a gas mixture of 30 per cent CO_2 and 70 per cent O_2. The number of inhalations necessary to produce curative effects varies from patient to patient and shows a slight variation from treatment to treatment with the same patient, ranging from about 17 to 45 deep respirations. The number of treatments necessary to produce clinical cures varies from 15 to about 150. The treatments are usually given three times a week.

The mode of action of the CO_2 treatment, for didactic purposes, can be considered on two levels. On the clinical level I have observed four different modes of beneficial reactions: (1) Simple decreasing and disappearance of the symptoms; (2) Direct abreaction of pathogenic emotions; (3) Indirect abreaction, and (4) Spontaneous analysis and reintegration.

By the term indirect abreaction I refer to the phenomenon of discharging pathologic emotions in connection with symbolic dreams or pseudohallucinations. The indirect abreaction, by means of dreams, is illustrated by the case of a girl who had spastic colitis of five years' duration. She felt nervous, was afraid of people, felt that no one understood her, and could not look into people's eyes because she felt uneasy while she was doing so. During one of her early treatments she screamed, covered her face with her hands, and turned violently from side to side while under anesthesia. When she recovered her composure she remembered that in her dream she had seen many ugly faces leering contemptuously at her.

During the further course of the treatment similar dreams

were produced by the patient with the difference that the faces in her dreams became more and more friendly and the patient was less and less afraid of them until one day she awakened from the treatment smiling. She then stated that the faces in her dream were very pleasant looking people. From that time on the patient was no longer afraid of people, she could look freely into the eyes of anyone and her pathologic social inhibitions had disappeared.

A good example of indirect abreaction in connection with pseudohallucinations occurred in the case of a patient who became an alcoholic as a consequence of an anxiety neurosis. This patient, upon awakening from the CO_2 anesthesia, looked at the psychiatrist with an expression of horror and said: "Your face looks horrible; I would like to slap it." The patient apparently was under a great tension, her fists opened and closed, and apparently she had to restrain herself forcibly from hitting the doctor. The patient kept saying: "Your face keeps changing all the time; one second you have a horrible face and the next second you have your normal face." This phenomenon probably should be understood in terms of "Gestalt Psychology." The patient was visibly upset when these pseudohallucinations terminated in about two minutes. She returned three days later trembling, crying, and apparently under extreme tension. At that time she stated that eight hours after having left the psychiatrist's office the last time she suddenly remembered whose face appeared superimposed on the psychiatrist's; to her great horror she recognized her mother's face. At the same time, she realized she had a great hatred for her dead mother of whom, consciously, she thought with great love and sorrow. Reassurance and one more treatment restored the composure of the patient.

The above described experience constitutes a transition to the fourth mode of action of the CO_2, that is: the spontaneous analysis and reintegration to normal personality pattern.

Patients of this group do not show any considerable emotional discharge during the treatment.

However, many hours after the treatment, these patients recollect forgotten or suppressed pathogenic experiences and discover their causal relations to the actual symptoms.

The mode of action of the CO_2 treatment on the somatic level consists of at least two groups of known phenomena: (1) the neurophysiologic changes, and (2) the endocrinologic changes produced by the CO_2.

The neurophysiologic changes in the function of the nerve were determined by Lorente de No as follows: (a) CO_2 produces an increase in the membrane potential of the nerve which increase in the membrane potential is accompanied by a rise of the threshold of stimulation of the nerve; (b) CO_2 increases the height and prolongs the duration of the action potential; (c) CO_2 produces an increase in the duration of the negative afterpotential; (d) CO_2 decreases the fatigability of the nerve cell. CO_2 increases the ability of the nerve to conduct trains of impulses because the presence of CO_2 delays the appearance of the signs of fatigue.

On a neurophysiologic basis the mode of action of CO_2 can be understood if we assume that a neurotic condition is a failure of homeostasis.

In the neurotic failure of homeostasis, I assume, an incessant reverberation in the feed-back mechanisms occurs in which the output of the system is reinforcing the input so that which should have been a negative feed-back has become a positive feed-back. CO_2, therefore, cures psychoneurotic conditions in which by repeated administrations it has permanently increased the threshold of stimulation in the pathologically reverberating circuits and, by turning positive feed-back circuits into negative feed-back circuits, it has achieved homeostasis.

There are animal experimental data to show that CO_2 produces endocrinologic changes in the test animals. These changes are not well known as yet and their role in the human neuroses is even less known. The changes are a preliminary increase in the function of the anterior lobe of the pituitary gland and an increased function of the adrenal cortex. Both increased functions are accompanied by hypertrophy of these glands. The increase in function of these glands is followed by a decrease in the function of the same glands. During these changes in the pituitary and in the adrenal glands, the thyroid gland shows a decrease in its function without accompanying anatomic change.

How the endocrinologic changes produced by the inhalation of the CO_2 enter into the mode of action of the CO_2 treatment is unknown. In several cases, however, I observed an improvement in the texture of the skin, the lustre of the hair, and brittle nails became healthy.

In several instances women with small breasts reported that their breasts increased in size. Above all, the normalizing of the menstrual cycle is a fairly common phenomenon during the CO_2 treatment.

Further endocrinologic research is desired to elucidate the above described changes.

THE GRANTHAM LOBOTOMY FOR THE RELIEF OF NEUROTIC SUFFERING

Frank J. Ayd, Jr., M.D.

Neurotic suffering is symptomatic of a variety of psychiatric disorders in which the personality of the patient is relatively intact even after years of illness. It may be due to persistent anxiety or depression, agonizing obsessions, recurrent doubts, irresistible compulsions, or torturing phobias. The primary cause of neurotic suffering often is irremediable and the resistance of these disorders to the usual method of psychiatric treatment is well known. In these cases, therefore, relief from neurotic suffering becomes the prime objective of treatment.

The relief from neurotic suffering that can be obtained by adequate psychosurgery is well recognized. However, psychosurgery for this purpose has seldom been employed in patients with fairly well preserved personalities, because of the personality changes, intellectual deficits, and convulsions that may follow the standard lobotomy operations.

In 1951, Grantham announced a new method of selective destruction of the ventromedial quadrant of the prefrontal lobe by electrocoagulation which eliminated many of the undesirable effects of the standard lobotomy procedure. Initially, Grantham performed his operation for the relief of pain in cancer patients. He observed the most beneficial results in those patients in whom anxiety was predominant. Since then, he has operated on approximately 200 psychiatric patients with some excellent results. McIntyre, Mayfield and McIntyre, in 1954, reported their favorable experience with the Grantham lobotomy in 30 psychotic and neurotic patients. These preliminary reports suggested that the Grantham lobotomy was superior to conventional psychosurgery for the relief of neurotic suffering.

Clinical Material

To evaluate the therapeutic effectiveness and advantages of the Grantham lobotomy this operation was performed on 30 non-hospitalized patients ranging in age from 24 to 75. These patients were severe, chronic neurotics or psychotics in whom neurotic symptomatology was paramount. All were seriously incapacitated by illnesses of three to 30 years duration. Their illnesses had been refractory to one or more of the following therapies: psychotherapy, group therapy, psychoanalysis, insulin and electro-shock, subcoma insulin, and hospitalization. In addition these patients had not benefited from Thorazine (300 mgm. to 800 mgm. daily) or Serpasil (3 mgm. to 10 mgm. daily) which they received for a period of two months to one year. Included in this group were 12 chronic mixed psychoneuroses, five chronic obsessive-compulsive neuroses, nine involutional depressions, two pseudo-neurotic schizophrenias, one paranoid schizophrenia, and one catatonic schizophrenia.

Selection of Patients

In the selection of patients for psychosurgery three factors are important: (a) the degree of anxiety and its incapacitating effects, (b) its intractability, and (c) the intactness of the personality. In view of the gravity of the decision to be made, in addition to repeated psychiatric examinations, special tests such as Rorschach and Funkenstein should be done whenever possible. If these preoperative investigative procedures disclose severe anxiety or depression, the patient is considered a proper candidate for lobotomy, providing there are no associated serious psychopathic traits.

A. *Psychoneuroses:* Twelve chronic psychoneurotic patients in this study suffered primarily from anxiety which was expressed in a variety of ways. They complained of persistent tension and apprehension, easy fatigability, feelings of inadequacy and inferiority, inability to concentrate, fear of insanity or some disease such as cancer, irritability, insomnia, crying spells, and depression. They suffered from repeated alarming anxiety attacks and psychosomatic disturbances. For years these patients sought relief from their symptoms by frequent visits to general practitioners, internists, and psychiatrists. In a fruitless search for a physical cause for their symptoms they had repeated cardiograms, x-rays, and other laboratory tests. Some were hospitalized at least once for surgery. They tried innumerable drugs, hypnosis, psychotherapy, psychoanalysis and in a few cases shock therapy. Because they had not responded to any previous treatment and permanent disability seemed inevitable, these patients were considered apt candidates for the Grantham lobotomy.

B. *Obsessional Neurosis:* No two obsessive-compulsive patients are alike. Therefore, obsessional patients must be carefully assessed for psychosurgery. In this study there were five intensely anxious obsessional neurotics whose distress was due primarily to obsessional thinking and phobias rather than to irresistible compulsions. They were tortured by recurring thoughts of harming someone. They suffered with religious scruples. Fears of every sort haunted them. They lived in constant doubt and had to go over things again and again. Frequently, they could not cope with the ordinary stresses and vicissitudes of life. Although they dreaded insanity and commitment to a psychiatric institution, they often asked if it was safe for them to live outside of a hospital. They were chosen for modified psychosurgery because they had not been helped by years of psychotherapy and psychoanalysis and there was no hope for a spontaneous remission.

C. *Depressive States:* Different varieties of depressive reactions may occur in the involutional period. Those which occur in the chronically anxious patients are characterized by intense anxiety and depression. These patients frequently are made worse by electroconvulsive therapy which relieves the depression but causes mounting anxiety and agitation. Many of these patients recover from their depressed state with conservative treatment. In some patients, however, the anxious depression becomes chronic.

In this study there were seven chronically anxious patients who became depressed during the involutional period. They complained of hot flushes, dizziness, headaches, rapid heart, indigestion, anorexia, constipation, and insomnia. Their mood was anxious and depressed and crying spells were frequent. They were sensitive and troubled by feelings of guilt, remorse, and unreality. They lacked confidence. They had no interest in their usual pursuits and thought of suicide. ECT had been administered to five of these patients. One patient had had 90 shock treatments and another over 200 treatments. All feared shock therapy because it made them so anxious. Because these patients had not responded to ECT, hospitalization, and other psychiatric treatment, they were selected for a modified lobotomy.

The effectiveness of ECT for involutional depression is well documented. However, there are some involutional depressives who respond initially to ECT but subsequently relapse. In these patients repeated convulsive treatments produce a transient elevation of the mood but no change in their melancholic ideation. In this study there were two chronic involutional depressives, who had not responded to repeated courses of ECT. They complained of unrelenting feelings of despondency and disinterest in anything but themselves. They spoke continuously of how they felt. They were self-deprecatory and self-derogatory. Hence they were selected for modified psychosurgery.

D. *Schizophrenic Reactions:* In this study, modified psychosurgery was considered for those schizophrenic patients who were not deteriorated. These patients were more disabled by the intensity of their neurotic suffering than by delusions and hallucinations.

Technique

Bilateral burr holes are made in the frontal area 6 to 8 cm. from the glabella and 2½ cm. lateral to the midline. The frontal horn of each lateral ventricle is injected with 10 cc. of air. Insulated electrodes are inserted into the frontal lobe parallel to the sagittal sinus and anterior to the frontal horn of the lateral ventricle until they contact the floor of the skull. The electrodes are then withdrawn 2 cm. and their position checked by lateral and anteroposterior roentgenograms. If the electrodes are not parallel or if the tip of either electrode is not in the correct position in the ventromedial quadrant, they are reinserted until their proper position is confirmed by x-ray. Electrocoagulation is then performed by turning on the current for 30 seconds at position 10 on the Universal Bovie electro-surgical unit.

Post-Operative Course

A. *Surgical:* In the immediate post-operative period (24 to 72 hours) most patients run a slight elevation of temperature up to 102 degrees. This rise of temperature is important prognostically since it occurred in most of the patients with a favorable therapeutic result. The majority of those patients with slight or no improvement did not have a post-operative elevation of temperature.

There are no marked variations in pulse or blood pressure following the Grantham operation. Improved patients had a decrease in their basal blood pressure of 10 to 20 mm. Hg. which begins to return to the pre-operative level after four to six months.

Post-lobotomy convulsions have not occurred in this group of patients. One man had a severe post-operative infection with meningitis. One woman hemorrhaged on the operating table but her post-operative course was uneventful. Most individuals were ambulatory 48 hours post-operatively. All but five patients were discharged from the hospital on the third to the fifth post-operative day.

B. *Psychiatric:* After recovery from the anesthetic most patients are mentally alert, and usually the benefits of the operation are apparent immediately. Psychiatric examination on the second and third post-operative day reveals an absence of confusion, disorientation, and retrograde amnesia, permitting an early evaluation of the patient's mental state. Impressive relief from anxiety and depression is observed in improved patients, while little or no change can be detected in those who are unimproved. Only one patient who appeared improved in the immediate post-operative period subsequently relapsed. All the others maintained their initial improvement for the six months to one year follow-up period.

A mild euphoric reaction occurred in two women. This euphoria appeared on the second post-operative day and subsided without special treatment within a week. A delirioid reaction occurred on the third post-operative day in two men who had been receiving barbiturates for several months prior to surgery. The clinical picture in these two cases closely resembled barbiturate withdrawal. Recovery from this delirioid reaction occurred within two weeks.

In this series of patients no serious adverse personality changes occurred. There was no release of undesirable neurotic or psychopathic traits. One elderly woman became more critical of, and hostile toward a relative with whom she has never had satisfactory interpersonal relations. Another elderly woman was quite irritable and argumentative, but this was controlled by Thorazine. Inertia, apathy, abnormal behavior, overtalkativeness, outspokenness, lack of initiative, wetting, excessive appetite, and loss of sexual control or moral inhibition did not occur in any of these patients.

Therapeutic Results

A Definition of Terms: 1—Marked improvement indicates dramatic relief of neurotic suffering, especially anxiety or depression. These patients were greatly improved over the pre-operative level, being able to cope adequately with situations which formerly evoked intense emotional reactions.

2—Moderate improvement means that there was less spectacular relief of neurotic suffering. These patients still have some neurotic symptoms, but they concern the patient less.

3—Slight improvement signifies some reduction in tension. Otherwise, these patients are essentially the same as pre-operatively.

4—Unimproved indicates that the patient derived no benefit from surgery.

The Grantham lobotomy produced marked improvement in 18 patients, moderate improvement in six, and slight improvement in two. Four patients were unimproved (Table I). This high rate of improvement is partially due to the selection of only the most suitable candidates for the operation.

TABLE 1

THERAPEUTIC RESULTS

Diagnosis	Marked	Moderate	Slight	Unimproved
Psychoneurosis, Mixed	7	4		1
Obsessional Neurosis	1	1	1	2
Involutional Anxious Depression	7			
Involutional depression	1	1		
Schizophrenia				
Pseudo-Neurotic	1			1
Paranoid	1			
Catatonic			1	
TOTAL	18	6	2	4

RORSCHACH STUDIES

A pre-operative Rorschach was administered to 22 patients. In general, these tests revealed the effects of prolonged anxiety in the retention of rigid intellectual controls with a resultant decline in spontaneity. Except for the obsessive-compulsives, who expressed their anxiety in a ceaseless striving for quantity, their productivity was below that of the normal. Their thinking was stereotyped and perseverative. They were prone to make hasty generalizations with inadequate articulation of the stimulus. They were unable to delay their impulses to allow them to engage in creative inner living. A weakening of control in the affective realm rendered them highly irritable but lacking in capacity for genuine emotional rapport. The Rorschach pattern did not disclose any positive signs for predicting the clinical outcome.

Funkenstein Test

Pre- and post-operative Funkenstein tests were performed on 21 patients. Pre-operatively 16 patients were in Groups VI and VII, four in Group I, and one in Group IV. The physiologic reaction of these patients to Mecholyl was moderate to marked. Epinephrine precipitable anxiety occurred in eight patients.

One month post-operatively, the Funkenstein tests revealed a mean fall in the basal blood pressure of 13 mm Hg. The physiological reactions of these patients to Mecholyl were more normal. Six of the eight patients with epinephrine precipitable anxiety pre-operatively, had the same reaction post-operatively. Thirteen of the 16 patients in Groups VI and VII pre-operatively fell into Group II or III post-operatively. Two other Group VI patients were in Group I post-operatively. Two of the four patients in Group I were in Group III after lobotomy. The remaining patients were in the same Funkenstein group pre- and post-operatively.

Advantages of Grantham Lobotomy

There are many advantages to the Grantham lobotomy which make this operation superior to conventional psychosurgery for neurotic suffering. This operation causes little destruction of the cortex. The lesion produced in the ventromedial quadrant is relatively small in contrast to the extensive area of destruction caused by conventional psychosurgery. This minimal damage to the cortex and the limited subcortical lesion substantially reduce the hazard of post-operative personality changes and convulsions.

Since the lesion in the ventromedial quadrant is small, it may not transact all of the fronto-thalamic fibers. The patient may only partially benefit from the operation. If necessary, therefore, the operative lesion may be enlarged by a second or third operation. Two patients in this study were unimproved after the first Grantham lobotomy. A second operation produced moderate improvement in one and slight improvement in the other.

Ventromedial quadrant electrocoagulation places little stress upon the patient's physical constitution. Physical disorders which would make conventional psychosurgery hazardous are not a contraindication to the Grantham lobotomy. The patients in this study had a variety of cardiovascular and pulmonary diseases which did not increase the operative risk.

Psychosurgery is not a procedure of last resort. It is a part of the total therapeutic program. It should be followed by psychotherapy and other rehabilitative measures. The rapidity with which a patient recovers from the Grantham operation, along with the absence of the psychic disturbances that follow standard lobotomy, permits the initiation of psychotherapy and rehabilitation in the immediate post-operative period. This is a decided advantage over other forms of psychosurgery.

Since the Grantham lobotomy usually does not cause personality changes and the recovery period is so rapid, lengthy hospitalization and special nursing care is unnecessary. The patients herein reported were in ward beds. The majority were ambulatory on the second or third post-operative day and were well able to tend to their personal needs. All but five patients were discharged from the hospital on the third to the fifth post-operative day. These factors make the Grantham operation economical, a consideration of prime importance to the private patient whose finances have been depleted by an expensive chronic illness.

This operation does not create any serious cosmetic problems, especially for the women. The operative scar is just behind the hair line. After the bandages have been removed, the women can conveniently cover the shaved area by rearranging their hair style. For the female patient this is of the utmost importance. In this study the women were not self-conscious about their appearance and this encouraged early socialization.

Summary

Thirty chronic neurotic and psychotic patients in whom neurotic suffering was paramount have been treated by the Grantham lobotomy. Pre-operatively, these patients had been refractory to the usual methods of psychiatric treatment. The Grantham operation produced marked improvement in 18 patients, moderate improvement in six, and slight improvement in two. Four were unimproved.

This paper covers the selection of patients, the post-operative course, and the advantages of this psychosurgical procedure. It indicates that the Grantham lobotomy is a tremendous step forward in the treatment of neurotic suffering.

TREATMENT OF ANXIETY STATES WITH MEPROBAMATE (MILTOWN)

WALTER A. OSINSKI, M.D.

In June, 1954, a drug, meprobamate (Miltown*), was called to my attention. The drug was discovered and studied pharmacologically by Dr. Frank M. Berger, who was also responsible for developing mephenesin.

Meprobamate is 2-methyl-2-n-propyl-1,3-propanediol dicarbamate. Pharmacologic experiments showed that the drug exerts selective interneuronal blocking action, as does mephenesin. It relaxed skeletal muscle but did not affect monosynaptic reflexes, peripheral nerve, or the myoneural junction. Meprobamate was also reported to be longer acting and more reliable in its results; it did not produce the nausea and vomiting that were often concomitants of therapy with mephenesin. Strikingly different from the effects of mephenesin was a pronounced and long-lasting tranquilizing effect apparent on all animals studied.

Monkeys treated with meprobamate lost their natural fear and hostility and became friendly and amendable to petting and handling. Interestingly, they did not become "dopey" or indifferent to their surroundings, but remained alert and curious and fully retained their appetite. Neuropharmacologic investigations using electroencephalographic recordings showed pronounced influence of the drug on subcortical structures, with greatest slowing and synchronizing of potentials from the thalamus. This tranquilizing action of the drug interested me

* The trade name of Wallace Laboratories for meprobamate is Miltown. Meprobamate used in this study was supplied by Wallace Laboratories.

in testing its possibilities clinically with patients in the Psychiatric Department at Albany Hospital.

Scope of the Study

The patients studied were seen during the period Sept. 15, 1954, to May 1, 1955, and were mostly referred from general practitioners or from medical consultants. All patients studied showed extraordinary anxiety, tension, or "nervousness" either as the only complaint or as important among other complaints. Within the limits of this criterion of selection, all patients who came during the period of the study were included, regardless of the diagnosis and regardless of whether the illness was acute or chronic.

Patients who required hospitalization were not accepted, and the psychotics who were included were borderline and ambulatory. One hundred and thirteen patients were treated with meprobamate during this study.

Procedure. Patients were given a psychiatric interview on admission and were seen at intervals of one week, and later of two weeks, as progress permitted. Psychotherapy was in all cases minimal. Patients who did not show good results from meprobamate treatment in a reasonable period of time—usually two or three weeks—were transferred to other treatment. All patients, however, whatever the duration of treatment, have been included in the analysis of results.

Dosage. The standard dosage used was one 400 mg. tablet three times a day. A few patients received an additional tablet before going to sleep at night. In occasional instances the dosage was reduced to one tablet twice a day when this appeared adequate as a maintenance dosage.

Standards of Evaluation. Two criteria were used in evaluating the results of treatment with meprobamate: (1) the extent of relief from presenting symptoms and (2) the degree of improvement in social and work adjustment. The following definitions were followed in assigning final ratings: Very good improvement—substantial to complete relief of symptoms with good social and work adjustment. Good improvement—considerable relief of symptoms with significant improvement in social and work adjustment. Some improvement—some relief of symptoms but no improvement in social or work adjustment. No improvement—negligible or no response to treatment with meprobamate.

Results

Table I shows the conditions in which meprobamate was used and the results obtained. In patients classified as being in anxiety states, anxiety, "nervousness," and tension were the sole or clearly dominant presenting symptoms. The psychoneurotic conditions classified under "other" did not fit into any of the other categories and presented mixed symptoms such as anxiety and depression or other more complicated neurotic patterns.

The results shown in Table I indicate that meprobamate has a definite effectiveness in anxiety states. In other disturbed conditions the drug appears of value in proportion to the com-

TABLE 1

Response to Meprobamate Treatment of 113 Psychiatric Patients

Diagnosis	Total cases	Very good	Good	Some	None	% Very good or good	% Some improvement
Psychoneurosis							
Anxiety state	52	15	26	8	3	79	94
Phobic	4		2	1	1		
Obsessive-compulsive	6	1		4	1		
Conversion reaction	6			2	4		
Other	19	2	11	2	4	68	79
Personality disorder							
Alcoholic addiction	7	4	2		1		
Barbiturate addiction	2	2					
Manic-depressive	7	2	2	2	1		
Schizophrenia	4		1	3			
Involutional depression	2			2			
Various	4	2	1		1		
TOTAL	113	28	45	24	16	65	86

ponents of anxiety and tension that are present. These results confirm closely the observations of Borrus and Selling. Meprobamate was also of considerable value in the treatment of alcoholism and of barbiturate addiction.

The manic-depressives were treated with meprobamate only after prior treatment of the depression by electroconvulsive therapy. The results reported, therefore, describe the degree to which postelectroshock confusion and tension were relieved in these conditions. The schizophrenic group consisted of 1 acute paranoid, 2 acute unclassified, and 1 chronic undifferentiated. The 1 case showing a good response was in the acute unclassified category. The group listed as "various" consisted of 2 cases of cerebral arteriosclerosis and 2 of post-traumatic encephalopathy, all with anxiety. The completely unresponsive case was one of cerebral arteriosclerosis.

The following cases illustrate the manner in which symptoms of tension and anxiety were overcome by the use of meprobamate.

Case 1. This 33 year old white woman gave a history of always having been somewhat nervous, even as a child. Both her parents were considered to be excitable people, but there was no evidence of mental illness. She made an uneventful adjustment in high school, and after graduation obtained a job as a secretary.

During the five years prior to her coming to the psychiatrist she had noticed fatigability and poor appetite and on occasion developed headaches. During the three months before her visit she began to complain of tension feelings in the back of the neck, occasionally experienced dizzy spells, and was aware of nervousness, particularly under pressure. About this time she was not only quite active on her job but was also making preparations for her marriage. Although she did not express any concern about her contemplated marriage and did not believe herself to be unduly upset, she was quite disturbed about her symptoms, namely, fatigability, tension feelings in the neck, and feeling somewhat sluggish.

Psychiatric interview failed to reveal any significant pathology. However, during the interview she appeared quite tense and restless and displayed increased heart rate and perspiration. The mere discussion of the various factors that might be contributing to her present state of affairs did not bring about any change in her symptomatology. She was evaluated by a general practitioner, who considered that she might be suffering from a hypothyroid state, but this was not substantiated by clinical tests.

She was started on phenobarbital, 1/4 gr. four times a day, without significant change. She was then started on meprobamate, one tablet three times a day, and within one week was free from her acute tension symptoms. She began to sleep soundly. Her general feeling of apprehension and concern over her physical status quickly disappeared. When interviewed two weeks later she told the examiner that she did not feel it was necessary to continue the medication any longer. When medication was discontinued, she continued to get along uneventfully. She married and is now pregnant and does not display any evidence of the symptoms that were evident at the time of her first interview.

Case 2. This 31 year old white man was apparently well until about three years before coming to treatment, at which time he began to notice nervousness, inability to concentrate, and periodic episodes of depression. These symptoms occurred at a time when he was attending a religious school and was having considerable difficulty in accepting his intended role as a clergyman. Although he was passing his subjects satisfactorily and was being praised for his accomplishments, he remained very uncomfortable. In spite of these sypmtoms he continued to pursue his objective. One day while attending classes he suddenly fainted. He was taken to a physician who evaluated him from a physical standpoint and made a tentative diagnosis of idiopathic epilepsy. He was placed on diphenylhydantoin and phenobarbital but his symptoms continued. He had at least four more fainting spells and finally had to leave the school.

After returning home he obtained a job as a clerk but soon found considerable difficulty in relating himself to people, particularly his superiors. His tension symptoms began to mount. He became irritable and found it difficult to concentrate on his work. At this time he consulted a psychiatrist. He was quite dejected over the fact that he had lost almost six years of his life in study, and he considered himself a failure. Psychotherapy gradually resulted in the disappearance of his depressive symptoms but he continued to remain quite tense.

He was started on amobarbital sodium, 1 gr. three times a day, and on this regimen noted only moderate improvement. He was then placed on 50 mg. of chlorpromazine four times a day and his symptoms became much more intense. After one week this drug was discontinued and he was then placed on meprobamate, 400 mg. three times a day. After one week he told the psychiatrist that for the first time in approximately four years he had experienced the best relief of his symptoms.

He is now working on his job, is married, and is getting long uneventfully. He has noted that it is necessary for him to continue taking 400 mg. of meprobamate three times a day. Whenever he stops the medication his symptoms return to a moderate degree. He has continued to get along on the drug without formal psychiatric treatment.

Combined Therapy. In 21 cases other drugs were used in conjunction with meprobamate. In Table II the therapeutic response obtained after administration of meprobamate with other drugs is analyzed and the results are compared with those obtained after meprobamate only. Meprobamate was given in combination with amobarbital sodium in 11 of the cases of anxiety reactions, 3 of the cases of the "other" psychoneuroses, and 1 of the cases of cerebral arteriosclerosis. The combined treatment accounted for four of the very good and seven of the good responses in the anxiety reactions, one very good and two good reactions in the "other" psychoneuroses, and the one very good result in allaying anxiety in cerebral arteriosclerosis.

TABLE 2
Meprobamate Used with Other Drugs

Medications used	Total cases	%	Very good	Good	Some	None	% Very good or good	% Some benefit
Meprobamate alone	92	81.4	21	33	23	15	58.9	83.7
Meprobamate with amobarbital sodium	15	13.3	6	9			100.0	100.0
Meprobamate with other drugs	6	5.3	1	3	1	1	66.6	83.3
Total	113	100.0	28	45	24	16	64.6	85.8

Meprobamate was used with amphetamine in 4 cases, resulting in one very good and one good response in the group of anxiety reactions, one complete failure of response in a case of alcoholism, and a good response in 1 of the depressives and 1 of the cases of post-traumatic encephalopathy. One phobic patient who had previously been receiving chlorpromazine received meprobamate in addition, but with continuing minimal effect.

An interesting observation was that in the course of this study, certain patients who did not respond to either amobarbital sodium alone or meprobamate alone showed a striking response to a combination of the two drugs when 0.1 Gm. of amobarbital sodium was given with 400 mg. of meprobamate. While the small number of cases treated with a combination of meprobamate and other drugs included in this study are insufficient to permit generalizations, they do seem to indicate that further experimentation might prove rewarding.

Duration of Treatment. Of the 73 cases that showed good to very good results, 65 per cent were on meprobamate treatment from one week to three months (14 from 6 to 30 days, 21 from 31 to 60 days, and 13 from 61 to 90 days). The remaining 22 cases in this group took meprobamate for from three to seven months, mostly on maintenance doses to sustain the good results achieved earlier.

Side Effects. Of the 113 patients treated with meprobamate, 6 at first complained of sleepiness. This effect wore off with time in all cases. Ten patients reported that they were troubled by dizziness, as a result of which 7 were transferred to other medication. Other side effects were not reported.

Previous Therapy. To compare the results obtained with meprobamate with those obtained under previous therapy, Table III was compiled, those cases without previous therapy being omitted.

Other drugs used concomitantly with amobarbital sodium were chlorpromazine, chlorpromazine and reserpine together, estrogen, bromide, and nicotinic acid. The last of these combinations was the only one to show any response. Other drugs used with electroconvulsive therapy were chlorpromazine (5 cases with some response, 2 with poor response), dextroamphetamine (1 case, good response), estrogen (1 case), Tuinal and amphetamine (1 case), and amobarbital sodium with chlorpromazine (1 case), all with poor response.

In this group of 94 cases suffering from a variety of psychiatric conditions, 93 per cent proved refractory to a number of widely used drugs. Sixty per cent of these refractory cases showed a good or very good response to meprobamate therapy. The results appear even more striking when the comparison is limited to those cases suffering from anxiety reactions. Of 40 cases suffering from anxiety states that proved refractory to previous treatment, 70 per cent showed a good or very good response to meprobamate therapy.

Some of the cases mentioned in Table III that were refractory to previous therapy but responded to meprobamate treatment required the joint administration of two drugs for optimum results. Thus, four of the very good responses and 10 good responses were from meprobamate combined with amobarbital sodium, and one very good and three good responses from meprobamate combined with dextroamphetamine. One case did

TABLE 3
COMPARISON OF RESULTS OF MEPROBAMATE AND PREVIOUS THERAPY

No. of cases	Drug or treatment	Previous therapy Response Good	Some	Poor	Meprobamate therapy Response Very good	Good	Some	None
44	Amobarbital sodium	1	2	41	13	21	6	4
8	Amobarbital sodium with other drugs		1	7	2	2	3	1
3	Phenobarbital			3		3		
1	Reserpine			1	1			
6	Electroconvulsive therapy	3	2	1		2	4	
21	Electroconvulsive therapy with amobarbital sodium	1	5	15	3	8	4	6
11	Electroconvulsive therapy with other drugs	1	4	6	1	4	4	2
94	Total	6	14	74	20	40	21	13

not respond to the joint administration of meprobamate and dextroamphetamine, and another case showed only minimal improvement from meprobamate and chlorpromazine.

Discussion

A number of excellent drugs have become available recently for the treatment of the emotionally disturbed. Probably greatest attention has been directed to chlorpromazine, a potent drug developed in France and widely used in Europe and in this country in neuropsychiatric states. Its particular value is with severe psychotics. In milder cases, however, the possible occurrence of serious side effects must be weighed against the therapeutic benefits.

Reserpine, the other most widely used tranquilizer, is fundamentally a hypotensive agent. Patients on reserpine therapy often pass through a stage of excitation during the first two or three weeks of treatment which may be distressing to both the patient and his relatives. Others may become listless and depressed. Meprobamate, which differs from both reserpine and chlorpromazine in chemical structure, does not have a specific effect on blood pressure, does not cause listlessness, agitation, or depression, and so far has not caused serious side effects. While experience with this new drug is not yet of long standing, indications suggest that in the treatment of anxiety states, meprobamate is just as effective as chlorpromazine or reserpine, and has the additional advantage of being safer and better tolerated.

The tranquilizers used previously have a definite influence on the autonomic regulatory mechanism of the body. Meprobamate does not seem to affect this mechanism, thus making it possible to achieve therapeutic results without disturbing the delicately adjusted autonomic equilibrium of the body. The good therapeutic results obtained with meprobamate in cases that proved refractory to treatment with a number of conventional remedies suggest that meprobamate has a mode of action that differs from that of chlorpromazine, reserpine, and the barbiturates.

Summary and Conclusions

Meprobamate was administered to 113 ambulatory patients treated at the Psychiatric Department of Albany Hospital. Meprobamate showed definite effectiveness in psychoneurotic anxiety states, and appeared to have a selective action in conditions in which anxiety and tension are prominent factors. A large number of cases that had proved unresponsive to various other forms of treatment including reserpine and chlorpromazine responded well to therapy with meprobamate.

The combination of meprobamate with amobarbital sodium in certain cases seemed to be of greater value than either drug given alone. A few patients reported drowsiness or dizziness, the former subsiding spontaneously upon continued administration. Other side effects were not reported. While meprobamate appears at least as effective as other tranquilizers, it seems to be safer and better tolerated and has the added advantage that it does not affect the autonomic functions of the body.

Acknowledgment

I am obliged to Dr. W. L. Holt, Head of the Department of Psychiatry, Albany Hospital, for many valuable suggestions and for help and advice throughout the course of this investigation.

ABREACTION—CATHARSIS:

A Critical Reappraisal

HAROLD PALMER, M.D.

The term "Catharsis" was first introduced into psychiatry by Breuer in the late nineteenth century, whereupon it was readily adopted by Freud, who at that time was collaborating with Breuer. Both of these investigators used the term to connote a therapeutic ritual whereby the patient is encouraged to confide in his physician by talking about himself and his problems in a thorough-going and painstaking biographical fashion. Apart from its use in modern psychiatry, Aristotle seems to have been the first person to have made use of it in connection with therapeutic value of drama.

The term "Abreaction" was first introduced by the same two investigators, Breuer and Freud, to denote a special class of emotional event which is peculiarly liable to occur in the course of a therapeutic catharsis, whenever the patient recalls vividly, traumatically engendered experience which originally had been associated with intense emotion, but for one reason or another had become "repressed" (or as Janet would have said, "dissociated") at the time of its original arousal. It follows naturally that the emotion which accompanies abreactions is most commonly fear; but it may be anger, sexual lust, or intense grief. The term "abreaction" connotes the purging of the "repressed" emotion and is seemingly of critical significance in all cathartic procedures, including that of Freudian psychoanalysis. Viewed from another angle, which resides within the French school of discourse, there is implicit in most abreaction the abolition of a state of "dissociation", and the "resynthesis" of the forgotten memory within the normal stream of consciousness.

It will be seen therefore that the two terms "catharsis" and "abreaction" are not synonymous; but clearly one can hardly be induced without the other occurring. Also, it is very important to stress the fact that in the course of manipulating these terms, and the clinical notions with which they are concerned, we are combining within one and the same discourse, ideas and terms derived separately from the French and German schools of psychiatry; this is apt to beget illogicalities and confusion of a variety so characteristic of our speciality as various notions migrate from one language and cultural setting to another.

Meanwhile, whether we think with Janet or with Freud, we may allow that a "dissociated" self is a sick self, and that "repression" weakens the ego as regulator to the self. We may allow that most psychotherapy is cathartic in mode and accept the likelihood that abreaction, even if in attenuated form, is beneficial. Some would urge the special value of exploiting either of these techniques in a "group" setting.

The systematic attention given to abreaction by military psychiatrists was aided and intensified by the discovery of pharmacological modes of its induction, which occurred in relation to the great increase of traumatic neuroses in warfare. For the tendency of a memory to become "repressed" or "dissociated" varies directly with the anguish which accompanies it, and the most severe anguish any of us can experience is the belief that death is imminent and inevitable.

Meanwhile, in spite of their long history within our speciality, it has never been satisfactorily established scientifically in what setting the therapist should induce and how he should manipulate "catharsis", nor how he should manipulate and exploit "abreaction." This state of affairs is largely due to the dual origin of modern psychiatric ideas from Vienna and Paris. What we must guard against is failure to scrutinize the claims of such esoteric schools as that of "psychoanalysis" to operate these clinical procedures pre-emptively and determine their mode of presentation.

Figuratively speaking, it might be said that Freud devoted the major part of his life attempting to find the answers to these two questions, and that psychoanalysis enshrines his answers. This technique eschews explicitly induced abreactions and exploits the situation of "transference" which develops in the course of psychoanalytic catharses. Largely as a consequence of the domination achieved by Freudian psychoanalysts over the thinking of psychiatrists, the phenomena and possible utility of specifically induced abreaction have suffered neglect. Moreover Freud very prudently warned against the hazards to which psychiatrists are exposed when employing specifically induced abreactive techniques; indeed psychoanalysis and the training of the analyst are designed primarily to guard against these dangers. This tendency in psychiatric speculative enquiry to be dominated by Freudian notions has resulted also in a tendency to jettison the notion of "dissociation" and its complementary notion of "resynthesis", both of which derive from Pierre Janet and the French school, in favour of the adoption of the Freudian notion of "repression" as constituting a central topic around which psychiatry should build its speculative hypothesis concerning the dynamic structure of mind.

The most important consequence of this relative eclipse of French causal hypothesis by those enunciated by the Viennese Jew has been the substitution of historical cause for teleological or moral cause in the philosophy of psychiatrists. This epochal change has been so tremendous in its impact on European (and its offshoot Anglo-American) culture that its importance must not be under-emphasized.

It was only as a consequence of the work of military psychiatrists with shell-shocked soldiers in World War II that the significance of this moral challenge achieved concrete recognition. For Freudian psychoanalysis utterly failed to induce the will to fight in military casualties however much they succeeded, under conditions favouring excusal from military duty, to render soldiers symptom free. Other workers, utilising abreactive techniques and concerned with the moral factor of military duty, claimed some success.

Meanwhile we may note in passing that subsequently it was discovered that the passage of an electrical force through the forebrain, within a certain critical amplitude range, induced abreactive phenomena somewhat similar to those first described by Breuer and Freud. These phenomena, together with their allegedly therapeutically beneficial accompaniments, have received concrete connotation within the therapeusis of "Non-convulsive electro-cerebral stimulation"; the claims advanced for this form of therapy have been investigated, however, by Catterall and others, but they were unable to confirm them.

Aside from the special consideration of abreaction, seemingly few would dispute the value of cathartic techniques, considered in general; these range from social tete-a-tete to the confessional and the fully-fledged course of Freudian psychoanalysis. The claims of abreaction as a specific mode of therapy, however, meanwhile remain controversial. It is unfortunate that it possesses such hazards and such a dramatic quality, as these make it suspect to the sober-minded as the likely tool of the mountebank; moreover not every psychiatrist claims to be able to employ it correctly, nor, therefore, possesses the right to criticize its value.

Meanwhile, the problem of its place in clinical psychiatry has been brought forward in relation to "group therapy" which in general may be said to involve a "cathartic" process, in the course of which striking "abreactive" phenomena are liable to occur. Not only, however, does group therapy see the therapeutic value of abreaction compel renewed debate, but it confronts us with a new setting for the phenomenon—group setting—within which incidentally we may note that as with all cathartic procedures, there also develops a "transference" situation. Moreover, that which is abreacted in the course of these group therapies differs when compared with individual techniques, so that anger and hostility rather than fear and lust dominate the therapeutic issue, with shame and revenge holding about the same position they held both in psychoanalytically induced and abreactive revelations.

It is of interest to note, in passing, that the role of the psychiatrist in a Freudian psychoanalysis is passive whereas in an abreactive seance it is authoritarian. In group therapy the psychiatrist's role is permissive. Attention has already been drawn to the moral implications of this apparent set of facts.

All three techniques are concerned to break up stereotypes of thinking, feeling and behavior, and all are characterized by the therapist ordering the mind of his patient and interpreting it for him. But whereas in the case of abreaction therapy this interpretation is teleological, in the case of psychoanalysis it is historical; group therapy invoking both causal interpretations.

Finally there is this special property of abreaction therapy which is of enormous significance to those clinicians who employ eclectic "total push" methods, viz. that whereas psychoanalysis and group therapy are to a large extent immiscible with physical modes of therapy, there is no incompatibility whatsoever between abreactive therapy and the physical therapies.

Within this examination of what appears to me to have been one of the main starting points of modern psychotherapy, it now seems reasonable to state my own views concerning its legitimate field of application and at the same time refer very briefly to my views concerning the other two principal cathartic procedures of "Freudian psychoanalysis" and "group therapy" respectively.

I am of the opinion that abreaction therapy has an appropriate place in the treatment of any Anxiety State which reasonably can be assumed to have been engendered by massive traumatic "real" experience, or by a series of experiences cumulatively and symbolically related to one another, but I am doubtful whether abreaction can profitably be used on more than one or two occasions. As has been implied above, there is always increase of scope for abreaction therapy in warfare and the period immediately following a war.

It is only to be expected that some psychiatrists, having learnt to manipulate this form of therapy with facility and confidence, may utilize it as one of their main lines of establishing contact with the patient, in comparable fashion to that in which most of us have our own favourite instrument of therapy. Experimental work with these forms of therapy is of course a matter to be considered entirely separately from its proved clinical value and there is for instance a tremendous amount of research work yet to be done in connection with ego structure, some of this work bearing on the pictorial arts.

I am of the opinion that cathartic techniques are fundamental to the whole process of psychotherapy, but I see no considerable means scientifically of determining to what extent thorough-going Freudian techniques are required. One's reverence for Freud and his contribution to psychiatry, and one's respect for one's colleagues, make it somewhat difficult to enunciate one's view at this short distance of time from Freud's decease. It sometimes appears, however, that psychoanalysis is on the retreat in Europe and that it may have reached the crest of its wave in the United States, whose shores it reached somewhat later, and that when it has exhausted its impetus in the newer countries it will eventually contract in respect of its therapeutic claims. I believe, however, that there will remain scope for individual assistance by means of analytic techniques to a considerable range of inadequate and psychopathic personalities. To what extent such help can be scientifically proved to depend on the technical psychoanalytic procedures as opposed to the general support which these lame persons obtain in this fashion seems to me will long remain debatable. The cathartic aspects of religion, art and ceremonial (especially the dance) have of course long been recognised; that such processes may achieve new forms of expression seems axiomatic. Nor must we forget the tete-a-tete, and the good bottle of Vouvray, which is at the centre of Europeanism, available to all who understand the secret of sharing their emotions with others. To these two traditional (and nowadays accepted) techniques of specific abreaction and psychoanalysis, we must now add "group therapy"; this is not only cathartic, but induced specific abreactive episodes. Unfortunately the rise of group therapy appears to presage the creation of a new "school."

In connection with the problems created by these esoteric "schools" in psychiatry, the great achievement of the physical remedies in my opinion lies in the destruction of the claims of "abreactionists", "psychoanalysts", and "group therapists" and any other "ists" to the pre-emptive right to help sick souls. Thereby it has made possible the establishment of fashionable and reputable eclecticism.

Within any modern eclecticism, I believe there remains a place for abreaction therapy, the most efficient mode of which in my opinion is excitatory abreaction using Ether; this however is but a special variety of cathartic techniques, involving special problems of "transference" but lacking the mystical dynamic of group therapy. Its unique property resides in its capacity for presentation with a teleologically orientated authoritarian technology.